Genetics of Allergy
and Asthma

CLINICAL ALLERGY AND IMMUNOLOGY

Series Editor

MICHAEL A. KALINER, M.D.

Medical Director
Institute for Asthma and Allergy
Washington, D.C.

1. Sinusitis: Pathophysiology and Treatment, *edited by Howard M. Druce*
2. Eosinophils in Allergy and Inflammation, *edited by Gerald J. Gleich and A. Barry Kay*
3. Molecular and Cellular Biology of the Allergic Response, *edited by Arnold I. Levinson and Yvonne Paterson*
4. Neuropeptides in Respiratory Medicine, *edited by Michael A. Kaliner, Peter J. Barnes, Gert H. H. Kunkel, and James N. Baraniuk*
5. Provocation Testing in Clinical Practice, *edited by Sheldon L. Spector*
6. Mast Cell Proteases in Immunology and Biology, *edited by George H. Caughey*
7. Histamine and H_1-Receptor Antagonists in Allergic Disease, *edited by F. Estelle R. Simons*
8. Immunopharmacology of Allergic Diseases, *edited by Robert G. Townley and Devendra K. Agrawal*
9. Indoor Air Pollution and Health, *edited by Emil J. Bardana, Jr., and Anthony Montanaro*
10. Genetics of Allergy and Asthma: Methods for Investigative Studies, *edited by Malcolm N. Blumenthal and Bengt Björkstén*

ADDITIONAL VOLUMES IN PREPARATION

Allergic and Respiratory Disease in Sports Medicine, *edited by John M. Weiler*

Genetics of Allergy and Asthma

Methods for Investigative Studies

edited by

Malcolm N. Blumenthal
**University of Minnesota Hospital
Minneapolis, Minnesota**

Bengt Björkstén
**University Hospital
Linköping, Sweden
and Tartu University
Estonia**

Marcel Dekker, Inc.   **New York•Basel•Hong Kong**

ISBN: 0-8247-9480-X

The publisher offers discounts on this book when ordered in bulk quantities. For more information, write to Special Sales/Professional Marketing at the address below.

This book is printed on acid-free paper.

MARCEL DEKKER, INC.
270 Madison Avenue, New York, New York   10016

Current printing (last digit):
10 9 8 7 6 5 4 3 2 1

Printed in the United States of America

Series Introduction

The fun in creating a series of books is to try to estimate where the interest in a field will be and to create a book that will be there at the right time. Such is the convergence of interest and the publication of this book on the genetics of asthma and allergy. We have all recognized that genetics has a profound influence on asthma, allergies, and IgE production; however, the exact mechanisms eluded clarification until now. Several years ago, when I wrote a chapter on asthma and tried to summarize the field, the best I could do was to state that "Asthmatics beget asthmatics." Now we can localize the genetic controls, and are developing an understanding as to how these genetic influences create the environment where asthma and allergies develop.

Getting Malcolm Blumenthal to take on the task of developing a timely and comprehensive text on this area was the most important step in producing this book. Malcolm is a scholar in this area, and had the political skills to enlist the help of the best investigators and authors in the field. He demonstrated these political skills by getting Bengt Björkstén to coedit the book.

This book not only summarizes the field of genetics, but also brings the study of the application of these observations to the practical world of the physician caring for asthmatic and allergic patients. It is timely, concise, and will prove useful for physicians trying to keep abreast of advances in the sciences related to their clinical interests.

Michael A. Kaliner

Preface

From the earliest days of study of the evolutionary process, there has been great interest in the genetics of species survival and disease transmission. Asthma and allergies are common conditions that are increasingly prevalent. They are well characterized and influenced by both environmental factors and heredity. In addition, the offending allergens can be identified and a pathogenic model defined. Thus, these conditions are excellent models for studying the genetics of a complex disease.

What causes asthma and allergies? How do they develop? What is wrong? Who is likely to suffer from them? What can be done to help these people? Can we prevent asthma and allergies? These questions have been asked for centuries, but, until recently, we have not had enough knowledge to answer them adequately. Rapid advances in molecular biology—as well as in our understanding of the biology of the immune system and how it relates to disease and tolerance—together with newer statistical methods have allowed us to gain significant insight into the development of these diseases. Methods and results obtained from the study of asthma and allergies may soon be applied to the study of other complex diseases.

This book is about the control of the biological traits of asthma and allergies by genes and their environmental interactions, and about the impact of this information on the population. To fully understand the genetics of asthma and allergies, one also has to understand their biology and the influence of environmental factors. Investigation of these areas is being performed in a variety of different disciplines at an extremely rapid rate. It is impossible to publish an up-to-date summary of the status of this rapidly expanding area. In this book, our goal is to provide the reader with current information regarding the genetics of asthma and allergies by presenting an overview of the methods being used to approach their study, the relevant biology, and our present knowledge of the genetics of these conditions. We begin by reviewing the history of the study of the genetics of asthma and allergies, beginning in ancient times. The following chapters in Part I discuss our present knowledge of human genetics and the immune system. Stephen Rich reviews human genetics and its application to the study of human characteristics (Chapter 2). Deborah Meyers describes the tools that are available for human genetic studies: phenotypes, sampling design, candidate loci, genetic markers, positional cloning, and an introduction to genetic analysis (Chapter 3). The functioning of the immune system, especially regarding the IgE system and the development of allergic conditions in different organs, is presented by Erwin Gelfand and Donald Leung (Chapter 4). Bengt Björkstén reviews the tools or methods used to study the immune system in allergic conditions. In Chapter 5, he addresses the gathering of historical information as well as in vitro and in vivo assays, stressing the importance of using a well-defined methodology. Newton Morton brings together the tools of human genetics and the methods of studying the immune system to describe in detail how to define the genetics and epidemiology of asthma and allergies (Chapter 6). Morton discusses the consequences of treating asthma and allergies as quantitative or qualitative, the impact of ascertainment through probands, strategies for gene mapping, and possibilities for combining different studies by meta-analysis. His chapter offers some insight into the ways we might further our understanding of all complex diseases.

Chapters 7 and 8 review the epidemiology of asthma and allergy, providing the reader with information about the importance of these conditions in terms of recent trends in asthma incidence, prevalence, morbidity, and mortality. The risk factors, rates of incidence, and trends over time are summarized by Kevin Weiss and Peter Gergen in Chapter 7. These authors emphasize the changing epidemiology of these conditions and, where feasible, compare trends over time internationally. Chapter 8 focuses more closely on the epidemiology of environmental risk factors influencing the development of asthma and allergy, particularly in childhood.

The genetic control of asthma and allergies has been studied using a variety of intermediate, as well as more complex, phenotypes. The chapters in Part II summarize in detail the results of investigations defining the genetics of asthma and allergies by looking at the various components (intermediate phenotypes) of these complex immune diseases. In Chapter 9, David Marsh, Thorunn Rafnar, Balaram Ghosh and Shau-Ku Huang present a review of the molecular genetic basis of the specific immune response to allergens. The regulation of IgE synthesis is discussed by Christine McMenamin and Patrick Holt in Chapter 10. An immunological explanation is provided for the critical period in early childhood and the genetic differences in immune responses to ubiquitous allergens. They emphasize the cellular and molecular mechanisms involved in the in vitro and in vivo regulation of IgE responses to dietary and inhaled antigens delivered to mucosal surfaces. In Chapter 11, Penny Lympany and Tak Lee provide an update of the role of the inflammatory response in atopy and asthma and of the way in which molecular biological techniques have been used in these studies. Lung function in asthma as well as recent advances regarding ventilation, dynamics, and gas exchange, and the genetic influences on them, are covered by Göran Hedenstierna in Chapter 12. In Chapter 13, Eugene Bleecker and Deborah Meyers review the genetics of bronchial hyperreactivity as a parameter of asthma and inflammation of the lung.

It appears that asthma and allergies are the result of multiple cell types and numerous cellular control mechanisms. The ultimate clinical picture is most likely determined by many genetic and environmental factors. The development of the complete phenotypes of asthma and allergies most likely involves the combination of a variety of simple and intermediate phenotypes. The genetics of these complex immune-related conditions (complex phenotypes), including asthma, rhinitis, urticaria and angioedema, anaphylaxis, atopic dermatitis, and contact dermatitis are reviewed in Chapter 14, along with a discussion of the problems, both scientific and ethical, that occur in studies of this type.

This book offers the reader a contemporary summary of the genetics of asthma and allergies and provides the information needed to 1) perform further investigative studies to understand the basis of these conditions and 2) understand the present and develop new methods of managing them. This should lead to better understanding and control of immunologically related conditions, such as asthma and allergies, which appear to be increasing in incidence, prevalence, morbidity, and mortality. This book provides information that helps answer the questions raised by the British biostatistician Bradford Hill: What is wrong? Who is going to develop it? What can be done about it?

Genetic studies are providing information regarding the pathogenesis of asthma and allergic disease, which will result in better understanding of these conditions. As a result, health professionals will be able to formulate their management in a rational way. It should be stressed that this information will ultimately benefit the individuals afflicted with these conditions. The identification of the genes and the role nongenetic factors play in the development of asthma and allergies will provide knowledge they need to manage their condition.

Malcolm N. Blumenthal
Bengt Björkstén

Contents

Series Introduction   *iii*

Preface   *v*

Contributors   *xi*

1. **Historical Perspectives**   **1**
   Malcolm N. Blumenthal

PART I   APPROACHES TO THE GENETIC STUDIES OF ASTHMA AND ALLERGY

2. **Human Genetics**   **19**
   Stephen S. Rich

3. **Tools for the Study of Genetics**   **47**
   Deborah A. Meyers

4. **Regulation of IgE Production and the Development of Allergic Responses in Different Organs**   **63**
   Erwin W. Gelfand and Donald Y. M. Leung

5. **Clinical Methods to Study the Immune System in Asthma and Allergy**   **91**
   Bengt Björkstén

6. Genetic Studies of Asthma and Allergy: Statistical Methods   111
    Newton E. Morton

PART II   EPIDEMIOLOGY OF ASTHMA AND ALLERGY

7. The Epidemiology of Asthma: Risk Factors, Rates, and
    Trends   137
    Kevin B. Weiss and Peter J. Gergen

8. Risk Factors for Sensitization and Development of
    Allergic Diseases   171
    Bengt Björkstén

**PART III   GENETICS OF INTERMEDIATE PHENOTYPES
               OF ASTHMA AND ALLERGY**

9. Specific Immune Responses to Purified Allergens   197
    *David G. Marsh, Thorunn Rafnar, Balaram Ghosh, and
    Shau-Ku Huang*

10. Regulation of IgE Synthesis In Vitro and In Vivo   211
    Christine McMenamin and Patrick G. Holt

11. Inflammation   241
    Penelope A. Lympany and Tak H. Lee

12. Ventilation, Dynamics, and Gas Exchange   281
    Göran Hedenstierna

13. Bronchial Hyperresponsiveness and Regulation of Total
    Serum IgE Levels   307
    Eugene R. Bleecker and Deborah A. Meyers

**PART IV   GENETICS OF ASTHMA, ALLERGY, AND
              RELATED CONDITIONS**

14. Genetics of Asthma, Allergy, and Related Conditions   327
    Malcolm N. Blumenthal

Index   *357*

Contributors

Bengt Björkstén, M.D. Professor and Chairman, Department of Pediatrics, University Hospital, Linköping, Sweden, and Adjunct Professor of Pediatrics, Tartu University, Estonia

Eugene R. Bleecker, M.D. Professor, Department of Medicine, University of Maryland School of Medicine, Baltimore, Maryland

Malcolm N. Blumenthal, M.D. Professor and Director, Asthma and Allergy Program, Department of Medicine, University of Minnesota Hospital, Minneapolis, Minnesota

Erwin W. Gelfand, M.D. Chairman, Department of Pediatrics, National Jewish Center for Immunology and Respiratory Medicine, Denver, Colorado

Peter J. Gergen, M.D., M.P.H. Director, Office of Epidemiology and Clinical Trials, Division of Allergy, Immunology, and Transplantation, National Institute of Allergy and Infectious Diseases, National Institutes of Health, Bethesda, Maryland

Balaram Ghosh, Ph.D. Assistant Professor, Department of Medicine, Johns Hopkins Asthma and Allergy Center, Johns Hopkins University School of Medicine, Baltimore, Maryland

Göran Hedenstierna, M.D., Ph.D. Professor, Department of Clinical Physiology, University Hospital, Uppsala, Sweden

Patrick G. Holt, D.Sc., F.R.C.Path Department of Clinical Sciences, TVW Telethon Institute for Child Health Research, West Perth, Western Australia, Australia

Shau-Ku Huang, Ph.D. Assistant Professor, Department of Medicine, Johns Hopkins Asthma and Allergy Center, Johns Hopkins University School of Medicine, Baltimore, Maryland

Tak H. Lee, M.D., Sc.D., F.R.C.P. Professor, Department of Allergy and Respiratory Medicine, Guy's Hospital, London, England

Donald Y. M. Leung, M.D., Ph.D. Professor of Pediatrics, University of Colorado Health Sciences Center, and Head, Division of Allergy and Immunology, National Jewish Center for Immunology and Respiratory Medicine, Denver, Colorado

Penelope A. Lympany, B.Sc., Ph.D. Department of Allergy and Respiratory Medicine, Guy's Hospital, London, England

David G. Marsh, Ph.D. Professor, Department of Medicine, Johns Hopkins Asthma and Allergy Center, Johns Hopkins University School of Medicine, Baltimore, Maryland

Christine McMenamin, Ph.D. Department of Clinical Sciences, TVW Telethon Institute for Child Health Research, West Perth, Western Australia, Australia

Deborah A. Meyers, Ph.D. Associate Professor of Medicine, Center for Medical Genetics, Johns Hopkins University School of Medicine, Baltimore, Maryland

Newton E. Morton, Ph.D., M.D.(Hon.) Professor, Department of Human Genetics, University of Southampton, Southampton, Hampshire, England

Thorunn Rafnar, Ph.D. Assistant Professor, Department of Medicine, Johns Hopkins Asthma and Allergy Center, Johns Hopkins University School of Medicine, Baltimore, Maryland

Stephen S. Rich, Ph.D.   Professor, Public Health Sciences (Epidemiology), Bowman Gray School of Medicine, Winston-Salem, North Carolina

Marsha M. Thompson, M.D., Ph.D.   Assistant Professor, Pulmonary Division, Department of Pediatrics, University of New Mexico, Albuquerque, New Mexico

Kevin B. Weiss, M.D.   Director, Center for Health Services Research, Rush Presbyterian St. Luke's Medical Center, Chicago, Illinois

Genetics of Allergy and Asthma

1

Historical Perspectives

Malcolm N. Blumenthal
University of Minnesota Hospital
Minneapolis, Minnesota

I. INTRODUCTION

The type of health we all enjoy is a result of the interaction of our bodies with our environment. Initially medicine, magic, and mystery were all one and the same thing. They were attempts to understand the unknown. This was especially true for maladies such as infectious diseases (i.e., plague) and allergic conditions (i.e., asthma or anaphylaxis). In these early times, individuals would develop the plague—an acute and often fulminant illness characterized by chills, prostration, fever, tachycardia, headache, vomiting, and delirium. Asthmatics would develop coughing, wheezing, and shortness of breath. During anaphylaxis, an individual would develop swelling of the entire body as well as shock. All of these would occur without an apparent cause or reason. Mystery, magic, and a little science were used to explain these phenomena.

The plague, when described in ancient times, was thought to be caused by the wrath of God. When information became available, it was noted that the clinical picture was a result of an interaction of the host with bacteria in its environment. It was soon realized that the immune system gave the individual protection against foreign environmental agents such as bacteria (1,2).

Descriptions of asthma and allergic reactions such as anaphylaxis also date back to early historical times (1,3–5). When better defined, these conditions were noted to involve an interaction of the host with factors in the environment, much like the plague. Pollen, dust, and animal dander are a few of the environmental factors that could trigger an episode of asthma. It also became apparent that the immune system was involved—but unlike in plague, the development of an immune response often resulted in adverse symptoms rather than protection against the foreign substance. Familial, if not genetic, factors have been known for many years to be involved in the development of allergic conditions such as asthma, eczema, and hay fever.

Our knowledge regarding the pathogenesis of asthma and allergies has, unfortunately, been woefully inadequate until recent times. This is because in order to understand the biology of a condition such as allergy, you have to know its genetics; however, to understand the genetics you have to know the biology. As a result of the knowledge gathered in different areas of study, we are increasing our understanding of the biology of allergic conditions. Information regarding these conditions has been obtained from a variety of disciplines, including immunology, statistics, biochemistry, physiology, molecular biology, and psychiatry. These disciplines are providing us with the tools and models to understand asthma and allergies—especially with regard to the role genetic and environmental factors play in the development of these conditions.

Asthma and allergies are good models with which to study the genetics of human diseases involving the immune system. They are common, involve both genetic and well-characterized causative environmental factors, have a well-defined clinical picture, have defined immune responses, and have an established model to use for study. Problems in the investigation of these conditions involve those of determining the proper phenotypes and parameters to be studied, the existence of polygenic factors, environmental factors, the selection of subjects, statistical analysis, and study design. The characteristics of the triggering agents, such as allergens, must also be examined. Despite these problems, advances are being made in our understanding of the genetics of allergies and asthma. Our present understanding of asthma and allergy is based on developments in the areas of genetics/heredity as well as the immune system.

II. HEREDITY/GENETICS

Heredity is the passing on of characteristics from parents to offspring. Genetics is the science of heredity. Although many traits and diseases (e.g., asthma and hay fever) have been known to be familial for many years, the science of human genetics is young. In ancient times, traits were traced through generations. Blood was thought by Aristotle to be the basic element of heredity in humans. He believed that blood flowed from parents to offspring carrying hereditary traits (1,6). The principles of heredity were used to produce improved plants and animals.

Three well-known doctrines of evolution (adaptive racial change) have been formulated: the Balthmic, which attributes change to an "inherent adaptive growth-force; the Lamarckian, which attributes evolution to the transmission of acquirements; and the Darwinian, which attributes it to natural selection (7). The Balthmic theory of evolution supposed that evolution has occurred in obedience to and under the immediate direction of a Deity. It is a theory of evolution by the occurrence of miracles. The Lamarckian theory stresses that acquirements are transmissible. It suggests that conditions that produce health in a succession of parents will ultimately lead to a race that is healthy, whereas contrary conditions will render the race sickly. For example, according to this theory, many generations of physically active workers would lead to descendants that are physically active. This theory suggests that all beneficial factors that act on a species are causes of evolution whereas all injurious factors would cause degeneration. The Darwinian theory is founded on two ascertained factors and two that are inferred (8). It insists on the universal occurrence of variation as a law of nature and asserts that the number of individuals of any species that survive and give birth to a full quota of offspring is not the same as the number that come into being. The inference of Darwinian theory is that, as a rule, the individuals that survive and have offspring are those that are better fit to the environment, and the "average of the race" is raised in successive generations, resulting in evolution. The publication of Darwin's *Origin of Species* provided the stimulus for the systematic study of heredity (8).

The observations of many generations of plants by Gregor Mendel led to his formulation of the first law of heredity (9), which led to the founding of the science of genetics. Mendel's work demonstrated two basic laws of heredity: (1) the law of segregation, which states that the pairs of genes from each parent separate, so that only one gene of each pair is transmitted by a sperm or by an egg; and (2) the law of independence, which states that each pair of genes is inherited independently of the other pairs. This latter law is not always followed in nature. Genes are inherited independently if they are on different chromosomes. However, if they are on the same area of the chromosome (i.e., linked), they tend to be inherited together.

On the basis of these early investigations, the modern study of inheritance began at the turn of the 20th century. Investigators initially used plants and then animals to develop and understand inheritance. These studies resulted in the realization that these newly discovered laws of biological inheritance may be applied to humans.

It became evident in the early 1900s that genes are located on chromosomes (10). The studies demonstrating the occurrence of mutations were performed in the 1920s (11). In the 1940s George Beadle and Edward Tatum reported that genes produce their effects through enzymes (12). Oswald Avery noted in 1944 that nucleic acid (DNA) was the key material in the genes (13). James Watson and Francis Crick in 1956 built a model showing the structure of DNA (13,14). The work of these investigators forms the foundation of the field of molecular genetics. Arthur Kornberg showed that DNA could reproduce outside a cell (15). The genetic code was solved in 1966, and subsequently there has been an explosion of studies providing the tools to define the basis of heredity (15). This has included the development of a methodology for recombining DNA molecules in vitro, and for cloning the resulting recombinant molecules in bacteria and yeast cells. The details of our present knowledge of genetics will be reviewed in Chapter 2.

Today enough is known with certainty to justify the inclusion of heredity into any study of human disease. It is a major area of study that is needed to understand the biology of human disease such as asthma and allergies. Knowledge of the laws that control the reproduction of living beings is essential to provide us with the methodology to help us understand and manage diseases.

III. IMMUNOLOGY

The term "immunology" is derived from the Latin words "immunitas" and "immunis," which had their origin in the legal concept of an exemption. Initially, in Rome, they described the exemption of an individual from service or duty and later, in the Middle Ages, the exemption of the Church and its properties and personnel from civil control. Antoinette Stettler traces the first use of this term in the context of disease to the 14th century, when Colle wrote *Equibrus Dei gratia ego immunis evas*, in referring to his escape from the plague epidemic. However, Silverstein in his book *The History of Immunology* states that Roman Marcus Annaeus Lucanus (A.D. 39–65) used the word "immune" in his epic poem "Pharsalia" to describe the resistance to snakebite of the Psylli tribe of North Africa. Although the term was used intermittently in relationship to the body's immune system for many years, it did not achieve widespread use until the smallpox vaccine became common (1).

A. Infectious Factors in Environment Causing Disease

1. Environmental Infectious Factors in Disease

Our present concept of immunology is built on studies in bacteriology. Among ancient peoples, epidemic and even endemic diseases were regarded as supernatural in origin and were thought to be sent by gods as punishment for the sins of man. The Greeks believed in the divine origin of epidemic diseases. At the time of the siege of Troy, the Greeks lost faith in their gods—and along with it, their belief in the divine origin of disease. Thucydides in 430 B.C. concluded that certain plagues were contagious. At the time of Moses, the Hebrews believed that leprosy was contagious. Quarantines were established in Marseilles and Venice in the 14th century. This was perhaps influenced as much by the religious feeling that a period of purification was needed as by the perceived need to avoid the environmental agent. On the basis of this idea, it was thought that a period of isolation would prevent the spread of disease. Hippocrates suggested that air when changed enough could become deleterious to individuals. In ancient times, the treatment—and, more important, the prevention—of these diseases was sought, for example, by sacrifices to appease the anger of the god. Despite this, self-immunization against the venom of serpents by introducing small quantities of poisons into cuts or scratches in the skin has been reported to have occurred in ancient times. Variolization, the inoculation against smallpox with dried material, was discovered in China over 20 centuries ago. Unfortunately, this effort to produce immunity prior to an infection not only induced active infection but initiated new epidemics. Different people were found to respond differently (1,5,16). Over the years it has become apparent that host factors, both genetic and nongenetic, as well as environmental factors influence the type of immune response and health an individual experiences. As a result, investigators became involved in studying precise technical methods and description of the etiological agents of infection, while others studied the mechanisms of the host's immune response to them.

2. Microbe Identified

It became evident that for some conditions—later defined as infectious diseases—there were agents in our environment that caused them. The discovery of bacteria in 1677 by Anton van Leeuwenhoek provided evidence that organisms affecting the host would cause diseases. Subsequent investigations have identified viral, fungal, and other infectious agents as etiological agents in the production of diseases (2,16,17).

3. Birth of Immunology—Identification of Immunity

The science of immunology grew out of the common knowledge that those who survive an infectious disease seldom contract the disease again during their lifetime. Thucydides recorded that when the plague was raging in Athens, the sick and dying would have received no nursing at all had it not been for the devotion of those who had already had the plague and recovered from it, since it was known that no one ever caught it a second time (1). In the late 1700s, Jenner's work laid the foundation for modern immunology (1,18). This was further developed in the late 19th and early 20th centuries by Pasteur as well as Koch, Metchnikoff, von Behring, and their associates (1,19,20).

4. Mechanism of Immunity

The first physician to study the immune or prophylactic power of cowpox in preventing subsequent smallpox was Edward Jenner. This was extended because of the germ theory of disease. Jenner converted the controlled observations into a scientific principle of prophylaxis. At the end of the 18th century he began his studies of immunity to smallpox, which resulted in the establishment of a method of protection against smallpox and a generally applicable principle of active immunization by an attenuated virus (1,18).

Almost 100 years passed between the period of Jenner and the establishment of the science of immunology by Pasteur, who recognized the relationship between vaccine, attenuated organism, and immunity (1,20). Even though little was known about the ways bacteria caused harm, Pasteur evaluated methods to prevent them by immunization. Although Jenner discovered the immune reaction to smallpox and Pasteur was successful in the practical achievement of securing immunity, the mechanisms whereby such proteins caused immunity remained obscure.

During the last decade of the 19th century, two schools of immunological doctrine developed. The first was the humoral theory, which stressed the importance of the action of the blood and tissue fluids. The second was the cellular theory, which emphasized the central role that various cells such as the phagocyte played in the immune response (1,19).

5. Humoral Immunity

The humoral theory originated over 2000 years ago with the teachings of Hippocrates, Celsus, and Galen (1). They stressed the importance of humors in the health of an individual. The development of serum therapy and the demonstration that blood had a bactericidal action gave further credence to this idea (1,2). This involved the development of toxins and antitoxins and the subsequent identification of antibodies and complements. All these findings were compatible with the theories expressed by Hippocrates that diseases were due to imbalances between blood, blood bile, yellow bile, and phlegm—all humoral components (1,5).

a. Antibodies Identified.   In the late 1800s, toxins and a substance that could neutralize or destroy them, thus preventing disease, were characterized. Pfeiffer demonstrated that immunity was due to the development of a specific neutralizing substance, or antitoxin, in the blood of the immune animals, and that such antitoxin immunity can be transferred to another animal. This substance was called an antitoxin. Soon after, the term "antibody" was developed to describe a more general and noncommittal "anti" substance found in the blood serum or body fluids of animals. This antibody, produced by the body against a specific foreign substance, would react specifically with the given foreign substance in some demonstrable way. Investigators started to describe a variety of different types of antibodies (1,18,21). Understanding of the presence of humoral antibodies and their importance in defense against infections resulted from the discovery of the precipitin reaction, and from Ehrlich's work on the antidiphtheria antibodies and diphtheria toxin (1,18,22). Ehrlich's studies led to the theory of the chemical nature of the antigen- antibody reaction including the side chain theory of antibody production. He postulated that immunological specificity is due to unique stereochemical relationships between active sites on antigens and antibodies. Doubts regarding Ehrlich's theory arose when reports circulated showing that antibodies could be produced against a wide variety of even benign, naturally occurring animal and plant substances. These substances included many items to which the host would normally never be exposed. It was thought to be unreasonable that an individual could make specific antibodies spontaneously against so great a number of foreign substances. During the middle of the 20th century it became clear that there was clonal selection of antibody formation and that DNA could control antibody structure (21). The amino acid sequences of immunoglobulin chains were subsequently described and it became evident that all immunoglobulins are structurally similar, but they are diversified and can be arranged into many groups and subgroups on the basis of variation in antigenic properties and amino acid sequences. Many immunoglobulin genes are inherited (germline genes). They are rearranged and diversified during B-cell development and even further by additional mechanisms during B-cell response to antigenic stimulation. These genes belong to different families, each isolated on a different chromosome and consisting of many gene segments.

Immunoglobulins are produced before antigens are ever encountered; however, before an immunoglobulin chain can be expressed, the appropriate gene segment has to be recombined. This rearrangement takes place as B cells develop from stem cells in the bone marrow. Our present understanding of the formation of antibodies is a result of studies demonstrating that the variable combinations of a number of minigene segments form antibody light and heavy chains (Chapter 4).

b. Complement Identified. In 1888, Nuttal suggested the existence of a protective substance in normal serum. This substance was further characterized and called alexin by Muchner and ultimately complement by Ehrlich. Jules Bordet further identified it and demonstrated its significance (1,16). Subsequent studies defined the complement system as a complex system of proteolytic enzymes, regulatory proteins, and proteins capable of causing the lysis of cells (23,24). The process of activation of the cascade of complement components is highly regulated. These several regulatory proteins (i.e., C1 esterase inhibitor, C3b inactivator) function to prevent uncontrolled complement activation. This system has a variety of biological functions and is an important humoral factor in immunity. Abnormalities in the genetics of regulatory proteins are often associated with distinct clinical diseases (i.e., hereditary angioedema) (24).

6. Cellular Immunity

In the 19th century, the controversy of the importance of humoral versus cellular immunity developed. Metchnikoff suggested clearly in 1884 that leukocytes might play an important role in the body's defense against infectious disease by virtue of their phagocytic capacities (1,19). He stated that the function of the phagocyte was to defend the host. Metchnikoff defined evolutionary mechanisms as a response to Darwinism. He compared Darwin's struggle of the species to the struggle within the organism. Metchnikoff suggested that the organism was an intrinsically disharmonious entity striving for harmony. Immunity and the inflammatory process were therefore necessary for establishing the organism's identity. He suggested that the phagocyte was responsible for harmonizing the potentially discordant cellular element during development. Once the organism is mature, these same mechanisms are used to protect the host's integrity and defend against pathogens. In other words, inflammation and immunity were viewed as the general process by which the organism was defined as it developed and protected as an adult. He felt that phagocytes were the main determinants of the cellular aspects of immunity. A controversy then developed between supporters of the humoral and cellular theories. Others, such as Sir Almroth Wright and S. R. Douglas, felt that both the cellular and humoral factors were important but interdependent (2,25).

This controversy was exemplified by Wright's message to the practitioners of medicines in Shaw's play *A Doctor's Dilemma* (26):

> Sir Almroth Wright, following up on one of Metchnikoff's most suggestive biological romances, discovered that the white corpuscles or phagocytes, which attack and devour the disease germs for us, do their work only when we butter the disease germs appetizingly for them with a natural sauce which Sir Almroth named opsonin.

Despite Metchnikoff's work, the importance of the cellular system was not established until the 1920s with investigations of Zinsser et al. regarding delayed hypersensitivity and further studies up to the present time. These included investigations of Gell, Hinde, Turk, Landsteiner, Chase, Billingham, Bret, Medawar, Waksman, Good, and Burnet (1,19). All these investigators emphasized the importance of the cellular system through work on tissue transplantation, immunological tolerance, and immunological deficiency diseases. The importance of the lymphocyte and the other cellular components of the immune system is now established.

B. Noninfectious Factors and the Immune System

Initially, the relationship between immunity and infections was the main focus of study in immunology. In the beginning of the 19th century, Bordet (1,21,27) and others demonstrated that antibody formation also occurred following the injection of nonmicrobes and their toxins. In addition, it became apparent that antibodies that appeared to bear no relationship to the state of resistance against the invading organism would often be produced in the course of bacterial disease.

The widely held view that antibody production was designed specifically to protect the infected host was questioned with the observation that sometimes the excess of antigen to the body results in severe adverse symptoms and even death. This phenomenon, in which an immunological response leads to reaction damage to cells of the body, was referred to as hypersensitivity. The original data on which this idea is based were provided by Portier and Richet for anaphylaxis (28) and by Arthus for the local Arthus reactions (29). Clemens von Pirquet with Béla Schick in 1902 described the serum sickness syndrome (18,30,31). It was von Pirquet who coined the word "allergy" in 1906 (31). He wrote, "For this general concept of changed reactivity, I propose the term 'Allergy.' 'Allos' implies deviation from the original state, from the behavior of the normal individual." Allergy was defined as an adverse immune reaction, and the formal study of allergy as a discipline began.

C. Genetics of the Immune System (Immunogenetics)

Inherited differences among individuals, or genetic polymorphism, has been noted to involve the immune system. Early studies were performed in the area of transplantation (1,5). Attempts to replace missing or defective tissues and organs have been reported since the Middle Ages. When tissue grafts failed, the recipient was said to be "immune." At the end of the 19th century, tumors were also investigated, particularly to determine whether it was the individual or something related to the cancer tissue itself that accounts for rejection. Transplantation studies resulted in identifying the importance of the major histocompatibility complex (32–34). Landsteiner showed that humans could be divided into several groups depending on their agglutinins specific for the erythrocytes of other humans (35). This was the basis for the ABO system of blood types. Von Dungern and Hirszfeld reported on different blood groups in humans (A, B, AB, O), which obeyed the normal Mendelian rules of inheritance (1). Scheibel demonstrated in 1943, using diphtheria toxoid in guinea pigs, that the specific immune response was genetically determined (36). Later it was demonstrated that immunoglobulins possess genetically determined antigenic markers as allotypes. Additional studies demonstrated that the maturation of an antibody response generally involved the sequential utilization of those genes that encode for the constant region of heavy chains (37). McDevitt and Chinitz as well as Benacerraf and Germain later showed that the immune response was associated with the major histocompatibility system (38,39). The study of the immune system (immunogenetics) developed through investigations of not only the histocompatibility system and the blood groups, but also the generation of immunological diversity, the formation of the immunoglobulin molecules and of the mechanisms for disease with regard to predisposition and resistance. As a result of all these studies, it has become apparent that the development of the immune system is influenced by genetic factors.

IV. ALLERGY

A. Description of Allergies

Descriptions of allergic conditions such as asthma, rhinitis, anaphylaxis, and food reactions date back to ancient times. Their relationship to the immune system was established in the last part of the 19th and first part of the 20th century. The conception that the immune system, which had been shown to protect our bodies, could cause adverse reactions was difficult to accept.

1. Allergy

It was not until the beginning of the 20th century through the work of Arthus, von Pirquet, and Schick that there was reanalysis of the well-established observations that the presence of humoral antibodies were important in defense against infections with the observations that other immune reactions involving humoral antibodies mediated adverse reactions (18,28–32). This resulted in the development of the term "allergy" by Clemons von Pirquet referring to adverse immune reactions (31). This term, although initially used to described humoral or antibody-mediated reaction, has also been used for cellular adverse reaction such as the tuberculin reaction. In this book, allergy will be defined as an adverse immune reaction.

2. Atopy

The term "atopy" was proposed by Coca and Cooke in 1923 to identify what were commonly known as clinical allergies involving reaginic or skin-sensitizing antibodies that are subject to hereditary influence (40). Atopy is derived from the Greek word meaning "out of place" or "strange disease." It is a term that has been redefined by many investigators since. It has been used to refer to (1) all allergic phenomena regardless of whether an antibody could be demonstrated; (2) clinical conditions associated with the presence of an identifiable IgE or response antibody; or (3) the presence of a specific skin-sensitizing, reaginic, or IgE antibody regardless of the presence of an identifiable clinical condition. In this book we will define atopy as an adverse immune reaction involving IgE antibodies.

3. Asthma

Asthma was described in ancient times and has been mentioned in the Bible. The term "asthma" appears very early in medical literature but referred to dyspnea in general. The word "asthma" is derived from a Greek word that means panting. The first valid description of asthma in terms of difficulty of breathing was by Aretaeus in c. A.D. 81–138. This was followed by other descriptions of asthma by Hippocrates, Galen, and Celsus. Environmental factors were noted to be associated with the development of asthma. Cardan, in 1545, diagnosed asthma triggered by feathers. Van Helmont in the 17th century described attacks of asthma caused by house dust and by eating fish fried in oil. Von Pirquet noted patients who, after horse serum therapy, developed urticaria and asthma (1,4). As defined by the Committee on Diagnostic Standards of the American Thoracic Society in 1962 (41), asthma is "a disease characterized by an increased responsiveness of the trachea and bronchi to a variety of stimuli and manifested by widespread narrowing of the airways that changes in severity either spontaneously or as a result of therapy."

4. Rhinitis

Allergic rhinitis is defined as inflammation of the nasal mucous membrane that is characterized by periods of nasal discharge, sneezing, and congestion that involves an IgE mechanism. It has been reported to be associated with asthma and atopic dermatitis. Rhinitis was also described in ancient times. Rhazes, in the 6th century, gave the first known description of hay fever in his dissertation on the cause of the coryza that occurs in the spring when the roses give forth their scent. Rose catarrh, or rose fever, was reported by Botallo in 1565 and by Binninger in 1651. John Bostock accurately described a syndrome from which he suffered, which he termed hay fever in 1819 (1,4,18). The identification of pollen as cause of this disease was reported by Morrill Wyman (42). He also noted a family predisposition. Blackley performed a systematic study to evaluate causative agents of hay fever and asthma stressing the importance of pollen (18,43).

5. Anaphylaxis

Anaphylaxis is considered an IgE-mediated, allergen-induced reaction in animals characterized by systemic reactions involving various tissues of the body, including the cardiovascular and gastrointestinal system as well as the respiratory tract and skin (44). Menes' (2641 B.C.) death was reported to have resulted from an anaphylactic reaction to venom. Magendi in 1839 followed by Flexner and T. Smith described animal models of what we would now call anaphylaxis (1,4). Credit for classic descriptions of anaphylaxis was reported by Portier and Richet (28). Clinical reports of anaphylaxis were noted initially to be due to horse serum used for administration of diphtheria and tetanus antitoxins. Rosenau and Anderson reported cases of anaphylaxis after horse serum, which at times led to death (18,45). Subsequently, many foreign materials—especially drugs and stinging insects—have been reported to cause anaphylaxis (44).

6. Urticaria and Angioedema

Urticaria is characterized by a cutaneous elevation that typically is as a wheal with erythema and blanches with pressure. It is frequently associated with itching. Angioedema is thought to involve a similar process but involves the deep dermal and subcutaneous tissue. Hippocratic writings described urticaria from mosquito bites and from gastrointestinal disturbances. Sydenham in 1685 described urticaria as similar to the stinging of nettles. Heinrich Quincke was credited with giving the first description of angioedema in 1882, though Bray states that Stolpertus first described it in 1778 (4,46).

7. Eczema

Eczema has been described since ancient times but has never been satisfactorily defined clinically. The term "eczema" comes from a Greek root meaning "to bubble, boil, burst forth." There has been controversy about the proper definition of eczema or atopic dermatitis. Initially *eczema* was applied to skin diseases of almost all varieties including lesions of smallpox and leprosy. Willan provided one of the early comprehensive definitions of eczema as a "condition generally due to the effects of irritation whether externally or internally applied and occasionally produced by a great variety of irritants in persons whose skin is constitutionally very irritable" (46). At present it has been characterized as a cutaneous response to various noxious stimuli in which erythema and vesiculation is seen in the acute stages and scaling and thickening of the skin in the chronic stages.

8. Atopic Dermatitis

Atopic dermatitis has been defined as a chronic, heritable, especially pruritic form of eczema (dermatitis), which possesses distinctive features in respect to localization of the lesion and is frequently associated with asthma and allergic rhinitis (47,48). In addition, most—but not all—atopic dermatitis patients produce identifiable IgE antibodies. Atopic dermatitis has a variety of clinical manifestations, which can be seen in infants, teens, and adults. Hanifin and Rajka have published diagnostic features of atopic dermatitis, which have been useful to investigators as well as practitioners (48). Seymour et al. further defined eczema in children below the age of 5, especially in infants (49). In the past, terms used for atopic dermatitis have included atopic eczema, eczema, dermatitis, Besnier prurigo, and neurodermatitis.

Through the years allergic conditions such as asthma, eczema, and anaphylaxis have been difficult to define. There is general agreement that there is no agreement on many of these definitions. It has not been shown to date whether many of these conditions we call allergy—such as asthma, atopy, and eczema—are a single disease involving a common pathway regulated by a particular gene(s), a group of similar-appearing diseases involving common pathways regulated by a variety of genes, or groups of conditions with similar clinical pictures that are a result of a variety of different mechanisms regulated by a variety of genes. Does asthma involve one or multiple phenotypes? The further study of the genetics of these conditions should resolve these questions.

B. The Immune System as It Relates to Allergy/Atopy

The study of adverse reactions of the immune system, or allergies, probably began with Jenner's observation of the accelerated vaccinal reaction in certain previously vaccinated persons (1,2). In 1837, Magendie described the sudden death of dogs that had been repeatedly injected with egg albumin. Flexner in 1894 reported that animals that were apparently uninjured by an initial dose of dog serum would succumb to a second dose administered after a lapse of some days or weeks (1). The first systematic study of anaphylaxis was undertaken by Portier and Richet in 1902 using the aquatic animal *Physalia* (28). The publication of Arthus in 1903 served to focus attention on the immune system and its involvement in the state of hypersensitivity, which develops after a certain interval following the parenteral injection of protein. He described these reactions after local injection as "local anaphylaxis" (29). It is now known that the Arthus reaction differs from passive anaphylaxis or systemic anaphylaxis as neutrophils are essential components, and complement participates in this reaction. Koch tuberculin reaction, thought initially to be a response to tuberculin toxic effect, was reevaluated in view of the work by Arthus and called an allergic reaction. Subsequently it was described as a tuberculin-type hypersensitivity, then delayed-type hypersensitivity, and ultimately cellular immunity (1,18). Therefore, the initial identification of the role of the immune system in causing adverse clinical reactions was described with regard to the Arthus reaction, anaphylaxis, and infections.

With this background, the beginning of the development of the field of allergic investigation in relation to the immune system and human conditions took place in 1905 when von Pirquet and Schick published their observations of serum sickness and subsequently introduced the term "allergy" (31). A connection between hay fever and asthma and the immune system was suggested by Blackley, who in 1873 reported skin reactivity to grass pollen with hay fever (18,43,50). Later, Alfred Wolff-Eisner in 1906 provided further evidence of skin-sensitizing antibody in these reactions and stressed the relationship between hay fever and a hypersensitivity state or reaction in the immunological sense (1,2,51). In 1910 Samuel Meltzer did the same thing for asthma in his description of "Bronchial Asthma as a Phenomenon of Anaphylaxis" (1,3,52). Oscar Menderson Schloss established the practicability of using the scratch test as a diagnostic procedure in human forms of hypersensitiveness (53). Initial studies by Blackley in 1873 (18,43,50) and more extensive studies by Noon and Freeman in 1911 developed the treatment of active immunization against hay fever by using pollen solutions (54,55). The intradermal testing procedure was subsequently developed by R. Cooke in 1915 (18). In the 1960s Johansson and Ishizaka described the immunoglobulin group IgE and demonstrated that it was the globulin that was called reaginic antibody (56–58). Further characterization of the immune system and its relationship to allergy is providing information to develop a model of allergic conditions such as asthma and allergic rhinitis. This includes characterization of cytokines and T and B cells, as well as the role of inflammation in the development of allergic conditions. Phenotypes can now be developed to study the pathogenesis of these conditions that involve genetic and environmental factors.

C. Allergy and Genetics

Early reports suggested a relationship between allergy and familial and genetic factors. Hippocrates (460–375 B.C.) suggested a relationship between these diseases and heredity (1). Wyman (1812–1903) described a family predisposition for autumnal catarrh (42), while Floyer noted in 1698 that asthma was familial (3). The heredity basis for angioedema was reported by Osler in 1888 (59,60). Other forms of familial urticaria have been described (61–64). By most definitions eczema or atopic dermatitis has a familial and heritable component (46–48).

Through the years it has become evident that familial if not genetic factors are involved in allergic conditions such as asthma, hay fever, eczema, and urticaria (65). The systematic study of the genetics of allergic conditions was started by Cooke and Vander Veer in 1916, who described the heritability of the clinical manifestations of sensitization or allergies such as bronchial asthma, hay fever, and urticaria (66). Since then, many studies have confirmed their findings (67,68). With the development of a variety of techniques in various disciplines, including immunology, biochemistry, molecular biology, and statistics, the specific genetics of allergic conditions are being defined.

V. MULTIDISCIPLINARY APPROACH TO THE UNDERSTANDING OF THE GENETICS OF ASTHMA AND ALLERGIES

In the beginning, many aspects of asthma and allergies were described in terms of mystery and magic. Through the years, on the basis of information gathered from many different disciplines, a working model of the immune system and its relationship to disease has evolved. It is becoming more and more apparent that the artificial separation between previously defined areas of the sciences is disappearing. One discipline needs the other for cross-fertilization, which in the end results in progress. Information from a variety of apparently unrelated fields, including biochemistry, biophysics, biology of cancer, cell biology, hematology, genetics, medicine, microbiology, molecular biology, pathology, pediatrics, statistics, and surgery, as well as immunology and allergy, is needed to understand the biology of asthma and allergies. Asthma and allergies result from an interaction of the host's genetic composition with nongenetic and environmental factors. This book will review the factors involved in the development of allergies using information obtained from a variety of different areas, which is allowing investigators and clinicians to improve their understanding and management of allergic conditions.

ACKNOWLEDGMENT

This work was supported in part by NIH Grant 5U01 HL49609.

REFERENCES

1. Silverstein M. A history of immunology. San Diego: Academic Press, 1989.
2. Swartz MN. *Yersinia, Francisella, Pasteurella* and *Brucella.* In: Davis B, Dulbecco R, Eisen H, Ginsberg, eds. Microbiology, 4th ed. Philadelphia: JB Lippincott, 1990: 601–614.
3. Unger L. The history of bronchial asthma. In: Bronchial Asthma. Springfield, IL: Charles C Thomas, 1945:10–34.
4. Major RH. Classic Descriptions of Disease, 3rd ed. Springfield, IL: Charles C Thomas, 1955.
5. Major RH. A History of Medicine, Vol. 1. Springfield, IL: Charles C Thomas, 1954.
6. Farrington B. Aristotle: Founder of Scientific Philosophy. London: Weidenfeld & Nicolson (Educational), 1965.
7. Reid CA. The Principles of Heredity. New York: EP Dutton, 1905:1–28.
8. DeBeer G. Charles Darwin: Evolution by Natural Selection. Garden City, NY: Doubleday, 1967.
9. Stern C, Sherwood E, eds. The Origin of Genetics: A Mendel Source Book. San Francisco: WH Freeman, 1966.
10. McKusick VA. Anatomy of the human genome. Hosp Pract (Hosp Ed) 1981; 16: 82–100.
11. Goodenough U. Genetics, 3rd ed. Philadelphia: WB Saunders, 1983.
12. Beadle G, Tatum E. Genetic control of biochemical reactions in neurospora. *Proc Natl Acad Sci USA* 1941; 27:499.
13. Crick FHC. The genetic code. Sci Am 1962; 207:66–77.

14. Watson JD. The Molecular Biology of the Gene, 3rd ed. Menlo Park, CA: WA Benjamin, 1976.
15. Edlin G. Human Genetics. Boston: Jones and Bartlett, 1990:86–101.
16. Brock TD, ed. and trans. Milestones in Microbiology. Englewood Cliffs, NJ: Prentice-Hall, 1961. Reprinted by the American Society for Microbiology, 1975.
17. Spink W. Infectious Diseases. Minneapolis: University of Minnesota Press, 1978.
18. Major RH. A History of Medicine, Vol. 2. Springfield, IL: Charles C Thomas, 1954.
19. Tauber A. The immune self: theory or metaphor. Immunol Today 1994; 15:134–136.
20. Tauber A. The immunological self: a centenary perspective. Perspect Biol Med 1991; 35:74–86.
21. Berzofsky J, Beekower IM. Immunogenicity an antigen structure. In: Paul WE, ed. Fundamental Immunology, 2nd ed. New York: Raven Press, 1989:169–208.
22. Samter M, Cohn S, eds. Excerpts from Classics in Allergy, 2nd ed. Carlsbad: Symposia Foundation, 1979.
23. Frank M, Fries L. Complement. In: Paul WE, ed. Fundamental Immunology, 2nd ed. New York: Raven Press, 1989:679–701.
24. Oltvai ZN, Wong EC, Atkinson JP, Tung KS. C1 inhibitor deficiency: molecular and immunologic basis of hereditary and acquired angioedema. Lab Invest 1991; 65:381–388.
25. Wright AE, Douglas SR. Proc Roy Soc Lond Ser B 1903; 72:364.
26. Shaw GB. Doctor's Dilemma: A Tragedy by Bernard Shaw. Minneapolis: Cornelius, 1966. (Reprint).
27. Bordet J. Studies on Immunity. Gay FP, trans. New York: Wiley, 1909.
28. Portier P, Richet C. Chapter de l'action anaphylactique de certains benins. C R Soc Biol Paris, 1902; 54:170.
29. Arthus M. Injections repetees de serum de cheval chez le pain. C R Soc Biol Paris, 1903; 55:817.
30. Von Pirquet C, Schick B. Die serum krankheit. Vienna: Deuticke, 1906. [English transl.: Serum Sickness. Baltimore: Williams & Wilkins, 1951.]
31. Von Pirquet C, Clemens. Munch Med Wochenschr 1906; 53:1457. Prausnitz C, trans. Gell PGH, Coombs RRA, eds. Clinical Aspects of Immunology. Philadelphia: FA Davis, 1963.
32. Kissmeyer-Nielsen F, Thorsby E. Human transplantation antigens. Appendix: current methods in histocompatibility testing. Transplant Rev 1969; 4:1–76.
33. Walford RL. The isoantigenic system of human leukocytes: medical and biological significance. Ser Haematol 1969; 2(2):1–96.
34. Hansen T, Sachs D. The major histocompatibility complex. In: Paul WE, ed. Fundamental Immunology, 2nd ed. New York: Raven Press, 1989:445–448.
35. Landsteiner K. The specificity of serological reactions, rev. ed. New York: Dover Publications, 1962.
36. Scheibel IF. Hereditary differences in the capacity of guinea-pigs for the production of the diphtheria antitoxin. Acta Pathol Scand 1943; 20:464–484.
37. Max EE. Immunoglobulins: molecular genetics. In: Paul WE, ed. Fundamental Immunology, 2nd ed. New York: Raven Press, 1989:235–290.

38. McDevitt HO, Chinitz A. Genetic control of the antibody response: relationship between immune response and histocompatibility (H-2) type. Science 1969; 163: 1207–1208.
39. Benacerraf B, Germain RN. The immune response genes of the major histocompatibility complex. Immunol Rev 1978; 38:70–119.
40. Coca AF, Cooke RA. On the classification of the phenomena of hypersensitiveness. J Immunol 1923; 8:163–182.
41. American Thoracic Society Committee on Diagnostic Standards for Non Tubercular Respiratory Disease. Definitions and classification of chronic bronchitis, asthma and pulmonary emphysema. Am Rev Respir Dis 1962; 85:762–768.
42. Wyman M. Autumnal Catarrh. New York: Hurd and Houghton, 1872.
43. Blackley CH. Experimental Researches on the Causes and Nature of Catarrhus Aestivus (Hay Fever or Hay Asthma). London: Bailliere, Tindall and Cox, 1873.
44. Marquardt DL, Wasserman SI. Anaphylaxis. In: Middleton E, Reed C, Ellis E, Adkinson NF, Yunginger JW, eds. Allergy Principles and Practice, Vol. 2, 3rd ed. St. Louis: CV Mosby, 1988:1365–1376.
45. Rosenau M, Anderson JG. Hypersusceptibility. JAMA 1906; 42:1007–1010 (abstract).
46. Vaughan WT, Black JJH. Skin diseases. In: Practice of Allergy, 3rd ed. St. Louis: CV Mosby, 1954.
47. Hanifin JM. Atopic dermatitis. In: Middleton E, Reed C, Ellis E, Adkinson NF, Yunginger JW, eds. Allergy Principles and Practice, Vol. 2, 4th ed. St. Louis: CV Mosby, 1988:1581–1604.
48. Hanifin JM, Rajka G. Diagnostic features of atopic dermatitis. Acta Dermatol Venereol 1980; 92(Suppl):44–47.
49. Seymour JL, Keswick BH, Hanifin JM, Jordan WP, Milligan MC. Clinical effects of diaper types on the skin of normal infants and infants with atopic dermatitis. J Am Acad Dermatol 1987; 17:988–997.
50. Blackley CH. Hayfever: Its Causes, Treatment and Effective Prevention: Experimental Research, 2nd ed. London: Bailliere, Tindall and Cox, 1880.
51. Wolff-Eisner A. Das heufieber: sein wesen und seine behandlung. Munich, 1906.
52. Meltzer SJ. Bronchial asthma as a phenomenon of anaphylaxis. JAMA 1910; 55: 1021–1024.
53. Schloss OM. A case of allergy to common food. Am J Dis Child 1912; 111:341.
54. Freeman J, Noon L. Further observations on the treatment of hayfever by hypodermic injection of pollen vaccine. Lancet 1911; 180(2):814–817.
55. Noon L. Prophylactic inoculation against hayfever. Lancet 1911; 180(1):1572–1573.
56. Ishizaka K. Ishizaka T. Physiochemical properties of reaginic antibody. 1. Association of reaginic activity with an immunoglobulin other than gamma A- or gamma G-globulin. J Allergy 1966; 37:169–185.
57. Ishizaka K, Ishizaka T. Physiochemical properties of reaginic antibody. 3. Further studies on the reaginic antibody in gamma A-globulin preparation. J Allergy 1966; 38:108–119.
58. Johansson SGO, Bennich H. Immunological studies of an atypical (myeloma) immunoglobulin. Immunology 1967; 13:381–394.

59. Osler W. Hereditary angioneurotic edema. Am J Med Sci 1988; 98:362–367.
60. Quincke H. Über akutes umschreibenes H-autoderm. Monatschr Prakt Dermatol 1882; 1:129–131.
61. Kaplan AP. Urticaria and angioedema. In: Middleton E, Reed CE, Ellis EF, Adkinson NF, Yunginger JW, eds. Allergy Principles and Practice, 4th ed. St. Louis: CV Mosby, 1988:1553–1580.
62. Alper CA, Abramson N, Johnston RB, Jandl JH, Rosen FS. Increased susceptibility to infection associated with abnormalities of complement-mediated functions and of the third component of complement (C3). N Engl J Med 1970; 282:350–354.
63. Black JT. Amylodoisis, deafness, urticaria, and limb pains: a hereditary syndrome. Ann Intern Med 1969; 70:989–994.
64. Warin RP, Champion RH. Urticaria. London: WB Saunders, 1974:113–119.
65. Pillsbury DM, Shelly W, Kligman A. Dermatitis and eczema. In: Dermatology. Philadelphia: WB Saunders, 1965:363–458.
66. Cooke RA, Vander Veer A. Human sensitization. J Immunol 1916; 1:201–305.
67. Blumenthal MN. Family, twin and population studies of allergic responsiveness. In: Marsh DG, Lockhart A, Holgate ST, eds. The Genetics of Asthma. Oxford: Blackwell Scientific Publications, 1993:133–141.
68. Gerrard JW, Blumenthal MN. Genetic factors. In: Weiss EB, Stein M, eds. Bronchial Asthma, 3rd ed. Boston: Little, Brown, 1993:26–31.

2

Human Genetics

Stephen S. Rich
Bowman Gray School of Medicine
Winston-Salem, North Carolina

I. INTRODUCTION

Human genetics is the application of the principles and tools of genetics to the study of human characteristics. The study of human genetics is, therefore, the investigation of human deoxyribonucleic acid (DNA). DNA is a polymeric, double-stranded molecule that is composed of adenine (A), thymine (T), guanine (G), and cytosine (C), which pair in specific ways to constitute the "blueprint" of our existence. The sequence of these bases forms the DNA molecule and, roughly speaking, can be considered as being translated into genes (the fundamental unit of heredity) and "nonsense" DNA.

The gene, representing the fundamental unit of inheritance, is itself composed of an ordered sequence of bases at a specific chromosomal site that is functionally defined by its protein product. The physical structure of a gene includes regions that may be involved in regulation of expression and contains regions that are used in producing a product (exons) and regions that do not "code" for a known product (introns). While DNA is double-stranded, the production of proteins is essentially mediated by ribonucleic acid (RNA), a molecule that is produced from the DNA template in the cell nucleus (transcription). A specific RNA (messenger RNA, or mRNA) is a processed RNA that serves as a template for the protein synthesis that drives the process of life.

The DNA that determines human variation and human disease is contained in the chromosomes. The human karyotype consists of 46 chromosomes—44 of these (the autosomes) occur in 22 homologous pairs, with each member of a pair containing the "same" genetic information. The remaining two chromosomes are the sex chromosomes—a female has two X chromosomes and a male has an X and a Y chromosome. Determination of the genetic factors that control susceptibility to disease or contribute to normal human variation in a characteristic centers on identifying how many genes control the characteristic, how they function, and where the genes are located.

In classic plant and animal genetic experiments, individual matings between male and female members can be used to identify specific genes and their location. In particular, the fruitfly, *Drosophila melanogaster*, has been a major experimental organism whose findings can often be used as the basis for human studies. Unlike the fruitfly, individually defined and manipulated matings between humans cannot be specified for prediction of outcome. In addition, the time to maturity and the life span in humans is too long to allow rapid observation of specific characteristics over generations. Thus, while the fundamental tools used for the study of humans may be similar or, in some cases, identical to those used in experimental organisms, the application of the tools to humans presents unique problems. This chapter highlights the general approach to the study of the genetics of human characteristics and, in particular, human disease.

II. ROLE OF GENETIC FACTORS IN HUMAN DISEASE

In order to better understand the approach to the investigation of human disease, several essential terms and concepts have to be defined. Genes are arranged in a linear array along the length of a chromosome. A genetic locus is considered to be a specific position on a chromosome of a gene. Although the position of a gene is relatively constant on a chromosome, the DNA sequence may differ at the site. This difference in DNA sequence of a particular gene may be detected in a number of ways, with each alternate form of the gene considered to be an allele. For a given individual, if both alleles are identical at a given locus, then the individual is said to be homozygous at that locus; alternatively, if the two alleles are different, that individual is said to be heterozygous at that locus.

The two alleles at a locus therefore define the genotype of an individual for that locus. In the broadest sense, the genotype of an individual is the sum total of all genetic effects defined by the individual (additive) effects of the alleles, the interactions among alleles at each locus (dominance), and the interactions among alleles at different loci (epistasis). The phenotype of an individual is the observed characteristic that is determined by the joint effects of the genotype and environmental factors and their interaction. In general, environmental risk factors can be classified as either "common" (shared household effects) or "random." Historically, the investigation of the manner in which environmental risk factors contribute to disease and the methods used to intervene in the exposure to these risk factors has been the substance of the field of epidemiology. In this context, a "susceptible" individual is one who will have a phenotype (disease) if the relevant exposure is present and will not have the phenotype (disease) if the exposure is absent. In genetic terms, the "susceptible" individual has a "susceptible genotype" and the outcome (phenotype) represents a genotype-environment interaction. Thus, a "susceptible" individual would not experience an allergic reaction in the absence of the allergen.

III. MAJOR TYPES OF HUMAN GENETIC DISEASE

Genetic factors that contribute to a phenotype can be of multiple forms; the characteristic may be due to a single gene, several genes, or many genes. Those diseases that are characterized as the result of a single mutant gene that has a large effect on the phenotype and are inherited in simple patterns are termed Mendelian. A Mendelian disorder is considered autosomal if the gene responsible is located on one of the 22 pairs of autosomes, or it is X-linked if the gene is located on the X chromosome. [A catalog of known single-gene disorders has been maintained by McKusick and periodically updated.] A dominant pattern of inheritance is one that requires only one copy (allele) of a mutant gene to express an abnormal (disease) phenotype, while a recessive pattern requires that two copies of a mutant gene be present to have a specific phenotype.

The patterns of inheritance for Mendelian traits have been determined from observational studies of disease transmission in families (or pedigrees). In general, an index case (or proband) is identified that brings the family into the study. For disease traits (qualitative characteristics), the proband is a person with disease (such as asthma or allergy). For traits that show continuous variation (quantitative characteristics), the proband may be an individual with an "extreme" phenotype (such as a high IgE level) or a random subject who is used to enroll the family into the study (regardless of his IgE level). Based on patterns of transmission of disease in families, many simple Mendelian traits have been classified according to their degree of dominance.

There are many cases of apparent simple Mendelian inheritance, however, when an individual who should present with a specific phenotype (disease) fails to do so. This may occur when an individual with a mutant gene fails to express the disease (in the case of an autosomal dominant disorder). Thus, the probability of exhibiting the disease when the susceptible genotype is present (the penetrance) is less than unity. This situation is considered a case of an incompletely penetrant trait. Penetrance for each genotype can be estimated and, when combined with the frequency of the susceptibility genes in the population, can be used to predict the prevalence of the disorder in the population. The explanation for reduced penetrance is not well resolved, but may be an indication that specific environmental factors (intra- or extrauterine) may play a role in the expression of genes and their resulting phenotypes.

A. Chromosomal Abnormalities

Abnormalities involving human chromosomes may be either structural (alterations in the chromosome itself) or numerical (alterations in chromosome number). Although the abnormality may be present in all cells of an individual, there may be a mixture of "normal" and "abnormal" cells; this is termed mosaicism.

Alterations in chromosome number typically emerge through nondisjunction—the failure of chromosome pairs to disjoin at anaphase in either the first or second meiotic division. Since humans have 23 pairs of chromosomes, any exact multiple of the haploid ($n = 23$) number is termed euploid. Although triploidy and tetraploidy are common occurrences in the plant kingdom, only a few triploids have been born in humans. Any number of chromosomes that is not an exact multiple of the haploid number is termed aneuploid. The most common form of aneuploidy in humans is Down syndrome, or trisomy 21.

Alterations in chromosome structure primarily result from breakage and abnormal repair. The result of aberrant repair of chromosomal damage is primarily seen in the DNA sequence as a deletion, duplication, inversion, or translocation. Deletions represent a loss of a portion of a chromosome, with the structurally abnormal chromosome lacking the genetic information that was present in the lost fragment. A common example of a deletion is the cri du chat syndrome, in which a portion of the short arm of chromosome 5 is deleted (1).

Duplications are noted by the presence of an extra portion of a chromosome. While the occurrence of duplication in some genes is deleterious and leads to specific syndromes, duplication of DNA appears to be common in the genome. Repetitive DNA sequences are distributed throughout the genome, and variation in size and type of these sequences has served as the basis for mapping many disease susceptibility genes (2,3).

Inversions involve the fragmentation of a chromosome by two breaks in the chromosome structure followed by inverted sequence repair. If the inversion is in one arm of the chromosome and does not involve the centromere, there is no difference in the ratio of short/long arm length (paracentric inversion). If the inversion involves the centromere, the repair may alter the short/long arm ratio. The primary role of inversions in the genesis of human disease and syndromes lies in the consequence of recombination (crossing over) during meiosis I, when a loop must be formed and gametes may be formed that are either normal, balanced inversions or unbalanced inversions (containing both duplications and deletions).

Translocations represent the exchange of chromosomal material from chromosomes. The exchange may occur between two nonhomologous chromosomes (reciprocal translocation) or two acrocentric chromosomes that fuse at the centromere and lose the short arms (Robertsonian translocation).

Chromosomal abnormalities are a significant cause of birth defects and fetal loss (4); individuals with chromosomal abnormalities usually exhibit characteristic phenotypes that represent a series of genetic alterations. For this reason, individuals with specific chromosomal aberrations may have a cluster of clinical signs and symptoms that channel the phenotype into a characteristic appearance (syndrome). The utility of chromosomal abnormalities in gene mapping has increased due to the ability to identify small deletions in patients whose phenotype includes a characteristic of interest. Thus, a syndrome that includes asthma as a component of the phenotype and has a deletion recognized on a chromosome would enable further evaluation of that chromosomal region as a candidate region for susceptibility to asthma.

B. Single-Gene Disorders

Mendelian principles of segregation of alleles and independent assortment have established the foundation for the study of single-gene disorders. The underlying principal of segregation treats the gene as the basic unit of heredity, with two alleles (one derived from each parent) that have equal probability of being transmitted to an offspring. The pattern of inheritance for most single-gene Mendelian disorders has been determined from the characterization of the transmission (or segregation) of the disorder in families. The four major types of Mendelian transmission are autosomal dominant, autosomal recessive, X-linked dominant, and X-linked recessive.

Autosomal disorders occur with equal frequency in each sex and should be transmitted independent of the sex of the parent. All individuals with an autosomal dominant disorder should have an affected parent, unless the disease in the subject is due to a new mutation. Usually, affected individuals are observed in each generation of a pedigree. Autosomal recessive disorders also occur in equal frequency in members of each sex and are transmitted independent of the sex of the parent. In contrast to the autosomal dominant case, most individuals with an autosomal recessive disorder have two "normal" parents.

X-linked transmission produces characteristic segregation patterns since males have only one X chromosome (from the mother, and one Y chromosome from the father) while females have two X chromosomes (one from each parent); thus, X-linked dominant disorders preclude affected father–affected son transmission. On the other hand, all daughters of affected males should be affected. Offspring of affected females have equal probability of being affected due to equal probability of the "affected" or the "unaffected" X chromosome being transmitted. This pattern is indistinguishable from that of an affected female with an autosomal dominant trait. X-linked recessive transmission again precludes father-to-son transmission. For a rare trait, X-linked recessive transmission results in many more males than females being affected; the more rare the trait, the less likely the presence of an affected female.

For classical Mendelian traits, a single locus producing disease that segregates in a family would result in specific expectations of offspring phenotypes (affected, not affected) conditional on the mating type (disease status) of the parents. These fixed ratios of genotypes (phenotypes) among offspring could be evaluated statistically with the data observed from the collection of family material. In its original form, segregation analysis was used to test whether the phenotypic distribution (affected status) among offspring was compatible with Mendelian inheritance (5). Although this method was sufficient to identify a single (but not necessarily the same) locus that predisposes to a disease in families (such as cystic fibrosis), a number of limitations were inherent that limited its use for complex human disorders (such as asthma).

C. Polygenic Traits

In the analysis of human variation, the number of syndromes and single-gene disorders contributes only a small fraction to the total of naturally occurring variability. The differences between any two individuals in numerous measurable characteristics (height, weight, etc.) are essentially matters of degree with no "natural" dichotomy (such as "tall" or "short"). Continuous variation of this type introduce complexity into the understanding of genetic effects since the segregation of individual genes often cannot be followed for these quantitative characters.

In the case of most single-gene disorders, genetic segregation at a locus with two alleles results in three (sometimes distinct) genotypes. If there are many genetic loci that affect a characteristic, the simultaneous segregation of these genes would produce many "classes" of genotypes. As the individual genetic effects decrease in magnitude, the distinction between the classes diminishes and the difference between the classes approaches our error of measurement. This apparent continuity approaches true continuity since these quantitative characteristics are also subjected to variation from environmental (nongenetic) sources. In this manner, the distinction between Mendelian single-gene disorders and quantitative (continuous) characters revolves around the number of genes and the magnitude of their effects on the phenotype. The observed variation that is caused by the simultaneous segregation of many genes with relatively small effect is termed polygenic variation, and those genes of small effect are referred to as polygenes.

The distribution of most metric characters (such as IgE level) in the general population closely approximates a normal distribution, or the phenotypic distribution can be manipulated (by a mathematical transformation such as square root or logarithm) to achieve normality. The property of normality allows for the application of many statistical techniques to understand the genetics of quantitative traits. For a quantitative trait, we typically can measure only the individual value; the segregating polygenic loci cannot be observed directly. Thus, the properties of a population or a family that we can observe are the means, variances, and covariances among members for that trait (6). The use of family structure then enables determination of the degree of resemblance between relatives.

Since a large number of segregating loci contribute to the quantitative trait, the identification of individual genes cannot be made. Further, it should be noted that, in families, parents contribute one-half of their genes (and not genotypes) to their offspring. Thus, any interactions between alleles at a locus (dominance) or between alleles at different loci (epistasis) are lost in the transmission of genetic material to the next generation. In this fashion, only average effects of the genes from each parent determine the average genotypic value for offspring. These genetic effects are referred to as "breeding values" or "additive effects" of genes (6).

The total variation in a quantitative character is the variance of phenotypic values. The phenotypic variance itself can be partitioned into the genetic variance (composed of the additive, dominance, and epistatic variances), the environmental variance, and any genetic-environment interaction and covariance. The variance of additive effects (the additive genetic variance) represents that portion of the total (phenotypic) variance for a quantitative trait that is transmissible from parents to offspring. Thus, the proportion of the total variance that is attributable to the average effects of genes determines the degree of familial resemblance. The ratio of additive genetic variance to total phenotypic variance is termed the heritability. The higher the heritability, the greater the influence of polygenes on the measured phenotype (Fig. 1).

The magnitude of heritability ranges from zero to one and reflects the contribution of polygenes to a characteristic in a given population in a given environment. Thus, the heritability for IgE level in two populations may not

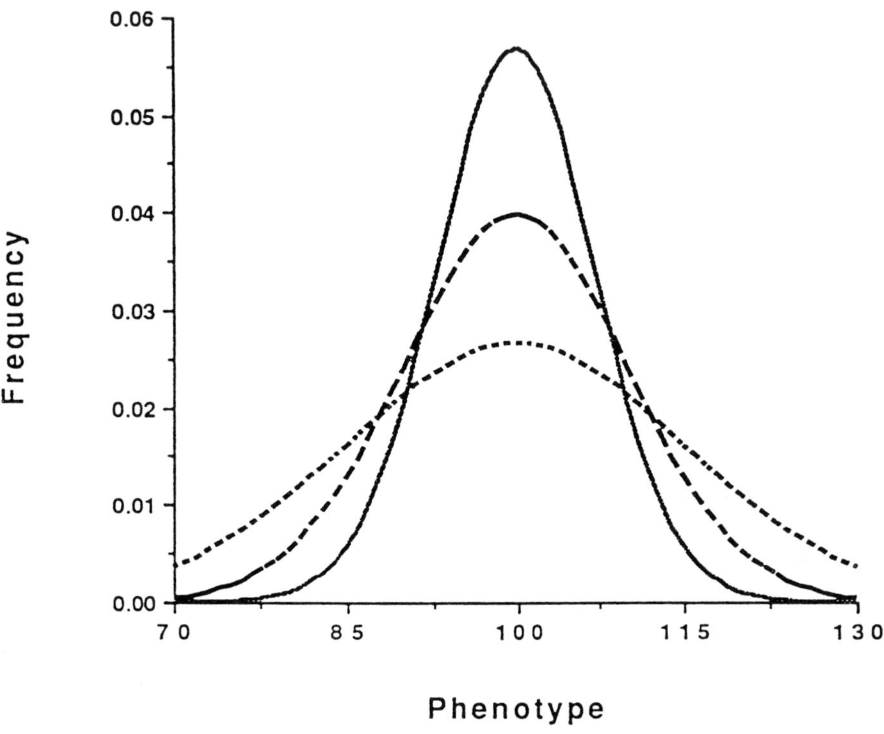

FIGURE 1   Frequency distribution of a phenotype (such as IQ). All individuals have the same genotypic (phenotypic) mean: individuals in the general population (dotted line); heritability of 50% (dashed line); heritability of 80% (solid line).

be comparable if the population structure (age, sex, ethnicity) and the environmental conditions (ragweed exposure) are different. In general, the traits in ex- perimental species of plants and animals that have the lowest heritabilities are connected with evolutionary conserved traits (fitness or reproductive characters).

D. Multifactorial Inheritance

A multifactorial trait is one that is determined by multiple factors—genetic and environmental—that aggregates in families without a clear pattern of Mendelian segregation. Multifactorial inheritance can be distinguished from polygenic inheritance in that polygenes are large in number but with individually small additive effects. Similar to the polygenic model, the resemblance between relatives for a multifactorial trait allows for the total phenotypic variance to be partitioned into components that reflect genetic and environmental differences. Analysis of quantitative traits (such as IgE levels) is performed in a manner consistent with a polygenic trait.

When the phenotype of interest is a disease (such as asthma), multifactorial inheritance takes a different approach. Phenotypes of this type may initially appear to be inappropriate for analysis under the multifactorial model since they exhibit discontinuous, rather than continuous, variation (7). However, the inheritance of disease can be modeled by the presence of an underlying continuity (or "liability") with a "threshold" that imposes a discontinuity on the expression of the trait. The extension from polygenic inheritance, therefore, is that the statistic of interest is the "heritability of liability" as measured by the resemblance (or correlation) of liability in relatives.

Although the multifactorial threshold model has been extensively used to study complex diseases, the underlying assumption of multiple genetic loci need not imply hundreds of genes each with small effect (as in the polygenic model). In particular, for some common diseases (asthma?) a few genetic loci with relatively large effect may be detected. These disorders that are clearly not Mendelian but do have a high degree of familial aggregation may be oligogenic (a few genes of large effect) rather than polygenic. Thus, the multifactorial basis of disease may be reduced to the interaction of an environmental "trigger" that forces the phenotype beyond the "threshold" defined in large part by a few genes of major effect. While it is difficult to conceive of an effective strategy to genetically map polygenes (owing to the large number of loci and the difficulty in detecting genes with small additive effects), there are strategies being developed that could be used to locate genes of major effect (oligogenes). Thus, complex disorders such as asthma, cancer, and cardiovascular disease may be approached by partitioning the underlying liability into individual genetic components.

IV. UNITS OF GENETIC ANALYSIS

Methods of human genetic analysis typically fall into two categories—population studies and family studies. The distinction between these two groups is not perfectly valid, since a population may represent a collection of families. For this purpose, however, population studies may be restricted to the random collection of families in a population or the collection of unrelated individuals for study. Family studies may include sibling pairs (including twins), sibships, nuclear families, or pedigrees. Although not discussed in detail here, the method of collection of data for analysis is of critical importance for some analytic approaches. The selection of individuals (or families) for study is referred to, in general, as ascertainment, with the ascertainment probability defined as the chance that an affected individual will be identified as a proband.

Two extreme situations of ascertainment are "complete" (with the ascertainment probability equal to 1 since all affecteds will be detected as probands) and "single" (the probability of an affected individual becoming a proband is small so that no family will likely have more than one proband). In practice, diseases are studied in families by collecting family members of affected children, resulting in "incomplete ascertainment." In all cases, the manner in which ascertainments are made should be well documented for appropriate inclusion of analysis (5). This is particularly critical in segregation analysis, a statistical method used to evaluate evidence for a single major gene that contributes to a phenotype. It is important to recognize, however, that it is the goal of the study that determines the optimal sampling and analytic strategies.

A. Twin Studies

About one in every 250 fertilizations, two daughter cells resulting from the cleavage of the zygote become separated and proceed to divide by mitosis to produce a separate individual. These two individuals are identical genetically and are called monozygotic (MZ) twins. When two different ova are available and are fertilized at the same time, the two individuals share (on average) their genes to the same extent as siblings and are called dizygotic (DZ) twins.

Studies of twins can often provide important evidence on the roles of genes and/or environmental risk factors in relation to genetic susceptibility to disease. In a group of twins with a given disorder, the cotwin in each pair is evaluated with respect to the disease in question. On the basis of the finding in the cotwin, the members of the pair are said to be either "concordant" (similar in phenotype) or "discordant" (different in phenotype). The greater the contribution of shared genes and/or shared environment to disease, the higher the concordance rate in MZ twins relative to DZ twins.

While a greater concordance rate in MZ twins over that observed for DZ twins is consistent with the importance of genetic factors, the presence of an MZ concordance rate of less than 100% underscores the importance of environmental factors in disease. For many complex disorders that involve both genes and environmental contributions to disease risk, the MZ twin concordance rate is significantly lower than 100%. In particular, many autoimmune disorders (such as insulin-dependent diabetes and systemic lupus erythematosus) that have a complex etiology involving HLA-mediated susceptibility with a likely environmental "trigger" have MZ twin concordance rates in the 25–60% range (8,9).

Analysis of twin concordance data typically involve the use of analysis of variance to estimate that portion of variation (the mean squares) that is attributed to "among pair" and "between pair" differences in either MZ or DZ pairs. These estimated mean squares are then equated to the expected mean squares for MZ and DZ twins, where the expected mean squares are functions of the genetic (additive and nonadditive) and the environmental (common and random) variance components (10). Based on the magnitude of the variance components, the heritability of the phenotype (disease susceptibility) can be estimated. Most analyses utilize twin pairs reared in the same environment, thereby confounding the effects of genes with those due to common (shared household) environment. Using a rare data set (of size several hundred) of twins reared together and twins reared apart, important insights into the role of shared genes and shared environment on phenotype can be obtained (11). Unfortunately, these data are useful only for quantitative (measured) characters (such as IgE level), since the frequency of disease (such as asthma) would result in only a few pairs of twins with one member affected. Use of families of MZ twins, however, may contribute significant insight to genetic mechanisms, however, since these families contain members with multiple genetic relationships (12).

B. Familial Aggregation

The determination that a specific disease aggregates in families is an important piece of evidence that genetic factors play a role in the etiology of the disorder. Although diseases that are caused by either genes or viral agents can cluster in specific families, the demonstration of familial aggregation of disease provides a foundation for further studies of disease transmission and gene localization.

One simple approach to defining familial aggregation is to contrast the prevalence of disease in first-degree relatives of probands (index cases) as compared to the prevalence in the general population. For diseases with complex etiology (such as epilepsy), the prevalence in relatives may be several times that seen in the general population, but may still be rare for selected subtypes of the disease (13). In particular, the stratification of risk to relatives by seizure etiology demonstrates potentially important clues to the role of genes and environment in the pathogenesis of epilepsy. The risk to relatives of probands with an acute symptomatic seizure (a historical event that is known to increase the risk for subsequent seizures) is not greater than the population rate, while the risk to relatives of probands with an idiopathic (or cryptogenic) seizure (absence of such an event) is significantly greater than the general population prevalence. While "seizures" may not demonstrate extensive familial aggregation, "idiopathic" seizures have a strong familial risk and seizure risk may be due, in part, to a genetic mechanism.

A second approach to familial aggregation is to treat "family history" as a risk factor (an exposure) in a case-control study. In this sense, a series of "cases" would be identified, probands who have clear clinical evidence of disease. A matched set of controls would be ascertained with clinical absence of disease. Each case and control would then be evaluated with respect to disease in family members, usually first-degree relatives. An analysis of association would then be performed to determine whether the existence of a family history provides increased risk of disease (14). Further genetic interpretation can be made if the risk to specific relatives can be estimated. The differential risk to siblings versus offspring can provide information concerning dominance effects, while information from second-degree and third-degree relatives can assist in discriminating likely models of transmission.

C. Disequilibrium Studies

As noted above, some of the characteristics of a case-control study have increased its use in genetic applications. In particular, all cases (probands) with disease can be ascertained in a population, but the larger number of controls need only be sampled at a much lower frequency. Use of genetic marker or candidate genes in cases and controls can also provide information concerning the importance of a chromosomal region or a specific expressed gene in the pathogenesis of disease. These latter applications contrast the frequency of alleles in cases with controls, resulting in a test of association and a related measure of genetic association, linkage disequilibrium.

Linkage disequilibrium is a statistical measure that provides evidence that specific haplotypes (combinations of genetic marker and disease alleles) are transmitted in a nonrandom fashion. The value of linkage disequilibrium is a function not only of the distance between the loci (marker and disease) but also of the allele frequencies in the population. In general, the stronger the disequilibrium, the closer the two loci are expected to be on the chromosome.

In many studies, significant differences in the allele frequencies, rather than disequilibrium statistics themselves, are used to judge whether a specific genetic marker locus is of importance in disease. One highly polymorphic multigene family has been extensively used in case-control studies involving autoimmunity. This group of genetic marker loci is the human major histocompatibility complex (MHC), or human leukocyte antigen (HLA) complex. The human HLA genes are located on the short arm of human chromosome 6 (6p21.3) and is divided into three groups of loci—class I, class II, and class III—that are mainly involved with antigen recognition (15). Each locus for class I (HLA-A, -B, and -C), class II (HLA-DR, -DQ, and -DP), and class III (C2, C4A, C4B, Bf) genes is highly polymorphic and has been used not only in HLA disease association studies but also in family studies. Many HLA associations have been demonstrated for autoimmune disorders [insulin-dependent diabetes mellitus (16), multiple sclerosis (17), rheumatoid arthritis (18), Graves' disease (19), etc.], and linkage to the HLA region has been shown in some cases [21-hydroxylase deficiency (20), idiopathic hemochromatosis (21)]. It should be recognized, however, that association and linkage are not synonymous, although evidence of association without linkage could represent an important role of a candidate locus (HLA) in the pathogenesis of disease (defective antigen presentation in a "susceptible" individual) without a susceptibility locus residing in the HLA region. This and other hypotheses would suggest a more complex pattern of inheritance that could involve interactions between host genotype and environmental risk factors.

D. Family Studies

The study of families has several unique properties in human genetics. First, the transmission of a phenotype (disease) in a family can be tracked and models of transmission can be formally tested. In this manner, evidence for the transmission of a gene with major effect can be documented (or refuted) and strategies to locate and identify that gene can be proposed. Second, under the assumption of the existence of a gene with large effect that provides susceptibility, families can be used to locate (or map) the susceptibility gene with respect to a series of genetic markers. The first task, evaluating evidence for a major gene, falls under the area called "segregation analysis." The latter task, locating a major gene, represents "linkage analysis."

1. Segregation Analysis

As discussed previously, segregation analysis in humans was originally restricted to the estimation of segregation frequencies; that is, it was used to test whether the phenotypic distribution (affected status) among offspring was compatible with Mendelian inheritance. This approach has been used to establish Mendelian inheritance for a number of single-gene disorders (22).

To extend the evaluation of family data into detection of a single major locus and a polygenic component simultaneously, while allowing for common sibling environment, the "mixed model" of analysis was developed (7). Under the mixed model, the classical segregation frequencies no longer have a defined utility; rather, a series of basic parameters that define alternative genetic models in terms of gene frequency, distances (on a scale of genetic liability) between genotypes, and heritability are estimated. Although the mixed-model analyses are most powerful for a quantitative trait, reduction of "liability" to "affection" status (affected or unaffected) is possible but with considerable loss of power.

In analysis under the mixed model, pedigrees need to be partitioned into component nuclear families due to numerical concerns. Clearly, there is loss of information when this partitioning takes place. To extend the mixed-model analysis to pedigrees, the "pointer" concept was developed (23). The pointer represents a relative in a pedigree (proband or secondary case) of extreme phenotype (affected if disease state is used) through whom the family was ascertained. Although there have been numerous studies to evaluate the utility of the mixed model and its implementation in genetic analyses, the statistical foundation for inference of specific genetic models lies in the formulation of the likelihood of a pedigree.

The likelihood (or probability) of a hypothesized (genetic) model that is evaluated on a set of families is proportional to the chance of observing those families (the transmission of the trait in the families) under that particular model. The components of the likelihood for a qualitative trait are penetrance (probability of a phenotype given a specific genotype), gene frequency, and the transmission probabilities. The likelihood of a set of families is defined as the product of the individual likelihoods for all the (independent) families. Thus, the most likely model that applies to the particular collection of families is that with the greatest likelihood.

One statistical approach that is used to evaluate alternative hypotheses (models) is the use of likelihood ratio tests (24). This approach forms a test statistic that is the ratio of the maximum likelihood value of the null hypothesis (genetic model) to the maximum likelihood value under the reference hypothesis that includes the null hypothesis as a subset. This reference hypothesis in many cases is that formed under the full (or mixed) model. Of fundamental importance in hypothesis testing, as the number of families increases, -2 times the natural logarithm of this ratio is distributed as a chi-square statistic with degrees of freedom equal to the difference in the parameter space for the two competing hypotheses. Thus, a likelihood ratio of zero would indicate that the data are not compatible with the null hypothesis, while a likelihood ratio approaching 1 would indicate that the data suggest that the "reduced" model is not significantly worse than the "full" model.

Segregation analysis under the mixed model has continued development to effects of additional loci and joint environmental effects. Another series of models that have been developed uses aspects of epidemiology (importance of environmental covariates) and their application of logistic regression analysis to model dependency (offspring "types" are dependent on their parent's "types"). These models, called "regressive models" (25), produce equivalent results to the mixed model for quantitative traits in nuclear families; however, the regressive model does not require partitioning of a pedigree into component nuclear families and allows for simultaneous inclusion and testing of environmental and genetic components.

With large sample sizes, segregation analysis can provide compelling evidence for the existence of a gene that predisposes to a phenotype or disease.

When families are partitioned on the basis of an indicator variable (clinical result or mating type), heterogeneity of the phenotype can be inferred. However, to confirm that a single gene exists that determines susceptibility, that gene ultimately has to be mapped in families.

2. Gene Mapping

A common method to map genes to specific chromosomal locations is linkage analysis. This application is based on the fact that loci that are physically close together on a segment of a chromosome tend to be inherited together (linked). If two loci are linked, the alleles at those two loci are not transmitted to a gamete independently (with equal probability of one-half) but are transmitted to the same gamete more than 50% of the time. Since the two loci are together on a chromosomal segment, crossing over may occur during synapsis at meiosis I. The result of this event is that the chromosomal segment retained in a gamete may be a combination of both parental chromosomes (Fig. 2). The closer the two loci are on a chromosome, the lower the probability of crossing over; thus, the frequency of crossing over (recombination) is a measure of the distance between the two loci. For small recombination frequencies, the distance between loci can be expressed in units of genetic distance called centiMorgans, cM. Thus, two loci that exhibit 1% recombination are said to be 1 cM apart. On average, a 1-cM genetic distance is equivalent to 1 million base pairs in physical distance.

To map disease susceptibility genes, two types of resources are required—informative families and polymorphic genetic markers. It has been demonstrated that for a nuclear family to be potentially informative for linkage between two loci, at least one of the two parents must be doubly heterozygous. For a genetic marker to be informative, it must appear in heterozygote form in a large number of individuals in the population. By convention, a genetic marker is said to be polymorphic when its most common allele is represented in at most 95% of the population. Although, by extension, a polymorphic marker would then have heterozygosity in the population of at least 10%, most DNA markers used in current mapping studies have heterozygosity values greater than 60%.

The method of linkage analysis most widely used is the lod score method (26). The lod score method provides two essential results—an estimation of the genetic distance between loci (in terms of the recombination fraction) and the statistical support for the null hypothesis of linkage between the two loci at the estimated distance. Briefly, the likelihood ratio statistic is formed by the ratio of two likelihoods, the first being the likelihood of the null hypothesis of observing the data given the loci are linked, and the second being the likelihood of observing the data given that the two loci are not linked (recombination of 50%).

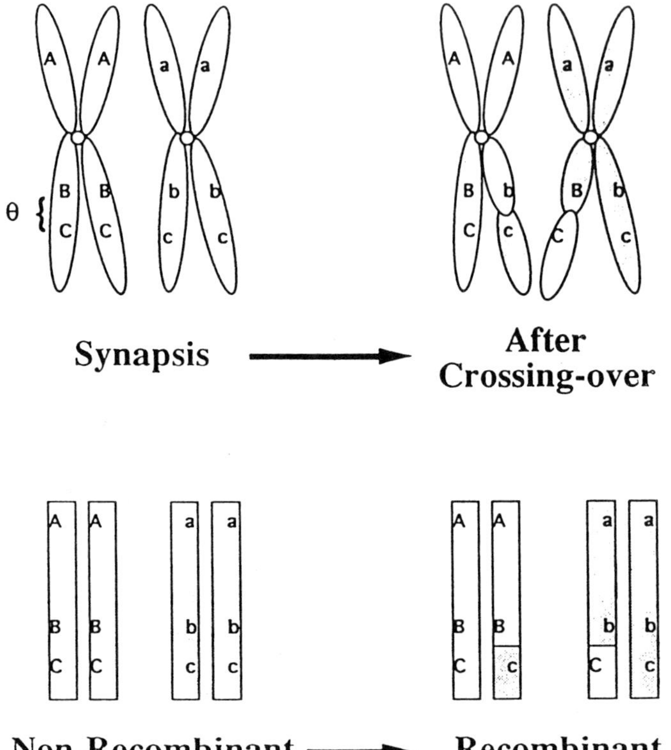

FIGURE 2 Crossing over between homologous chromosomes in meiosis I and resulting gametes.

The likelihood of each independent family is multiplied together to obtain the accumulated likelihood for a set of families from a given population. The logarithm of this total likelihood ratio is called the lod score. Since the logarithm of a product of independent likelihoods is computed, the sum of the log likelihoods provides the total lod score. In this fashion, the sum of the lod scores for independent samples (evaluated at specific recombination fractions) can be used to obtain the maximum likelihood estimate of the recombination fraction.

Historically, a lod score critical value of 3.0 or greater at a given recombination fraction has been used to determine whether statistically significant evidence in favor of linkage has been observed. This roughly translates into an odds of at least 1000:1 in favor of linkage at that recombination fraction.

Similarly, a lod score of -2.0 or less at a given recombination fraction has been used as significant evidence against linkage, approximately a 1:100 odds in favor of linkage (or 100:1 odds against linkage). These critical values were selected to minimize the appearance of linkage in a family (or pedigree) by chance segregation of a genetic marker with a disease locus.

Linkage analysis is a powerful tool that can be used to identify a specific chromosomal region that leads to the detection of a biological basis for disease (27). This strategy, in which a disease is identified, cloned, and sequenced based on its location to known genetic markers, is called "positional cloning" or "reverse genetics." This strategy is in contrast to "forward genetics," which begins with a known protein product and then identifies the location of the gene on the "human gene map."

For many diseases, however, the etiological basis of the phenotype may differ between families. In this case, the "same" phenotype may be caused by mutations at different (unlinked) loci. Diseases of this type are called genetically heterogeneous (or nonallelic heterogeneity). Linkage analysis can be used to evaluate evidence for genetic heterogeneity by computing individual lod scores in a set of families for a genetic marker and summing the lod scores for all families. Several test statistics have been proposed to evaluate evidence that the total lod score differs significantly from the sum of the maximum individual lod scores (28,29). A significant linkage heterogeneity result would indicate that some proportion of families in the data set are linked to the genetic marker in question, while the remaining families are not linked (30). A recent example of genetic heterogeneity occurs in the autosomal dominant disorder spinocerebellar ataxia (SCA), in which some families have been shown to have disease caused by a locus on chromosome 6 (SCA1) and other families significantly reject that location, even though there is clinical homogeneity (31).

With the growth and development of the map of human genetic markers, linkage analysis can be used in two additional ways to confirm the location of a disease susceptibility locus. The first approach is to simply use additional markers in the same chromosomal region to confirm the initial finding of linkage. This use of the linkage map can be used to eliminate potential chance results in a rapid procedure. The second approach is to consider more than two loci (disease and a marker) at a time. Use of multiple loci helps to resolve several limitations of linkage analysis—information content of matings (greater opportunity for each parent to be heterozygous for a set of markers), observation of recombination (greater opportunity for crossing over due to greater distance covered), and power gain from the formation of a "known" fixed map of genetic markers. A major role of the human genome project in this regard is the generation of linkage maps of known markers, thereby allowing the evaluation of evidence for the placement of a disease locus onto an established map. The application of likelihood methods using multiple genetic markers is called "multipoint" linkage analysis (32). In an analogous manner to standard (two locus) linkage analysis, the log likelihoods of each locus order need to be determined and compared for statistical support of one order over other competing orders (33).

Although linkage analysis is recognized as a powerful tool for mapping genes, the approach does have a serious limitation. The analysis of the family data assumes that the underlying genetic transmission model is known. For many complex diseases, the transmission of susceptibility may neither be known with certainty nor follow classical Mendelian segregation patterns. Thus, a second method of analysis for linkage can be used that does not require the specification of an underlying genetic model. This approach uses phenotypic and genotypic similarity in siblings as a method of comparison.

In general, sib pair methods can be classified into those using identity by state methods (34) or identity by descent relationships (35). In the affected sib pair method, comparisons of genotypes are made between siblings with disease. This method reduces misclassification in phenotype (due to either recombination at the disease locus, age at onset effects, or incomplete penetrance) and compares concordance in the genetic marker with concordance in disease (36). By necessity, the affected sib pair method requires highly polymorphic markers. The statistic to be calculated is simply a chi square that compares the observed number of affected sib pairs that share both marker alleles, one marker allele, or no marker alleles with that expected under absence of linkage (25% of sib pairs would share one, 50% would share two, and 25% would share no marker alleles). Under situations with linkage, there should be an excess in sharing two marker alleles and a deficit in sharing no marker alleles. This approach has been used to support evidence for linkage of insulin-dependent diabetes to the HLA complex (37).

Another recent approach uses all sib pairs, whether they are affected or not. This method, called the robust sib pair method, samples more individuals and determines the similarity in sib pairs as a "squared trait difference." Although originally constructed for analysis of quantitative traits, this method can be applied to dichotomous (disease) phenotypes (38). The criterion used for linkage in the robust sib pair method is the regression of the squared trait difference on the estimated proportion of genes shared identical by descent (IBD) at a marker locus or, alternatively, the correlation between the estimated proportion of genes that the sib pairs have IBD at each of two marker loci. If linkage exists between the trait and the genetic marker, the regression (or correlation) is expected to be significantly negative. If there is absence of linkage, the regression (or correlation) is expected to be not significantly different from zero.

The transmission models for complex diseases such as asthma and allergy are not known but are assumed to involve both multiple genetic and environmental risk factors. To evaluate the feasibility of mapping genes for a complex disease, a number of parameters relating to the risk of the disease in relatives of probands are required. Unfortunately, these data are often missing from the literature and, to a large extent, a formal analysis of power to detect disease susceptibility genes with respect to competing genetic hypothesis cannot be performed. In the absence of these data, additional indirect evidence and simulation studies can be performed to evaluate the power to detect a major gene(s) providing disease susceptibility.

Evidence in favor of genetic factors contributing to disease susceptibility can be obtained indirectly. Often, there is evidence of familial aggregation (increased risk of disease in siblings of probands), although this risk may be due to aggregation of genetic and/or environmental risk factors. The existence of large pedigrees with members who have the disease occurring in several generations also suggests evidence for a major gene contributing to risk. The occurrence of the disease in significant rates within an isolated population can also be used as evidence in favor of genetic factors.

The power to map a genetic trait by linkage analysis depends on a number of factors, including the available human material (individuals, siblings, families, pedigrees), the mode of inheritance of the disease, and the availability of informative genetic markers. For disease with families available, several alternatives are possible. In the absence of a known mode of inheritance, it is possible to consider a series of alternative genetic models based on existing family data. Using computer simulations, these data can be extrapolated to a likely collection of families of similar structure and availability. Using this approach, model-dependent methods of analysis can be employed, based on alternative (competing) genetic models. Families with several affected members also provide material for model-independent (nonparametric) methods of analysis, including affected sib-pair, robust sib-pair, and affected pedigree member (APM) methods.

It has been demonstrated that the prevalence of a disease in the general population can be expressed as a function of the allele frequencies of the trait and the three penetrances (or the probability of expressing the trait for the three trait genotypes). The risk of disease in a relative is then a function of the population prevalence and the genetic covariance between the proband and a relative, expressed by the additive and dominance genetic variances. The distribution of IBD scores for affected sib pairs can be determined as a function of the genetic variance components, the population prevalence, and the recombination fraction between the disease and genetic marker locus, θ. Using candidate genes, $\theta = 0$, so with linkage of the candidate to asthma or allergy, for example, the proportion of affected sib pairs sharing both alleles IBD (IBD

= 2) will always be greater than 1/4 and the proportion of sib pairs sharing one or no alleles IBD will always be less than 1/2 and 1/4, respectively.

The ratio of risk to a relative of type R (offspring, sibling, etc.) to that observed in the general population is defined to be the risk ratio, λ_R. This ratio will always be greater than unity should genetic factors be important and can be used to (1) model the likely modes of transmission for a complex disease and (2) determine power of a proposed linkage study. The probability that an affected sibling pair will share two alleles IBD at the genetic marker locus (or candidate gene) is a function of λ_S and the recombination fraction, θ.

For a disease with strong familial (genetic) influence, the recurrence risks in relatives (siblings) may be increased 10-fold over that in the general population ($\lambda_S = 10$). For a homogeneous, single-disease susceptibility locus, the power to detect linkage with 100 affected sib pairs approaches 100% for a dense map of genetic markers (θ approaches 0) and remains high for a more realistic genome-wide search. For diseases with weaker evidence for genetic effects ($\lambda_S = 6$), nearly 200 affected sib pairs would be required to allow equivalent power. Thus, the number of affected relative pairs is critically dependent upon the trait (disease), its frequency in the population, and the extent of genetic factors that contribute to disease susceptibility.

Given the rapidity of sample collection of sib pairs, one strategy to be considered in complex disorders could be the initial ascertainment of sib pairs for screening the genome. Although there is strength in no assumption of transmission model for disease, there is also weakness in that there is no estimate of recombination fraction. Thus, strong evidence in favor of a given region (such as significant concordance for multiple linked markers) could be followed by formal analysis of linkage by the lod score method under alternative competing transmission models, either obtained from the literature or by application of segregation analysis. This combined approach should provide significant strength of the diverse analytic methods to further our understanding of complex phenotypes.

V. HUMAN GENETIC STUDIES OF ASTHMA AND ALLERGY

Asthma is a common clinical disorder characterized by reversible obstruction of the bronchial airways, which is an increasingly serious cause of morbidity and mortality in the general U.S. population (39). It is defined by a spectrum of clinical findings—the presence of a clinical history of coughing, wheezing, and shortness of breath that is intermittent in occurrence; the presence of expiratory wheezes that is episodic; and pulmonary function less than 80% of predicted (based on FEV_1 and FEV_1/FVC ratio) that is reversed by at least 20% after use of bronchodilators (airflow reversibility). The prevalence of asthma in the U.S. population ranges from 3% to 5%, with both sexes equally affected, and blacks more commonly affected than other ethnic groups. Recent studies indicate that asthmatic symptoms, as well as asthma prevalence, may be increasing (40), although this is controversial (41). The presence of a genetic component to the susceptibility of asthma has also been suggested, based on numerous twin, family, and population studies.

Allergy is thought to be a major component of asthma and, therefore, serves as a correlated phenotype of asthma. Allergy was originally defined as a type of hypersensitivity peculiar to humans, which was subject to hereditary influence, and presented as the characteristic whealing reaction; further, there were characteristic circulating antibodies and clinical symptoms such as asthma and hay fever. Most patients with atopic allergy are characterized by long-term increased levels of IgE in response to minimal amounts of allergen leading to immediate or type I hypersensitivity. Most of the features of atopic disease, however, can be traced to the presence of allergen-specific IgE and the release of inflammatory mediators by cell-bound IgE in patients exposed to an allergen (42). The following is a summary of some of the applications of the tools used in human genetic studies of asthma and allergy. More detailed treatment of these topics and the analytic methods can be found in other chapters.

A. Specific Immune Response

The specific immune response in is dependent on a variety of different steps leading to the final clinical syndrome. Much of the interest in the genetic basis of the immune response to specific allergens has focused on genes in the human MHC. Early family studies, using complex allergens, had indicated that a genetic locus for sensitivity was likely to reside in the human MHC (43,44). Studies using simple purified allergens have supported the hypothesis that an immune response locus may reside in this region (45–47). Thus, research was focused on the search for a specific immune response gene in the MHC. Although strong associations between IgE response to specific allergens remain with MHC class II genes, there has been no evidence that the presence of specific novel sequences provides susceptibility that is genetically transmitted (48).

B. Mediator Release

The interaction of IgE with cells and their ability to release mediating substances has been the subject of few reports. Plasma histamine levels were shown to be normally high at young age and decrease with increasing age (49); however, atopic children had higher levels than normal children and there was a significant correlation between plasma histamine levels in atopic children, but not in normal children. Nevertheless, IgE-dependent basophilic histamine release has not been clearly established as being under genetic control in asthma.

An earlier twin study estimated correlations in histamine release from basophils in response to anti-IgE, f-*met* peptide, and the calcium ionophore A23187 (50). The correlation among MZ twins was significantly greater than among DZ twins for anti-IgE and A23187, but not for f-*met* peptide. These data suggest that anti-IgE release and calcium ionophore release of histamine were determined in part by genetic factors, while genes probably had little effect on the release of histamine from f-*met* peptide. The genetic factors that contributed to IgE-mediated release of histamine appeared to be independent of serum IgE levels. Thus, there is potential for genetic factors contributing to IgE-mediated release of inflammatory mediators from mast cell basophils.

C. Bronchial Hyperresponsiveness

Familial factors have been reported to be involved in the development of bronchial hyperresponsiveness, defined principally as the bronchial response to methacholine inhalation challenge. An early study (51) demonstrated the presence of a bimodal distribution for methacholine response, suggestive of a major gene responsible for this measure of bronchial hyperresponsiveness. After the bronchial response to methacholine challenge was measured in families, segregation analysis (52) indicated that pure environmental models could be rejected and that a familial component to the transmission of the bronchial response to methacholine could not be rejected; however, there was no evidence that the observed bimodal distribution in response in individuals with a family history of asthma was due to a single major gene. In a separate study, bronchial reactivity patterns appeared to be consistent with a genetic effect (53); however, there was no relationship between bronchial reactivity and serum IgE levels, consistent with the hypothesis of separate genetic control of hyperresponsivity and hyperproduction of IgE.

D. Serum IgE Level

Serum IgE level in normal and asthmatic populations has been shown to be controlled (at least in part) by genetic factors. Concordance of IgE levels in twins and the pattern of transmission of IgE levels in families are consistent with a significant genetic regulatory effect. Twin studies have resulted in a heritability estimated between 50% and 84% while family studies have suggested a major gene contributing to IgE levels (54–57). The mode of inheritance remains unresolved, possibly owing to unclear exposure history and/or genetic heterogeneity.

Earlier studies evaluated aspects of genetic transmission of IgE levels using segregation analysis in three large pedigrees, many of whose members had atopic sensitivities to ragweed (58). Results of the statistical analysis rejected the environmental model (of equal transmission frequency for all genotypes), suggesting a strong hereditary involvement in IgE distribution. The best-fitting single-locus model suggested that high IgE levels were determined by a dominant allele; however, when families were analyzed separately, there was evidence of significant heterogeneity due to one family favoring recessive inheritance of high IgE levels, one with no clear mode, and the third somewhat in favor of dominant inheritance. Several investigators have reported evidence indicating a recessive regulatory locus (59), such that an individual with the homozygous recessive genotype had persistently elevated levels of IgE. Bivariate segregation analysis of IgE levels (57) has indicated that an IgE regulatory locus contributed to the familial transmission of allergy, although the mode of inheritance was not clear.

E. Asthma

The development of asthma is complex and likely to be a function of genetic susceptibility and environmental exposure. Genetic predisposition has been most clearly demonstrated by a series of twin studies. Using a Swedish twin register (60), same-sex twin pairs identified over a 40-year period were evaluated with respect to asthma and related symptoms. Twin concordance for asthma in MZ twins was 19.0%, while the concordance in DZ twins was 4.8%, consistent with a strong familial (genetic) regulation of asthma. A more recent twin study evaluated concordance for asthma/wheezing among twins from the Australian National Health and Medical Research Council Twin Registry (61). The disease correlation was higher in MZ twin pairs ($r = 0.65$) than in DZ pairs ($r = 0.25$); further, the correlation was higher in male MZ twins ($r = 0.75$) compared with female MZ twins ($r = 0.60$). These results are again consistent with a genetic factor common to asthma and hay fever.

Familial aggregation studies have also implicated genes in the pathogenesis of asthma. When asthma is defined by the occurrence of wheezy episodes in response to allergens, exercise, or emotion, as well as with symptoms that suggested respiratory infection, the percentage of children with at least one asthmatic relative was significantly greater in the asthmatic probands than in the controls (62). When the histories were partitioned into extrinsic and intrinsic asthma among the relatives of control children, neither the prevalence of asthma nor the atopic status of the asthmatic relatives was influenced by the atopic status of the proband (63). These findings supported the hypothesis that asthma and atopy were inherited independently.

The role of specific candidate genes in asthma susceptibility has been equivocal. Older studies have suggested that there were associations between asthma and various HLA antigens; however, these reports could not be reproduced. Recent studies have centered efforts on allergen-specific responses, in hopes of reducing heterogeneity. An association between the IgE response to

Der p I and bronchial asthma has been reported (64), and studies in two populations have suggested that specific MHC class II haplotypes segregate with the occurrence of mite-sensitive allergic asthma. These and other results suggest the presence of an MHC-linked recessive locus that controls the IgE responsiveness to mite allergens and confers susceptibility to allergic asthma.

VI. SUMMARY

Asthma and allergies are conditions in which genetic factors have been shown to play a significant role in the pathogenesis of disease. Genetic factors also play a role in the development of a specific immune response to aeroallergens, IgE production, release of mediators, and the development of a hyperreactive airway.

The genetic basis of asthma and allergies remains unresolved. In this chapter, some of the tools and human resources needed to utilize genetic, molecular, biological, and statistical methods have been described. Using a highly polymorphic battery of DNA marker loci, it appears feasible to identify the genes involved in the development of bronchial asthma, allergies, and their associated phenotypes. Identification of these genes and their function will facilitate new treatment protocols and will lead to an understanding of the interactions between genes and environment that are relevant to asthma and allergy.

ACKNOWLEDGMENT

This work was supported in part by NIH Grant HL49609.

REFERENCES

1. Overhauser J, McMahon J, Oberlender S, Carlin ME, Niebuhr E, Wasmuth JJ, Lee-Chen J. Parental origin of chromosome 5 deletions in the cri-du-chat syndrome. Am J Med Genet 1990; 37:83–86.
2. Weber JL, May PE. Abundant class of human DNA polymorphisms which can be typed using the polymerase chain reaction. Am J Hum Genet 1989; 44:388–396.
3. Novick GE, Gonzalez T, Garrison J, Novick CC, Batzer MA, Deininger PL, Herrera RJ. The use of polymorphic Alu insertions in human DNA fingerprinting. EXS 1993; 67:283–291.
4. Fryns JP, Kleczkowska A, Kubien E, Petit P, Van den Berghe H. Cytogenetic survey in couples with recurrent fetal wastage. Hum Genet 1984; 65:336–354.
5. Morton NE. Genetic tests under incomplete ascertainment. Am J Hum Genet 1959; 11:1–16.
6. Falconer DS. Introduction to Quantitative Genetics, 2nd ed., New York: Longman Scientific & Technical, 1981.

7. Morton NE, Maclean CJ. Analysis of family resemblance. III. Complex segregation of quantitative traits. Am J Hum Genet 1974; 26:489–503.
8. Kumar D, Gemayel NS, Deapen D, Kapadia D, Yamashita PH, Lee M, Dwyer JH, Roy-Burman P, Bray GA, Mack TM. North-American twins with IDDM: genetic, etiological, and clinical significance of disease concordance according to age, zygosity, and the interval after diagnosis in first twin. Diabetes 1993; 42:1351–1363.
9. Deapen D, Escalante A, Weinrib L, Horwitz D, Bachman B, Roy-Burman P, Walker A, Mack TM. A revised estimate of twin concordance in systemic lupus erythematosus. Arthritis Rheum 1992; 35:311–318.
10. Eaves LJ. The utility of twins. In: Anderson VE, Hauser WA, Penry JK, Sing CF, eds. Genetic Basis of the Epilepsies. New York: Raven Press, 1982:249–276.
11. Tellegen A, Lykken DT, Bouchard TJ, Wilcox KJ, Segal NL, Rich SS. Personality similarity in twins reared apart and together. J Pers Soc Psychol 1988; 54:1009–1031.
12. Nance WA, Corey LA. Genetic models for the analysis of data from the families of identical twins. Genetics 1976; 83:811–826.
13. Anderson VE, Hauser WA, Rich SS. Genetic heterogeneity in the epilepsies. Adv Neurol 1986; 44:59–75.
14. Slattery ML, Kerber RA. A comprehensive evaluation of family history and breast cancer risk: the Utah Population Database. JAMA 1993; 270:1563–1568.
15. Trowsdale J. Genomic structure and function in the MHC. Trends Genet 1993; 9: 117–122.
16. Rich SS, Weitkamp LR, Barbosa J. Genetic heterogeneity of insulin-dependent (type I) diabetes mellitus: evidence from a study of extended haplotypes. Am J Hum Genet 1984; 36:1015–1023.
17. Hillert J. Olerup O. Multiple sclerosis is associated with genes within or close to the HLA-DR-DQ subregion on a normal DR15,DQ6,Dw2 haplotype. Neurology 1993; 43:163–168.
18. Ploski R, Vinje O, Ronningen KS, Spurkland A, Sorskaar D, Vartdal F, Forre O. HLA class II alleles and heterogeneity of juvenile rheumatoid arthritis: DRB1*0101 may define a novel subset of the disease. Arthritis Rheum 1993; 36:465–472.
19. Balazs C, Bokk A, Molnar I, Stenszky V, Farid NR. Graves' ophthalmopathy, eye muscle antibodies and HLA antigens. Exp Clin Immunogenet 1989; 6:190–192.
20. Abbal M, Belvedere MC, Livieri C, De Paoli F, Martinetti M, Severi F, Cambon-Thomsen A. Italian extended HLA haplotypes in congenital adrenal hyperplasia. Tissue Antigens 1988; 32:17–23.
21. Jouanolle AM, Yaouanq J, Blayau M, Perichon M, Fauchet R, Font MP, Le Gall JY, David V. HLA class I gene polymorphism in genetic hemochromatosis. Hum Genet 1990; 85:279–282.
22. Elston RC. Segregation analysis. Adv Hum Genet 1981; 11:63–120.
23. Lalouel JM, Morton NE. Complex segregation analysis with pointers. Hum Hered 1981; 31:312–321.
24. Edwards AWF. Likelihood: An Account of the Statistical Concept of Likelihood and Its Application to Scientific Inference, 2nd ed., London: Cambridge University Press, 1978.

25. Bonney GE. On the statistical determination of major gene mechanisms in continuous human traits: regressive models. Am J Med Genet 1984; 18:731–749.
26. Morton NE. Sequential tests for the detection of linkage. Am J Hum Genet 1955; 7:277–318.
27. Collins FS. Positional cloning: let's not call it reverse anymore. Nat Genet 1992; 1: 3–6.
28. Morton NE. The detection and estimation of linkage between the genes for elliptocytosis and the Rh blood type. Am J Hum Genet 1956; 8:80–91.
29. Smith CAB. Testing for heterogeneity of recombination fractions in human genetics. Ann Hum Genet 1963; 27:175–182.
30. Musarella MA, Anson-Cartwright L, Leal SM, Gilbert LD, Worton RG, Fishman GA, Ott J. Multipoint linkage analysis and heterogeneity testing in 20 X-linked retinitis pigmentosa families. Genomics 1990; 8:286–296.
31. Ranum LP, Rich SS, Nance MA, Duvick LA, Aita JF, Orr HT, Anton-Johnson S, Schut LJ. Autosomal dominant spinocerebellar ataxia: locus heterogeneity in a Nebraska kindred. Neurology 1992; 42:344–347.
32. Lathrop GM, Laouel JM, Julier C, Ott J. Strategies for multilocus linkage analysis in humans. Proc Natl Acad Sci USA 1984; 81:3443–3446.
33. Ott J, Lathrop GM. Goodness-of-fit tests for locus order in three-point mapping. Genet Epidemiol 1987; 4:51–57.
34. Penrose LS. The general sib-pair linkage test. Ann Eugen 1953; 18:120–144.
35. Haseman JK, Elston RC. The investigation of linkage between a quantitative trait and a marker locus. Behav Genet 1972; 2:3–19.
36. Green JR, Woodrow JC. Sibling method for detecting HLA-linked genes in disease. Tissue Antigens 1977; 9:31–35.
37. Barbosa J, King RA, Noreen H, Yunis EJ. The histocompatibility system in juvenile, insulin-dependent diabetic multiplex kindreds. J Clin Invest 1977; 60:989–998.
38. Wilson AF, Elston RC, Tran LD, Siervogel RM. Use of the robust sib-pair method to screen for single-locus, multiple-locus, and pleiotropic effects: application to traits related to hypertension. Am J Hum Genet 1991; 48:862–872.
39. McFadden ER, Gilbert IA. Asthma. N Engl J Med 1992; 327:1928–1937.
40. Bauman A. Has the prevalence of asthma symptoms increased in Australian children? J Paediatr Child Health 1993; 29:424–428.
41. Weitzman M, Gortmaker SL, Sobol AM, Perrin JM. Recent trends in the prevalence and severity of childhood asthma. JAMA 1992; 268:2673–2677.
42. Ishizaka K. Ishizaka T. Human reaginic antibodies and immunoglobulin E. J Allergy 1968; 42:330–363.
43. Levine BB, Stember RH, Forino M. Ragweed hay fever: genetic control and linkage to HLA haplotypes. Science 1972; 178:1201–1203.
44. Blumenthal MN, Amos DB, Noreen H, Mendell NR, Yunis EJ. Genetic mapping of Ir locus in man: linkage to second locus of HL-A. Science 1974; 184:1301–1303.
45. Marsh DG, Hsu SH, Roebber M, Ehrlich-Kautzky E, Freidhoff LR, Meyers DA, Pollard MK, Bias WB. HLA-Dw2: A genetic marker for human immune response to short ragweed pollen allergen Ra5. I. Response resulting primarily from natural antigenic exposure. J Exp Med 1982; 155:1439–1451.

46. Goodfriend L, Choudhury AM, Klapper DG, Coulter KM, Dorval G, DelCarpio J, Osterland CK. Ra5G, a homologue of Ra5 in giant ragweed pollen: isolation, HLA-DR-associated activity and amino acid sequence. Mol Immunol 1985; 22: 899–906.
47. Freidhoff LR, Ehrlich-Kautzky E, Meyers DA, Ansari AA, Bias WB, March DG. Association of HLA-DR3 with human immune response to Lol p I and Lol p II allergens in allergic subjects. Tissue Antigens 1988; 31:211–219.
48. Zwollo P, Ehrlich-Kautzky E, Scharf SJ, Ansari AA, Erlich HA, Marsh DG. Sequencing of HLA-D in responders and nonresponders to short ragweed allergen, Amb a V. Immunogenetics 1991; 33:141–151.
49. Fujisawa T, Komada M, Iguchi K, Uchida Y. Plasma histamine levels in normal and atopic children. Ann Allergy 1987; 59:303–306.
50. Marone G, Poto S, Celestino D, Bonini S. Human basophil releasibility. III. Genetic control of human basophil releasibility. J Immunol 1986; 137:3588–3592.
51. Townley RD, Bewtra AK, Nair NM, Brodkey FD, Burke KM. Methacholine inhalation challenge studies. J Allergy Clin Immunol 1979; 64:569–574.
52. Townley RG, Bewtra A, Wilson AF, Hopp RJ, Elston RC, Nair N, Watt GD. Segregation analysis of bronchial response to methacholine inhalation challenge in families with and without asthma. J Allergy Clin Immunol 1986; 77:101–107.
53. Longo G, Strinati R, Poli F, Fumi F. Genetic factors in nonspecific bronchial hyperreactivity: an epidemiologic study. Am J Dis Child 1987; 141:331–334.
54. Meyers DA, Bias WB, Marsh DG. A genetic study of total IgE levels in the Amish. Hum Hered 1982; 32:15–23.
55. Matsushita S, Sasazuki T. Genetic control of IgE immune response. Clin Rev Allergy 1989; 7:125–139.
56. Berciano FA, Crespo M, Bao CG, Alvarez FV. Serum levels of total IgE in non-allergic children: influence of genetic and environmental factors. Allergy 1987; 42: 276–283.
57. Borecki IB, Rao DC, Lalouel JM, McGue M, Gerrard JW. Demonstration of a common major gene with pleiotropic effects on immunoglobulin E levels and allergy. Genet Epidemiol 1985; 2:327–338.
58. Blumenthal MN, Namboodiri K, Mendell N, Gleich G, Elston RC, Yunis E. Genetic transmission of serum IgE levels. Am J Med Genet 1981; 10:219–228.
59. Willcox HNA, Marsh DG. Genetic regulation of antibody heterogeneity: its possible significance in human allergy. Immunogenetics 1978; 6:209–225.
60. Edfors-Bubs ML. Allergy in 7000 twin pairs. Acta Allergol 1971; 26:249–285.
61. Duffy DL, Martin NG, Battistutta D, Hopper JL, Mathews JD. Genetics of asthma and hay fever in Australian twins. Am Rev Respir Dis 1990; 142:1351–1358.
62. Sibbald B, Horn ME, Gregg I. A family study of the genetic basis of asthma and wheezy bronchitis. Arch Dis Child 1980; 55:354–357.
63. Sibbald B, Horn ME, Brain EA, Gregg I. Genetic factors in childhood asthma. Thorax 1980; 35:671–674.
64. Sporik R, Holgate ST, Platts-Mills TA, Cogswell JJ. Exposure to house-dust mite allergen (Der p I) and the development of asthma in childhood: a prospective study. N Engl J Med 1990; 323:502–507.

3

Tools for the Study of Genetics

Deborah A. Meyers
Center for Medical Genetics
Johns Hopkins University School of Medicine
Baltimore, Maryland

I. INTRODUCTION

The study of complex disorders such as asthma and allergy is an area of interest to geneticists. These disorders are not inherited in a simple Mendelian fashion, but there is an increased risk to relatives of affected individuals (1–4), suggesting a genetic component. These disorders are also more prevalent in the population than Mendelian disorders, which are relatively rare. Therefore, they are of greater concern from the public health viewpoint, and delineating the role of genetics in such disorders should have widespread significance. Our understanding of the pathophysiology would be advanced and, hopefully, lead to new and better treatment programs.

This chapter will review the "tools" that are available for genetic studies of asthma and allergy. These tools include the different phenotypes, populations, and types of families that may be studied as well as the various laboratory and analytical methods for genetic studies. An overview of the various tools is presented here; the reader should consult the appropriate literature and experts in specific areas for further information and to stay informed in the rapidly advancing field of genetics.

II. DEFINITION OF PHENOTYPE

First, it is necessary to decide on the phenotype to be studied. Although a phenotype such as asthma is difficult to define, it is necessary to determine how the phenotype is to be measured, i.e., what data need to be collected. In general, the same tests (laboratory and clinical) should be performed on all family members whenever possible. For several reasons, it is important that testing is performed in a standardized manner using well-accepted protocols. First, given the complexity of delineating genetic factors for a disorder with known environmental influences, the data collected need to be of the highest quality. Second, it will be easier to compare results with other studies if well-accepted measures of the phenotype are used. This is also true for the questionnaire data. For comparisons between studies, a questionnaire that has previously been validated and used in other studies should be utilized, if possible, with modifications as necessary. Questionnaires should be tested in pilot studies to determine the feasibility of using them in a given population of families.

Unlike some complex genetic disorders such as several of the mental disorders, there are numerous expressions of the allergic and asthma phenotype that can be studied either as quantitative or qualitative measures or both. Therefore, especially to perform quantitative analyses, it is important that strict laboratory criteria are used for these tests, and that they are performed in as reproducible a manner as possible.

A. Qualitative Measures

Often, an investigator is interested in studying the disease phenotype based on a definition that includes the results of the laboratory tests as well as data on symptoms and the effects of confounding variables such as smoking and allergen exposure. Although the probands may be ascertained because they have "classic" asthma, it is still necessary to classify the other family members as "affected" or "unaffected" for analysis of the clinical phenotype. Family members can be classified as having "asthma," "possible asthma," "uncertain airways disease," "chronic obstructive pulmonary disease," or "unaffected" (5). This is a common strategy for linkage studies of complex disorders where different classes are assigned different probabilities of being gene carriers (6). It will always be difficult to classify some family members, so a category of "uncertain airways disease" is needed to avoid misdiagnosis. For example, family members with a significant smoking history who are hyperresponsive are difficult to classify, because of the relationship between smoking, airways obstruction, and bronchial hyperresponsiveness (BHR) (7). Family members who meet only some of the criteria for asthma may be classified as "possible asthma." It is important to restudy families members over time who have the "possible" or "uncertain" phenotype as well as young "unaffected" individuals to determine whether they may be developing asthma. Generally, families should be recontacted every few years to update the phenotypic data.

B. Quantitative Measures

It is important to consider quantitative genetic analyses as well as using predetermined clinical cutpoints. There are difficulties with studying quantitative traits since the actual value for a given measure such as BHR (e.g., slope) or total serum IgE levels may vary with age, sex, and even time of the year tested. Although these variables are often included as covariates in the analyses, it is hard to determine whether such adjustments are adequate.

However, quantitative analyses should be performed to utilize the full extent of the family data, which is expensive and time-consuming to collect. For example, high total serum IgE levels correlate with the clinical expression of allergy and asthma (8–12). Several studies have shown that IgE levels are related to BHR, a major feature of the asthma phenotype that may reflect the presence of airways inflammation (8,9,12,13). Therefore, the results from family studies on the genetic regulation of total IgE levels are relevant to determining the role of genetics in both allergy and asthma.

Additional parameters that can be analyzed as either quantitative or qualitative variables include measures of BHR, bronchodilator reversibility, and airflow obstruction. Since clinical criteria for a "normal" versus "abnormal" test result may not reflect whether a given family member is a gene carrier, analysis of these variables as quantitative measures is important. These variables may be analyzed both as continuous measures and using published cutpoints. For example, segregation analysis of BHR using the slope permits evaluation of BHR as a continuum and not just as "normal" versus "abnormal" response based on a PC_{20} FEV_1. The resulting genetic model can then be used to define phenotypes, but the clinical relevance of the results should be considered. For example, in the study of total serum IgE levels by Meyers et al. (14,15), evidence for a rare recessive gene was found but the clinical relevance of such a finding is unclear. The results from analyses of several relevant parameters as continuous measures may be useful in defining the "affected" versus the "unaffected" phenotype.

III. SAMPLING DESIGNS

The purpose of a given study will influence the type of data to be collected. Association studies may be performed on a sample of unrelated individuals, but in general, family data are needed. Several different types of families may be studied, each with advantages and disadvantages. For any study, it is important to design a data base for storage and management of the data collected.

Although this is easily done using commercial data bases that are available for microcomputers, it is an important and crucial step since large amounts of data are usually collected.

A. Unrelated Individuals

Studies of unrelated patients may provide useful genetic information and are often performed before family studies are undertaken. Usually these studies are "association" studies to determine if there is a relationship between a clinical phenotype or a specific measure of the phenotype and a polymorphism or specific alleles of a candidate gene. There are numerous studies of components of the allergic phenotype and the HLA loci (reviewed in Chapters 9 and 14). For the asthma phenotype, Liggett et al. (16) have investigated polymorphisms in the β_2 receptor on chromosome 5 in unrelated patients. Once genes important in asthma and allergy are mapped, association studies of specific mutations in candidate genes will be needed. However, given the complexity of the phenotype, these studies may not be easy to perform and the results will need careful interpretation.

B. Twins

Twin studies also provide important information and are useful to perform before studying families. The heritability of the disease in question or components of the disease can be determined by comparing monozygotic twin pairs to dizygotic twin pairs. It is usually assumed that the twins share a common environment, which lessens the impact of environmental influences, although this may not be true for studies of adult twins. Of course, there are no age differences within a pair of twins. Often, studies are restricted to twins of the same sex, which is appropriate for studies of allergy and asthma since there are reported sex differences in prevalence of the disorders (reviewed in Chapter 14).

C. Nuclear Families

Basically, three types of families may be studied: nuclear families, extended pedigrees, or inbred populations. Nuclear families consist of children and parents. One may attempt to phenotype the entire family for the disorder in question or to study only affected sibs for the disease in question but to draw blood and perform genetic marker studies on the parents also. An advantage of studying nuclear families is that they are probably representative of the disease in the general population. However, if significant heterogeneity exists or if only a proportion of the families have a genetic form of the disorder, it is more difficult to detect linkage since evidence for linkage will be seen in only a proportion of the families. This disadvantage is also true for affected sib pairs. An advantage of studying only affected sib pairs is that it is likely that the sibs have a similar form of the disorder, and if there are significant age effects, it may be difficult to phenotype the parents. Age effects and the effects of smoking are both reasons why one may choose to study affected sib pairs for asthma.

Usually for genetic studies, families are not ascertained in a random manner (for example, studying all children in grade 3 at the local school and their parents and siblings). Many genetics disorders are too rare to use this approach. However, random ascertainment of families is possible for studying allergic disease, for example; however, if one is studying asthma, it is unlikely that sufficient numbers of affected individuals would be sampled. The method of ascertainment of families needs to be clearly specified. If families are being ascertained to determine the mode of inheritance of the disease in question through segregation analysis, the family may not be ascertained in a manner favoring a specific mode of inheritance. For example, if an investigator studies only families with an affected parent and child, the results would be biased in favor of dominant inheritance.

If linkage analysis is the aim of the study, families are often ascertained for the presence of multiple affected family members, hopefully "loading" the family in favor of genetics. This is often done after a genetic basis for the disorder has been determined in order to genotype the most informative families. A compromise situation is to ascertain a family through two affected sibs and study all parents, other sibs, and possibly additional relatives. Both segregation and linkage analysis can then be performed.

D. Extended Pedigrees

Extended pedigrees are often used for genetic studies especially for disorders with evidence for a dominantly inherited major gene. A family may be ascertained through a single proband and then extended to aunts, uncles, grandparents, and cousins as available. A single large pedigree may provide evidence for linkage reducing the problem of genetic heterogeneity. Of course, this family may not be representative of most families with this disorder, but if a gene is localized from such a pedigree, it can be tested in other families. Even if it is found to represent a rare form of the disorder, it is still an important step in understanding the genetics of the disorder. For example, the APP mutations on chromosome 21 are now considered to be a "rare" cause of Alzheimer's disease (17) but represent the first linkage and gene found for this disorder. For complex disorders that are relatively common, a possible difficulty in studying extended pedigrees is that there may be several genes segregating for the disorder within the pedigree. For a common disorder, it is possible that one gene is transmitted through the pedigree but that in another branch of the pedigree, a different gene may be segregating, having been introduced by a spouse marrying into the family. The power to detect linkage is reduced, although based on computer simulation studies, there may well still be sufficient power to detect linkage (18). However, it is important to phenotype all family members (including spouses) to try to determine if multiple genes may be segregating within the pedigree. For example, in a pedigree where a spouse has asthma, additional genes may be present.

E. Isolated Populations

Isolated populations with large extended pedigrees and inbreeding are another source of families for genetic studies as long as the disorder being studied is present in the population. Because of founder effects, a given population may have a low frequency of a trait or disease that is relatively common in the general population. Examples include the Amish population in the United States (19) as well as isolated island populations in other parts of the world. The Amish are a closed community in which individuals may leave but individuals from the outside community do not marry into Amish families (20). This represents a closed gene pool with a founder effect; i.e., the genes present and their relative frequency in the current members of the community are derived from the original founding couples. Because of their large family size, known genealogy, and relatively homogeneous environment, such populations are often used for genetic studies. Due to the founder effect, genes mapped in such populations may not be representative of the major genes found in the general population. However, as with studying large pedigrees without inbreeding, such findings are still of importance.

Other examples of closed populations include those that are physically isolated, such as island populations. A well-studied island population is that of the Tristan da Cunhans from an island in the South Atlantic (21). In 1961, the population of approximately 268 members was removed because of a volcano eruption. Almost all of the individuals except young children were studied while in the United Kingdom. They have returned to the island and are still of interest to geneticists since it remains a small, closed, and isolated population. Again, results from such studies may or may not be directly applicable to families in the general population but the results could provide useful insights into studies of noninbred families.

In summary, it is important for the investigator to carefully consider the types of families available for study and the manner in which the families will be ascertained. These decisions should be based on the aims of the study as well as the availability of various populations. Generally, it is important to study family members as completely as possible. Complicated statistical analyses will not compensate for lack of quality in the data collected.

IV. CANDIDATE LOCI

A. Pathophysiology

The reader is referred to Chapters 4 and 5 on mechanisms important in asthma. It is also important to understand the current knowledge of the disease process. This will allow one to design the appropriate studies to determine the relationships between these candidate genes and the asthma phenotype as seen in family studies. For example, studies of chromosome 5q should be considered since there are several genes that may be important in the regulation of IgE and the development or progression of inflammation associated with allergy and asthma. They include interleukin-3 (IL-3), IL-4, IL-5, IL-9, IL-13, granulocyte-macrophage colony-stimulating factor (GM-CSF), a receptor for macrophage colony-stimulating factor (CSF-1R), and fibroblast growth factor acidic (FGFA) (22–24). Therefore, family studies may be designed to evaluate the relationships between these candidate genes and measures of the asthma phenotype.

B. Other Resources

There are other approaches that may lead to useful information on candidate regions of the genome. For example, patients with chromosomal aberrations such as translocations and deletions may lead an investigator to an appropriate candidate region when the patient also has the phenotype being studied. An example is Alzheimer's disease where it was observed that individuals with trisomy 21 have an increased risk of develop-ing Alzheimer's disease. This led investigators to genotype members of families with multiple cases of early-onset Alzheimer's disease for markers on chromosome 21 where mutations in the APP gene have now been delineated (17).

Another approach that may lead to useful information for asthma in general is to study specific subtypes of the disorder, especially if they appear to have a strong genetic component. For example, in breast cancer, women with an early age of onset are more likely to have affected relatives, and linkage studies on these families led to the first mapping of a gene for this common disorder (25). It is not obvious that there are subtypes of the asthma phenotype with a strong genetic component but such studies are worth considering. Obviously, it is easier to perform genetic studies if the families studied have a more homogeneous form of the disorder.

Another approach is to utilize results of studies in other organisms. For example, mouse studies have suggested recessive inheritance of hyperresponsiveness to specific challenges (26,27). Obviously, it is easier to perform family studies in mice than in humans. Once such a locus (loci) is mapped in another species, the syntenic regions in the human genome should be studied. In addition, if genes are identified, then genes in humans with a similar function may be studied.

V. MOLECULAR GENETICS

A. Genetic Markers

The general purpose of linkage studies is to detect cosegregation between measures of a phenotype and markers known to be inherited in a simple Mendelian manner. Linkage studies may be done for candidate loci as well as highly polymorphic markers spaced throughout the genome. It is now feasible to search the genome with highly polymorphic markers, usually simple sequence repeat (SSR) loci at least every 5–10 cm (28,29). Polymorphic markers mapped to either side of a candidate gene may be used to evaluate a region of interest especially if there are no known polymorphisms within the candidate gene.

Several factors need to be considered when performing genotyping studies. First, the accuracy of the data is extremely important. Autoradiographs should be read by two independent readers; even if an automated system is used, an appropriate level of error checking needs to be part of the standard laboratory procedure. It is best if at least one of the readers is blind to family relationships. Laboratory staff must be blind to the phenotypes of family members. After input (usually twice) into a data base, the genotypes should be checked for any discrepancies within families that need to be resolved by repeat scoring or genotyping. Then it is often useful to perform two-point linkage analysis between the most recent marker typed and any other markers typed in that region. For example, if double crossovers are detected, it is likely that there are data errors. The genotypes that are rechecked should include the ones in question and a sample of the remaining ones. A bias may be introduced by rechecking only recombinant individuals since they can be changed to be only nonrecombinant. The same type of procedure should be followed when rechecking families after analysis between the marker and disease phenotype has been performed. Only the analytical staff should have both the clinical and genotyping data. Both data bases need to be maintained in a data base system where it is easy to update the genotypes or phenotypes and track the changes that were made.

B. Positional Cloning

It is beyond the scope of this chapter to describe the various methods used to isolate genes once a disease has been mapped (30). This techniques change rapidly and are not specific to the study of asthma. Therefore, investigators should consult with appropriate molecular geneticists for these studies. However, several general points should be noted. For Mendelian disorders, multiple markers are typed in the region of interest to identify "key" recombinant individuals to perform fine structure mapping, i.e., to determine by linkage analysis the smallest stretch of DNA where the gene is localized. However, this process is not as simple for complex disorders. Because of the genetic models utilized, it is not possible to identify recombinants with as much confidence as for a Mendelian disease (it may represent a phenocopy), and the recombination fraction is often overestimated (31). One would seldom be willing to classify an unaffected individual as a recombinant since it is likely that penetrance is not complete. Therefore, identifying genes after mapping studies have been completed is a more complicated process. In addition, it is important to understand the disease process to determine the function and type of gene that may exist in that particular chromosomal region. There are several strategies for fine-mapping genes for complex disorders; the molecular aspects will be discussed in this section and the appropriate analysis in Chapters 2 and 6 on genetic analysis.

Once evidence for linkage is obtained, additional highly polymorphic DNA markers in the region need to be typed in the families. Information on relevant markers is available through the Internet using various data bases such as Genome Data Base and Collaborative Human Linkage Center. Genetic maps of the region are available with data on markers (usually simple sequence repeats) including degree of heterozygosity and the primer sequence. It is difficult to determine the order of markers that are tightly linked because a large number of families need to be genotyped if recombination between the markers is rare. Also, it is important to distinguish between rare recombinants and errors in genotyping. Therefore, it is very helpful if the loci have been ordered by physical mapping techniques. One approach to physical ordering is the creation of contiguous DNA blocks (contigs). The chromosome is cut into small pieces, which are cloned and ordered. The order of markers can then be determined by determining which contigs contain certain markers. Genotyping these additional markers in regions of interest allows the investigator to determine where every crossover event has occurred in this region in the families with a disorder such as asthma or allergy. This allows one to determine the most likely location of the genes involved in the disease process. Known candidate genes in the region can then be studied by typing family members for polymorphisms within the candidate and determining whether there is cosegregation between the polymorphism and the disease. It may be necessary to sequence the candidate gene from a sample of affected and unaffected individuals to detect polymorphisms and possible relevant mutations. Families can then be typed for these polymorphisms to determine their relevance. If there are no candidate genes that have been mapped to the region of interest, then more involved molecular techniques such as chromosome walking are needed to detect genes. However, it is important to remember that techniques for "finding genes" depend on having the gene well localized, which is a major problem in complex disorders such as asthma and allergy. Generally, further investigation of genes already mapped to the area, even if some distance from the region detected by linkage analysis, is the preferred approach. Thorough searching of data bases and understanding the disease process allow one to determine whether there may already be candidate genes in the region.

In fine mapping, haplotypes of the family members for all markers in the region can be constructed to determine crossovers and the most likely location of the disease gene. One can determine whether certain haplotypes are more frequent than expected by chance in the affected individuals, which may represent a genetic background on which disease mutations occurred. This is especially useful when candidate genes are included in the haplotypes. As described in the next section, these haplotypes should also be studied in a sample of unrelated affected individuals to determine associations between haplotypes and the disease. All of these approaches are useful for fine mapping as long as one realizes that simple answers are not usually seen; for example, there will not be a perfect (or even almost perfect) relationship between a haplotype and the disease or between a mutation in a candidate gene and the disease even if the genes relevant to the disease are being studied. One expects multiple genes mapping to different regions and environmental factors to be important in complex disorders such as asthma and allergy.

VI. GENETIC ANALYSIS

A. Associations and Disequilibrium Studies

Population data are often used to compare the frequency of a given genetic trait such as a specific polymorphism in a candidate gene in individuals with and without the disease phenotype, as a first step in genetic studies. The sample of control subjects to use is not always an easy decision; the subjects need to be matched for any variable that may influence the results. Obvious matching factors are race, sex, and age but other factors specific to the disorder being studied should also be considered.

Associations may be seen for several reasons basically relating to the marker allele (or candidate marker allele) having a role in the pathogenesis of the disorder. Another explanation of an observed association is linkage disequilibrium. An association is seen in population data because there is tight linkage between the loci and a common genetic background for the affected haplotype is observed. Studies of linkage disequilibrium can be a powerful tool for determining the most likely location of a postulated gene once linkage has been detected (32). However, it is important to remember that disequilibrium is usually detected in an interval of 1–2 cm (33). Therefore, it is necessary to type many DNA markers in the region of interest to determine the small region where disequilibrium may be present. Family members and unrelated subjects are both useful for such fine-mapping studies. Creation of unique haplotypes in unrelated patients is not always possible, so it is important to consider obtaining DNA from the parents. Olson and Wijsman discuss sample size considerations in detecting linkage disequilibrium and show that in some cases very large samples are needed (33). They also stress the importance of being able to accurately genotype individuals for the disease locus. Again, in complex disorders such as asthma and allergy, this remains a major problem.

B. Heritability and Risks to Relatives

It is useful to estimate heritability for a given phenotype before undertaking additional studies such as a large study of families (possibly multicenter) to perform segregation and/or linkage analysis. In addition, there are various techniques for estimating risk to relatives (reviewed in Ref. 34), which are also useful to perform. If the estimates of heritability or risk to relatives are low, large-scale family studies would probably be needed, and the value of such studies needs to be determined. Estimates of risk to relatives are useful in postulating the number of genetic loci that may be involved (35).

Another approach is to analyze the family data using a method such as the haplotype-relative-risk method (36). This method uses data from the nuclear family where the parental genotype (or haplotype) not transmitted to the affected child represents the control individual. Since it is often difficult to ascertain and study an appropriate control population, this is a useful technique to consider.

C. Segregation Analysis

Segregation analysis is performed to determine whether a genetic model is consistent with the family data. For example, does the qualitative or quantitative trait being measured segregate as a Mendelian dominant? Often the regressive models (37) as implemented in S.A.G.E. (38) are used for these analyses. Covariates such as age and sex can be included as well as covariates specific to the disorder being studied, such as smoking status in studies of asthma. Analysis is then performed to determine whether the segregation of the trait is consistent with a major gene model with two alleles, with or without a polygenic component. Other models tested include environmental, sporadic, and polygenic models. The resulting likelihoods are then compared to determine the best-fitting or most parsimonious model. The estimates of the parameters from this model, such as the mean value for affected family members for a quantitative trait, can then be used for the linkage analysis.

More complicated approaches to segregation analysis can also be utilized and should be considered in studies of allergy and asthma since there are multiple measures of the phenotypes. For example, bivariate segregation analysis can be performed to address the question as to whether there is a single locus accounting for two related measures. In addition, two-locus segregation analysis is useful to determine whether a single trait is controlled by two major genes. The computer program PAP (39) can be used for many of these analyses.

D. Linkage Analysis and Mapping

For Mendelian disorders, linkage analysis is performed using the method of maximum likelihood (lod scores) based on the genetic model for the disorder obtained from the segregation analysis. Indeed, for many Mendelian disorders, especially those with complete penetrance, it is not even necessary to perform a formal segregation analysis. The mode of inheritance is clear from inspection of the family data. For disorders such as asthma, it is possible to perform complex segregation analyses of the important components of the disorder as well as the clinical phenotype to determine whether a major gene model (dominant, recessive) is appropriate. The results from these analyses may then provide a genetic model for linkage analysis using the likelihood approach. If the families are ascertained in a manner compatible with segregation analysis, it is appropriate to attempt such model fitting especially since there are several quantitative variables that can be analyzed, such as total IgE levels, degree of BHR and of reversibility, including age, sex, and smoking as covariates.

Two-point lod scores can then be calculated using the genetic model from the segregation analysis for quantitative and qualitative measures. The linkage analysis should include a test for evidence of genetic heterogeneity (40) since it is reasonable to assume that multiple genes are involved in a complex disorder such as asthma or its component phenotypes. Even without results from segregation analyses, lod scores may be calculated under both a dominant and recessive model. Lod scores are relatively robust to model misspecification if dominance is correctly specified (41). However, as with any statistical analysis, there is an increase in false positive results when multiple analyses are performed after the data have been collected. One possible solution to this problem is thorough computer simulation of the family data to determine an empiric p value for the actual results (42).

Because of the relationship between asthma and allergy, it may be necessary to include two-locus models in the analysis. Single-locus models have been shown to still have power to detect linkage even if the true underlying model is two-locus with epistasis (43). However, this is dependent on the frequency of each gene and magnitude of the effect of each gene on the expression of the phenotype. If both an "allergy gene" and an "asthma gene" are important in expressing the asthma phenotype, two-locus models should be utilized and may provide a considerable increase in power to map the genes in question (44).

The other approach to linkage analysis is to use nonparametric methods of analysis such as affected sib pair analysis and the affected pedigree member method (45–47). The affected sib pair method is based on identity by descent (45,46); it is a measure of whether the affected sibs each inherited the same marker alleles from their parents. Significance is based on whether there is an increased sharing of alleles versus that expected by chance. The affected pedigree member method, derived by Weeks and Lange (47), is based on identity by state relationships that are applicable to pedigree data. Significance is measured by the proportion of affected members of the pedigree who share marker alleles in common. This method is sensitive to the allele frequencies for the markers being studied; if a marker allele is quite frequent, it is more likely that affected members of a pedigree will all have this allele even if linkage is not present. In general, when linkage is present, these methods are expected to give results similar to the results of the likelihood analyses. Although these nonparametric methods are not based on a specific model of inheritance, definition of the "affected" phenotype is still crucial. The assumption is made that the affected sibs share disease gene(s) in common based on both having the affected phenotype.

It is important to remember that any postulated linkage needs to be confirmed and the identification of one major locus does not mean that other major loci are not also present. The failure to replicate a postulated linkage has become a serious problem in studies on the genetics of complex disorders. A major reason for failure to replicate, as discussed by Risch (48), may be the interpretation of a lod score calculated under an unlikely model. Lod score analysis assumes that the underlying genetic model for the disorder being studied is known. Clear evidence for a specific genetic model for asthma has yet to be delineated.

There are several obvious reasons for failure to confirm a postulated linkage. For purposes of replication, it is important to use the same definition of the affected phenotype and the same genetic model that were used in the original study. The presence of genetic heterogeneity is often given as a possible reason for failure to replicate. It seems unlikely that this should be a reason for failure to replicate across relatively homogeneous populations (such as Caucasian families from the United States and England). However, heterogeneity may be confounded with differing expression of genes because of exposures to different allergens. In addition, if several genes interact in disease expression (oligogenic inheritance), it may be very difficult to replicate a "true" linkage (49). In different sets of families, different proportions of the genes involved may be present and the "linked" gene may not be detected in all studies. Consistent results between the various analytical methods utilized for linkage analysis should be obtained. Basically, it is important to use a conservative approach to declaring linkage; findings should be published but remain tentative until confirmed.

Additional studies to define the asthmatic (and allergic) phenotype are necessary. Results from further epidemiological studies on the effects of age, sex, smoking, and allergen exposure on disease expression would provide valuable data for future genetic studies. Family studies of both allergy and asthma have already begun in a number of countries. It is very important that investigators from the various studies collaborate to replicate areas of possible linkage and to pool resources to search the genome for major genes for these disorders and to further understand the role of genetic and environmental factors.

REFERENCES

1. Marsh DG, Meyers DA, Bias WB. The epidemiology and genetics of atopic allergy. N Engl J Med 1982; 305:1551–1559 (Med Progress).
2. Townley RG, Bewtra MD, Wilson AF, Hopp RJ, Elston RC, Nair NM, Watt GD. Segregation analysis of bronchial response to methacholine inhalation in families with and without asthma. J Allergy Clin Immunol 1986; 77:101–107.
3. Clifford RD, Pugsley A, Radford M, Holgate ST. Symptoms, atopy, and bronchial response to methacholine in parents with asthma and their children. Arch Dis Child 1987; 62:66–73.
4. Hopp RJ, Townley RG, Biven RE, Bewtra AK, Nair NM. The presence of airway reactivity before the development of asthma. Am Rev Respir Dis 1990; 141:2–8.
5. Panhuysen C, Amelung PJ, Meyers DA, Bleecker ER, Postma DS. Family studies of asthma and allergy. American Thoracic Society, Boston, 1993.
6. Ott J. Genetic linkage analysis under uncertain disease definition. Banbury Rep 1990; 33:327–331.
7. Tashkin DP, Altose MD, Bleecker ER, Connett JE, Kanner RE, Lee WW, Wise R. The Lung Health Study. 3. Airways responsiveness to inhaled methacholine in smokers with mild to moderate airflow obstruction. Am Rev Respir Dis 1992; 145: 301–310.
8. Burrows B, Sears MR, Flannery EM, Herbison GP, Holdaway MD. Relationship of bronchial responsiveness assessed by methacholine to serum IgE, lung function, symptoms, and diagnoses in 11-year-old New Zealand children. J Allergy Clin Immunol 1992; 90:376–385.
9. Sears M, Burrows B, Flannery EM, Herbison GP, Hewitt CJ, Holdaway MD. Relation between airway responsiveness and serum IgE in children with asthma and in apparently normal children. N Engl J Med 1991; 325:1067–1071.
10. Johansson SGO, Bennich HH, Berg T. The clinical significance of IgE. Prog Clin Immunol 1972; 1:1–25.

11. Burrows B, Martinez FD, Halonen M, Barbee RA, Cline MG. Association of asthma with serum IgE levels and skin-test reactivity to allergens. N Engl J Med 1989; 320:271–277.
12. Halonen M, Stern D, Taussig LM, Wright A, Ray CG, Martinez FD. The predictive relationship between serum IgE levels at birth and subsequent incidences of lower respiratory illnesses and eczema in infants. Am Rev Respir Dis 1992; 146:666–670.
13. Airway inflammation in asthma. Am Rev Respir Dis 1990; 145:S1–S58.
14. Meyers DA, Beaty TH, Freidhoff LR, Marsh DG. Inheritance of serum IgE (basal levels) in man. Am J Hum Genet 1987; 41:51–62.
15. Meyers DA, Beaty TH, Colyer CR, Marsh DG. Genetics of total serum IgE levels: a regressive model approach to segregation analysis. Genet Epidemiol 1991; 8: 351–359.
16. Reihaus E, Innis M, MacIntyre N, Liggett SB. Mutations in the gene encoding the β_2-adrenergic receptor in normal and asthmatic subjects. Am J Respir Cell Mol Biol 1993; 8:334–339.
17. Tanzi RE, Vaula G, Romano DM, Mortilla M, Huang TL, Tupler RG, Wasco W, Hyman BT, Haines JL, Jenkins BJ, Kalaitsidaki M, Warren AC, McInnis MG, Antonarakis SE, Karlinsky H, Percy ME, Conner L, Growdon J, Crapper-McLachlan DR, Gusella JF, St George-Hyslop PH. Assessment of amyloid B-protein precursor gene mutations in a large set of familial and sporadic Alzheimer disease cases. Am J Hum Genet 1992; 51:273–282.
18. Hodge SE, Greenberg DA. Sensitivity of lod scores to changes in diagnostic status. Am J Hum Genet 1992; 50:1053–1066.
19. Meyers DA, Bias WB, Marsh DG. A genetic study of total IgE levels in the Amish. Hum Hered 1982; 32:15–23.
20. McKusick VA, ed. Medical Genetic Studies of the Amish. Baltimore: John Hopkins University Press, 1978.
21. Thompson EA. Pedigree Analysis in Human Genetics. Baltimore: Johns Hopkins University Press, 1986.
22. Chandrasekharappa SC, Rebelsky MS, Firak TA, Le Beau MM, Westbrook CA. A long-range restriction map of the interleukin-4 and interleukin-5 linkage group on chromosome 5. Genomics 1990; 6:94–99.
23. Kelly J. Cytokines of the lung. Am Rev Respir Dis 1991; 141:765–788.
24. Van Leeuwen BH, Martinson ME, Webb GC, Young IG. Molecular organization of the cytokine gene cluster, involving the human IL-3, IL-4, IL-5 and GM-CSF genes, on chromosome 5. Blood 1989; 73:1142–1148.
25. Hall JM, Lee MK, Newman B, Morrow JE, Anderson LA, Huey B, King MC. Linkage of early onset familial breast cancer to chromosome 17q21. Science 1990; 250:1684–1689.
26. Levitt RC, Mitzner W. Expression of airway hyperreactivity to acetycholine as a simple autosomal recessive trait in mice. FASEB J 1988; 2:2605–2608.
27. Levitt RC, Mitzner W. Autosomal recessive inheritance of airway hyperreactivity to 5-hydroxytryptamine. J Appl Physiol 1989; 67(3):1125–1132.
28. Weissenbach J, Gyapay G, Dib C, Vignal A, Morissette J. Millasseau P, Vaysseix G, Lathrop M. A second-generation linkage map of the human genome. Nature 1992; 359:794–801.

29. Genome Data Base. Baltimore: Welch Library, Johns Hopkins University.

30. Collins FS. Positional cloning: let's not call it reverse anymore. Nature Genet 1992; 1:3–6.

31. Risch N, Giuffra L. Model misspecification and multipoint linkage analysis. Hum Hered 1992; 42:77–92.

32. Edwards JH. Allelic associations in man. In: Ericksson AW, Forsius HR, Nevanlinna HR, Workman PL, Norio RK, eds. Population Structure and Genetic Disorders. New York: Academic Press, 1980:239.

33. Olson JM, Wijsman E. Design and sample-size considerations in the detection of linkage disequilibrium with a disease locus. Am J Hum Genet 1994; 55:574–580.

34. Khoury MJ, Beaty TH, Cohen BH. Fundamentals of Genetic Epidemiology. New York: Oxford University Press, 1993.

35. Risch N. Linkage strategies for genetically complex traits. I. Multilocus models. Am J Hum Genet 1990; 46:222–228.

36. Knapp M, Seuchter SA, Baur MP. The haplotype-relative-risk (HRR) method for analysis of association in nuclear families. Am J Hum Genet 1993; 52:1085–1093.

37. Bonney GE. Regressive logistic models for familial disease and other binary traits. Biometrics 1986; 42:611–625.

38. S.A.G.E. Statistical Analysis for Genetic Epidemiology, Release 2.1. Computer program package available from the Department of Biometry and Genetics, LSU Medical Center, New Orleans, LA, 1992.

39. Pedigree Analysis Package. Hasstedt SJ. Revision 4.0. Department of Human Genetics, University of Utah, Salt Lake City, 1994.

40. Ott J. Analysis of Human Genetic Linkage. Baltimore: Johns Hopkins University Press, 1991.

41. Clerget-Darpoux FC, Bonaiti-Pellie M, Hochez J. Effects of misspecifying genetic parameters in lod score analysis. Biometrics 1986; 42:393–399.

42. Weeks DE, Lehner T, Squires-Wheeler E, Kaufmann, Ott J. Measuring the inflation of the lod score due to its maximization over model parameter values in human linkage analysis. Genet Epidemiol 1990; 7:237–243.

43. Vieland VJ, Hodge SE, Greenberg DA. Adequacy of single-locus approximations for linkage analysis of oligogenic traits. Genet Epidemiol 1992; 9:45–59.

44. Schork NJ, Boehnke M, Terwilliger JD, Ott J. Two trait-locus linkage analysis: a powerful strategy for mapping complex traits. Am J Hum Genet 1993; 53:1127–1136.

45. Penrose LS. The general sib-pair linkage test. Ann Eugen 1953; 18:120–144.

46. Haseman JK, Elston RC. The investigation of linkage between a quantitative trait and marker locus. Behav Genet 1972; 2:3–19.

47. Weeks DE, Lange K. The affected-pedigree member method of linkage analysis. Am J Hum Genet 1988; 42:15–26.

48. Risch N. Genetic linkage: interpreting lod scores. Science 1992; 25:803–804.

49. Suarez BK, Van Eerdewegh P, Hampe CL. Detecting loci for oligogenic traits by linkage analysis. Proc Int Cong Hum Genet 1991; 63.

4

Regulation of IgE Production and the Development of Allergic Responses in Different Organs

Erwin W. Gelfand

National Jewish Center for Immunology and Respiratory Medicine
Denver, Colorado

Donald Y. M. Leung

University of Colorado Health Sciences Center
and National Jewish Center for Immunology and Respiratory Medicine
Denver, Colorado

I. INTRODUCTION

The discovery of IgE or reaginic antibody provided the basis for beginning the immunochemical and cellular unraveling of the mechanisms underlying immediate hypersensitivity responses. It is now well recognized that the major feature that distinguishes atopic patients from nonatopic individuals is their capacity to develop a sustained IgE response to environmental allergens. Through the unique property of IgE to bind to high-affinity receptors, $Fc\varepsilon R1$, on basophils and mast cells, crosslinking of membrane-bound IgE by allergen triggers the release of a variety of leukocyte chemotactic factors, cytokines, and an array of vasoactive mediators that are responsible for the clinical manifestations of immediate hypersensitivity reactions.

B lymphocytes undergo immunoglobulin (Ig) isotype switching and differentiation into Ig-secreting cells in response to antigen and costimulatory signals delivered by $CD4^+$ T-helper cells. As summarized in Chapter 10, cytokines play an important role in these processes. For IgE, interleukin-4 (IL-4), which is produced by T cells and mast cells, plays an essential role. Under certain conditions, IL-13 may also have a role in the induction of IgE synthesis. Many other cytokines can modulate IL-4-induced IgE synthesis both in vivo and in vitro. Interferon-γ (IFN-γ), IFN-α, IL-8, IL-10, IL-12, and transforming growth factor (TGF)-β all inhibit IL-4-induced IgE synthesis in vitro, whereas IL-5, IL-6, and tumor necrosis factor (TNF)-α have enhancing effects. Based on the knowledge regarding the induction and regulation of IgE synthesis and the role of allergen-specific T cells and regulating cytokines produced by these and other cells, we will examine the allergic immune responses in different anatomical sites and review various therapeutic approaches for intervention in the development of an IgE response.

II. BIOLOGY AND STRUCTURE OF IgE

A. Immunoglobulin E

IgE has a molecular weight of approximately 190 kDa, of which 12% is carbohydrate (reviewed in Ref. 1). It has the same basic four-chain structure found in other immunoglobulins, i.e., two light and two heavy (epsilon) chains. However, the molecular size of the ε polypeptide chain is 11 kDa more than the gamma, delta, or alpha polypeptide chains. This is because the ε chain has five domains (one variable and four constant region domains). Lymphocytes that secrete an Ig isotype other than IgM have generally undergone a DNA recombinational event in which a productively arranged VDJ gene segment is repositioned to a site immediately 5' of the expressed C_H gene, with looping out and deletion of intervening C_H genes (reviewed in Ref. 2). Such deletional switching is carried out in regions of tandem repeats, termed switch(s) regions, which are present 5' of each C_H gene, except Cδ. IL-4 is sufficient for the expression of 1.8-kb germline ε transcripts but not 2.2-kb productive ε mRNA (3). When B cells are stimulated with IL-4 together with either EBV (4) or anti-CD40 (5), both germline and productive ε mRNA transcripts are induced. In both cases, the combination results in deletional switch recombination that involves a direct joining of Sμ to Sε. Thus it appears that, at the molecular level, two separate signals are necessary to induce isotype switching to IgE. A first signal is B-cell activation, which induces a switch recombinase capable of switching to any active C_H gene. A second signal is provided by IL-4, which induces germline transcription of the Cε gene, making it a substrate for the recombinase.

In serum, IgE is present as a monomer and is found in very low concentrations. As a result of its unique property to bind with high affinity to FcεR1 on mast cells, basophils, and Langerhans cells, normal serum IgE levels are sufficient to sensitize these cells (1,6,7). Recent studies using genetic engineering techniques have allowed mapping of the IgE binding site for FcεR1 to a 76-amino-acid peptide that spans the C-terminal portion of the Cε2 domain and the N-terminal portion of the Cε3 domain in the native IgE molecule (8, 9). The IgE molecule can also bind to low-affinity IgE receptors (FcεRII or CD23) on lymphocytes, monocyte/macrophages, eosinophils, and platelets. The binding site for FcεRII has been localized to the N-terminal region of the Cε3 domain proximal to the FcεRI binding site (10).

B. Interaction of IgE with Cellular FcεR1 Receptors

The high-affinity FcεRI mediates mast cell and basophil degranulation. As such, it is a major determinant in the development of immediate hypersensitivity reactions. The binding of IgE to FcεRI, however, is not sufficient to activate mast cells and basophils. Exposure of receptor-bound IgE to a multivalent allergen is necessary to initiate cell activation (1). The FcεRI is a tetrameric complex composed of one α chain, one β chain, and one dimer of identical γ chains (reviewed in Ref. 11). The α chain is predominantly extracellular and is the part of the FcεRI that interacts with IgE. The β and γ chains are hydrophobic membrane proteins that are not involved in the IgE binding reaction. Transfection studies indicate that efficient surface expression of the IgE-binding α chain requires cotransfection of the γ cDNA and, to a lesser extent, the β cDNA. The β chain has homology to the CD20 molecule, a protein found on B cells that has ion channel properties. The γ chain has been found in FcεRI(–) cells. This has led to the interesting observation that other Fc receptors also use the γ chain. Recent studies indicate that phosphorylation of the γ chain may be a critical step in the activation of mast cells.

It has been known for many years that allergen-induced crosslinking of IgE antibodies on mast cell and basophil surfaces can trigger the release of preformed mediators such as histamine, proteases, heparin proteoglycans, eosinophil chemotactic factors, and neutrophil chemotactic factors (reviewed in Ref. 12). Later, it was recognized that the stimulation of these cells can also lead to the generation of newly formed, cell-membrane-derived lipid breakdown products such as leukotrienes C_4, D_4, E_4, prostaglandin D_2, and platelet-activating factor. Each of these preformed or newly formed mediators has been shown to have potent proinflammatory effects in vivo. These effects include increased vascular permeability and vasodilation, bronchial smooth-muscle contraction, increased mucus production, as well as increased chemotaxis of eosinophils, neutrophils, and mononuclear cells. Thus, many of the signs and symptoms of allergic responses can be attributed to these specific mast cell and basophil products with the particular clinical manifestations of a given hypersensitivity reaction, depending on the anatomical location of mediator release.

Recently, it has also been found that crosslinking of IgE on these same cells results in the synthesis and release of a variety of cytokines, including IL-1, IL-3, IL-4, IL-5, IL-6, granulocyte-macrophage colony-stimulating factor (GM-CSF), and tumor necrosis factor-alpha (TNF-α) (13–15). These cytokines play a critical role in the induction of late-phase allergic responses and regulation of IgE synthesis, promote mast cell differentiation and survival, and sustain chronic allergic inflammation by modulating leukocyte effector function and expression of cellular adhesion molecules.

C. Interaction of IgE with Cellular FcϵRII Receptors

Unlike FcϵRI, the low-affinity IgE receptor (FcϵRII or CD23) is distributed on a variety of cell types (Chapter 10, 16). There are two forms of the receptor, which differ by only a few amino acids in the terminal portion of the cytoplasmic domains (17). The FcϵRIIa form is observed only in B cells, whereas the FcϵRIIb form is observed on B lymphocytes, macrophages, platelets, and activated T cells. It remains controversial as to whether FcϵRII is present on eosinophils. There is no structural homology between FcϵRI and FcϵRII. The FcϵRII is a member of the calcium-dependent animal lectin family (18). Allergic diseases are associated with increased expression of FcϵRII on B lymphocytes, macrophages, platelets, and activated T cells. This may reflect, at least in part, the increased synthesis of IL-4 in allergic diseases, and the capacity of IL-4 to up-regulate expression of FcϵRII.

The exact function of FcϵRII is unclear. Since its discovery, the FcϵRII has been proposed to have a role in IgE regulation, either as the intact molecule or as a proteolytically cleaved soluble form (termed sFcϵRII or sCD23). It has also been proposed that FcϵRII may be involved in the endocytosis of IgE complexes (19). This results in highly efficient antigen presentation by the respective FcϵRII$^+$ B cells. More direct roles for FcϵRII in the pathogenesis of chronic inflammatory allergic reactions are suggested by the observation that interaction of allergens with IgE bound to FcϵRII on monocyte/macrophages, eosinophils, and platelets results in the release of a variety of inflammatory mediators (20,21).

III. CELLULAR COMPONENTS OF THE ALLERGIC RESPONSE

A. Induction of IgE Synthesis by T Cells

T cells play two important roles in the induction of IgE synthesis (Chapter 10). First, they can provide important and essential growth factors such as IL-4. Second, physical contact between T and B cells provides a second signal which, in combination with IL-4, results in the induction of IgE synthesis (22). Furthermore, IL-4-induced IgE synthesis is strongly inhibited by monoclonal antibodies directed against cell adhesion molecules.

Although initial studies focused on the requirement for cognate interaction between T and B cells [recognition by the T-cell receptor (TCR)/CD3 complex on CD4$^+$ T cells of major histocompatibility complex (MHC) class II antigen plus peptide on B cells] as a prerequisite for the induction of IgE synthesis, more recent studies indicate that noncognate T cell–B cell interaction, in which the T-cell receptor (TCR) does not recognize the B cell MHC class II antigen plus peptide complex, can also support IL-4-dependent IgE synthesis (23). Recent studies indicate that these T and B cell interactions are mediated by the B-cell antigen CD40 and its ligand expressed on activated, but not on resting, T cells.

B. Biology of T-cell CD40 Ligand–B-cell CD40 Interaction

CD40 refers to a 50-kDa glycoprotein expressed on the surface of a variety of cell types including B lymphocytes, follicular dendritic cells, thymic epithelium, and some epithelial carcinomas (24). It is a member of the TNF receptor family of molecules. Studies using monoclonal antibodies to CD40 have indicated a diverse array of biological activities resulting from signaling through CD40.

Importantly, highly purified B cells costimulated with rIL-4 and various MAbs directed against the B-cell antigen, CD40, induce the synthesis of high levels of IgE antibody, as discussed in Chapter 10 (5,25,26,44). Stimulation of B cells from nonatopic donors with anti-CD40 MAb, in the absence of IL-4, results in a small increase of IgG synthesis, but no IgE or IgM synthesis. When both anti-CD40 and rIL-4 are added, however, large amounts of IgE are synthesized.

CD40 stimulation alone, however, can enhance IgE production by in vivo–driven IgE-producing cells from atopic patients (26). Of interest, rIL-4 has been demonstrated to up-regulate CD40 expression on B cells. B cells from atopic donors have been found to have increased expression of CD40 on their cell surface (27). Thus, the capacity of anti-CD40 alone to enhance IgE production by B cells from atopic donors may reflect in vivo exposure to IL-4. These data suggest that the signals delivered for IgE production by IL4 and CD40 stimulation could serve as a model for activation of IgE synthesis seen in vivo in human allergic disease. More important, as noted above, the CD40/CD40 ligand interaction appears to be critical for IL-4-induced T-cell-dependent IgE synthesis.

The natural, human ligand for CD40 (gp39, CD40L) is a 33-kDa type II membrane glycoprotein expressed primarily on the surface of activated T-helper cells. The expression of CD40L during cognate T-cell/B-cell interaction is essential in the development of thymus-dependent immunity. This has been proven with the recognition that X-linked hyper-IgM syndrome results in severe reduction of Ig isotype switching and antibody responses, resulting from point mutations or deletions in the gp39 gene (32–36).

CD40L has numerous effects on B cells. Recombinant CD40L stimulates the proliferation of B cells in the absence of a costimulus (28) and induces Ig secretion in the presence of an appropriate cytokine (37). In terms of IgE secretion, addition of CD40L together with IL-4 to purified B cells induces IgE secretion. Indeed, a soluble form of CD40 inhibits T-cell-driven isotype switching to IgE in IL-4-treated B cells (38). In addition, EBV-transformed B cells transfected with CD40L can replace T cells in synergizing with IL-4 to induce IgE synthesis in B cells (31).

Engagement of CD40 by antibody and presumably CD40L results in increased protein tyrosine kinase activity (39). In a B-cell line, anti-CD40 also resulted in increases in lyn kinase activity and phosphorylation of phospholipase $C\gamma2$ and phosphatidylinositol-3-kinase indicating that activation of these kinases may play an important role in mediating the biological responses following ligation of CD40. Indeed, the activation of these kinases may be prerequisite for the ability of anti-CD40 antibodies or CD40L to induce, in the presence of IL-4, switching to $C\varepsilon$ as well as induction of IgE synthesis by purified B cells.

C. Modulation of IgE Synthesis by Cytokines

Although IL-4 is the major cytokine known to cause isotype switching to IgE synthesis, other cytokines and mediators have been found to modulate IL-4-induced IgE synthesis (Chapter 10). IL-5, a non-isotype-specific B-cell growth factor (49), and IL-6, a non-isotype-specific late B-cell differentiation factor, both up-regulate IgE synthesis induced by IL-4 in peripheral blood mononuclear cells (PBMC) (41). Endogenous IL-6, in particular, is critical for IL-4-induced IgE synthesis in PBMC, since anti-IL-6 antibody strongly inhibits the production of IgE in such cultures. TNF-α has also been reported to enhance IgE production, in both T-cell-dependent and -independent systems (42). Recently, a novel cytokine, IL-13, was found to induce IgE and IgG4 in human B cells in an IL-4-independent manner (43–45).

Interferon-gamma (IFN-γ), IFN-α, transforming growth factor-β (TGF-β), IL-8, PAF-acether, prostaglandin E_2, and the neuropeptides, vasoactive intestinal peptide (VIP) and somatostatin, have all been reported to inhibit IL-4-induced IgE synthesis in experimental animals and humans. Inhibition appears to be mediated by different mechanisms for each of the cytokines, implying indirect effects mediated through different cell types and/or factors produced following incubation with these cytokines.

D. Compartmentalization of T Cells Based on Cytokine Profile

The concept of a subdivision of $CD4^+$ helper T cells based on their cytokine profile was first proposed by Mosmann and Coffman in 1989 (46). T_{H1}, but not T_{H2}, cells produce IL-2, IFN-γ, and lymphotoxin, whereas T_{H2}, but not T_{H1}, cells produce IL-4, IL-5, IL-6, and IL-10 (Table 1). IL-3 and GM-CSF were secreted by both types. Although both T_{H1} and T_{H2} cells can enhance B-cell proliferation, T_{H2} cells but not T_{H1} cells support B-cell antibody secretion (46). This may be due to the ability of T_{H1} cells to kill B cells, probably via IFN-γ and lymphotoxin production, as well as the capacity of T_{H2} but not T_{H1} cells to produce IL-6, a B-cell-differentiation factor. T_{H1} cells appear to be primarily involved in delayed-type hypersensitivity responses (47).

The selective expansion of T_{H2} cells is thought to play a critical role in including IgE synthesis because of the selective ability of IL-4 secreted by T_{H2} cells to induce immunoglobulin gene switching to the ε locus (42,48). In addition to stimulating IgE synthesis via IL-4, T_{H2} cells also enhance two other important components of allergic responses. First, at least in mice, IL-3 and IL-4 are mast cell growth factors (49). Second, IL-5 induces the proliferation and differentiation of eosinophils (50).

The mechanisms that regulate the differentiation of resting T cells into T_{H1} versus T_{H2} cytokine secretion phenotypes are an active area of investigation. The nature of the antigen used for cellular activation, the cytokine milieu, the origin of the antigen-presenting cell, as well as the genetic background of the host all appear to play a role. For example, in mice, the cytokine environment has also been identified as having an important influence on the type of helper T cell generated. T_{H1} cells are preferentially generated when $CD4^+$ cells are cloned in the presence of IFN-γ or IL-12 (24,25,51). Conversely, Swain and co-workers (52) have reported that the presence of IL-4 during helper-T-cell effector generation in vitro enhances the development of IL-4 and IL-5

TABLE 1   T-Helper Cell Subset and Cytokine Profile

T_{H1} cytokines	T_{H2} cytokines
IL-1	IL-4
IL-2	IL-5
IFN-γ	IL-10
IL-6	IL-13
TNF-α	TGF-β
IL-13	

secreting effectors while suppressing the development of T cells that secrete IL-2 and IFN-γ.

Allergen-specific CD4$^+$ T-cell clones established from atopic patients have a T_{H2} lymphokine profile, provide help for IgE synthesis, and enhance eosinophil differentiation, whereas helper T-cell clones from the same patients, specific for nonallergenic antigens, have a T_{H1} profile (53–55). Furthermore, CD4$^+$ clones from nonatopic individuals, specific for the same allergens, have a T_{H1} profile (55). Antigens such as those expressed on parasites seem to be able to evoke a T_{H2} response regardless of the genetic background. In contrast, the genetic background seems to be critical for the generation of a T_{H2} response against allergens. It is also likely that the antigen-presenting cell itself can influence the differentiation of helper T cells. In this regard, Finkelman et al. (56) have reported that macrophages, by secreting IFN-α early in the course of an immune response, e.g., to an infectious agent, down-regulate the IgE response but enhance IgG2a synthesis in mice.

E. Role of T_{H1}/T_{H2} Cells in Human Allergic Disease

Although this dichotomy of T-helper cells is somewhat established in mice, a human counterpart of T_{H1} and T_{H2} cells has been difficult to demonstrate, at least in vivo. Of note, although mouse T-cell clones can frequently be classified into either the T_{H1}- or the T_{H2}-cell pattern of cytokine secretion, a number of laboratories have also found that other cytokine secretion patterns can be observed (57,58). Such patterns include the T_{H0}-cell pattern in which IL-2, IFN-γ, IL-4, and IL-5 are present. Other intermediate patterns have been seen particularly when unimmunized mice are used as donors for T-cell cloning. Repeated antigen stimulation, however, results in T cells that predominantly produce IL-4 or IFN-γ. These experiments provide evidence that there are precursor T cells that differentiate into T_{H1} versus T_{H2} cells (59,60).

These results also fit well with data obtained with many human T-cell clones. In this regard, most alloreactive or PHA-induced human T-cell clones derived from the peripheral blood of normal donors have intermediate patterns of cytokine production that do not fit clearly into T_{H1} or T_{H2} cells. However, T cells isolated from diseased tissues or peripheral blood of patients with active disease have been found to exhibit T_{H1}- or T_{H2}-like cytokine profiles. Thus, CD4$^+$ T cells isolated from thyroid glands of patients with autoimmune thyroiditis develop into T-cell clones that produce IFN-γ but not IL-4. In contrast, most T cells infiltrating the conjunctiva of patients with vernal conjunctivitis develop into T-cell clones producing high levels of IL-4 but not IFN-γ (61). Using in situ hybridization, Kay and co-workers have also reported increased mRNA expression of IL-3, IL-4, IL-5, and GM-CSF in skin biopsies of allergen-induced late-phase reactions in atopic subjects and asthmatic airways (62).

The potential importance of a dysregulation of IL-4 and IFN-γ production in allergic diseases is further supported by immunological characterization of PBMC from patients with atopic dermatitis (AD) and marked by elevated serum IgE levels (reviewed in Ref. 63). B cells and monocytes from AD patients express increased levels of the CD23 (low-affinity IgE receptor) surface antigen. Since IL-4 plays an important role in the induction of IgE synthesis as well as CD23 expression on B cells (64) and monocytes (65), these observations suggest that AD is associated with increased secretion of IL-4 in vivo. In this regard, several investigators have reported that the increased spontaneous production of IgE in vitro by PBMC from AD patients can be inhibited by the addition of anti-IL-4 (66,67). Furthermore, allergen-specific T cells cloned from AD skin lesions and AD peripheral blood demonstrate an increased frequency of T_{H2} cells (55).

PBMC from AD patients have also been found to have a decreased capacity to produce IFN-γ in response to a number of stimuli (66,68,69). A significant inverse correlation has been reported between IFN-γ generation in vitro and IgE serum concentrations in vivo in AD (69). Spontaneous IgE production by PBMC from AD patients can also be suppressed by the addition of IFN-γ (66). Taken together these data suggest that an imbalance of IL-4 and IFN-γ production may account for many of the immunological features found in patients with allergic disease and elevated IgE levels. The recent observation that mast cells also produce cytokines such as IL-4 provides a T-cell independent mechanism as well by which IgE synthesis may be enhanced following exposure of an individual to allergen.

F. T-Cell-Independent Systems of IgE Induction

Aside from T cells, there are a number of direct (T-cell-independent) B-cell activators that can act in combination with IL-4 to induce IgE synthesis. In this regard, it has been shown that stimulation with IL-4 and EBV induces T-cell-independent IgE synthesis in human B cells (70,71). IgE production in this system was shown to be due to de novo induction of isotype switching, rather than from expansion of a precommitted sIgE$^+$ B-cell population, which has undergone Cε switching in vivo, because sIgE-negative B-cell precursors could be stimulated by EBV and IL-4 to produce IgE.

Hydrocortisone has also been found to up-regulate IL-4-dependent IgE synthesis by normal unfractionated mononuclear cells (72,73). These observations have been extended to demonstrate that sIgE-negative B cells from nonatopic donors can be induced to synthesize IgE when incubated with a combination of hydrocortisone and rIL-4 (73). The mechanisms by which hydrocortisone synergizes with IL-4 are unknown. However, these in vitro observations provide an immunological basis for in vivo studies, which have demonstrated that during the first 2 weeks after systemic steroid therapy atopic individuals frequently have a rise in serum IgE (74).

Taken together, these data indicate that the second signal(s) required for IgE production can be delivered to B cells through different activation pathways. It is likely, however, that these different pathways will share the ability to activate switch recombination in B cells that have been incubated with IL-4 to render the Cε locus accessible.

IV. SENSITIZATION OF SPECIFIC TARGET ORGANS

As our understanding of the generic immune system has evolved, it has become clear that the complexity of human disease is in part a reflection of specialized immune responses suited to the specific needs of individual organs or tissues (Table 1). This concept was first introduced in 1974 by Guy-Grand et al. (75), who described preferential localization of IgA-producing B cells in gut Peyer's patches. It was subsequently realized that these specialized collections of lymphoid cells, along with lymph nodes draining the gut and the associated blood and lymphatic vessels, could be considered an integrated immunological unit termed "gut-associated lymphoid tissue" (GALT). Similar observations have been made in the skin and the lung.

A. Skin and Atopic Dermatitis

The term "skin-associated lymphoid tissue" (SALT) was first coined by Streilein in 1978 to describe those cellular elements that provided the skin with the capability to deal with antigenic challenges occurring at or within the skin's surface (76). The major cellular constituents of SALT are keratinocytes, Langerhans cells, mast cells, skin-infiltrating T lymphocytes, postcapillary venule endothelial cells, and regional lymph nodes linking the skin with the systemic circulation via different and efferent lymphatics. An examination of current concepts regarding IgE-mediated skin inflammation in allergen-induced late-phase responses and atopic dermatitis (AD) provides relevant examples of the manner in which these cells are integrated into allergic skin reactions.

There are several mechanisms by which the IgE molecule participates in the induction of an inflammatory cell response in the skin. Clinically significant allergen-induced reactions are associated with an IgE-dependent biphasic response (77,78). In cutaneous biphasic reactions, following exposure to allergen, mast cells bearing IgE directed to the relevant allergen become activated and release a variety of mediators, cytokines, and leukocyte chemotactic factors into local tissue within 15–60 min of allergen challenge. This immediate reaction is associated with pruritus, erythema, and capillary leakiness. Three to four hours after this immediate reaction begins to subside, there is onset of a late-phase reaction (LPR), characterized initially by expression of leukocyte adhesion molecules on postcapillary venular endothelium. This is followed by the infiltration of eosinophils, neutrophils, and mononuclear cells into the inflamed area. Granulocytes reach their maximum cell accumulation at 6–8 hr, and by 24–48 hr after onset of the reaction, the cellular infiltrate consists predominantly of mononuclear cells.

Recently, there have been several important insights into the immunological events that accompany allergen-induced LPRs. Kay and co-workers (79) have demonstrated that the cellular infiltrate in allergen-induced late-phase skin reactions expresses increased mRNA for IL-3, IL-4, IL-5, and GM-CSF, but no mRNA for IFN-γ. These results suggest that the T cells infiltrating into the allergen-induced LPR are equivalent to murine T_H2 cells.

It has also been demonstrated that LPRs are associated with the release of cytokines such as IL-1 and TNF (80). These cytokines play an important role in the induction of leukocyte adhesion molecules (81). Of note, the AD skin lesion as well as the cutaneous LPR is associated with the induction of leukocyte adhesion molecules such as ELAM-1 (E-selectin) and ICAM-1 (82, 83). More important, allergen-induced vascular adhesion molecule expression in cultured skin explants, devoid of infiltrating cells, can be blocked by neutralizing antibodies to IL-1 and TNF. Thus, the local release of such cytokines from mast cells, Langerhans cells, or macrophages is likely to represent an important event in the subsequent accumulation of inflammatory cells at the site of allergic reactions.

Langerhans cells and macrophages infiltrating into the AD skin lesion bear IgE antibody on their cell surface. Binding of IgE to Langerhans cells and macrophages occurs via both high-affinity and low-affinity IgE receptors (84, 85). Langerhans cells (LC) are bone-marrow-derived and belong to the family of dendritic antigen-presenting cells. They are important in initiating primary and secondary immune responses toward foreign proteins or peptides at the interface of epithelial surfaces and the environment. Such surfaces include nasal, buccal, and gastrointestinal epithelium, pulmonary mucosal surfaces, and epidermis. The observation that IgE is present on LC in patients with AD has suggested a possible role for LC in this disease. The degree of expression of FcϵR1 on LC is variable and often low in skin from normal individuals, in contrast to lesions of patients with AD (86). Recent immunohistochemical studies have shown positive staining and gene transcripts for the α, β, and γ chains of FcϵR1 on LC. Initial data suggest that similar to mast cells and basophils, the biochemical pathway activated by FcϵR1 aggregation on LC involves the activation of protein tyrosine kinases and increases in intracellular free calcium (87).

Macrophages can express low-affinity IgE receptors (CD23) in response to IL-4 (85). Allergens have been demonstrated to activate IgE-bearing macrophages in an IgE-dependent manner with the formation of leukotrienes, PAF, IL-1, and TNF (88,89). Patients with AD contain circulating autoantibodies to IgE that can also activate macrophages bearing IgE (90). The activation of IgE-bearing Langerhans cells and macrophages by allergens and autoantibodies to IgE could thus contribute to the skin inflammation associated with AD. Although IgE-bearing Langerhans cells and macrophages have been found in other inflammatory skin diseases such as psoriasis, these other skin conditions are not associated with the production of allergen-specific IgE. Thus, the expression of IgE-bearing Langerhans cells in these inflammatory skin conditions may not have the same pathogenic consequences as in AD.

Finally, it is thought that IgE-bearing Langerhans cells in AD skin play an important role in cutaneous allergen presentation. Of note, IgE-bearing Langerhans cells from AD skin lesions, but not Langerhans cells that lack surface IgE, are capable of presenting house dust mite allergen to T cells (91). These results suggest that cell-bound IgE on Langerhans cells facilitates binding of allergens to Langerhans cells prior to their processing and antigen presentation. Furthermore, CD4$^+$ T cells repeatedly stimulated by Langerhans cells appear to preferentially differentiate into IL-4-secreting T_{H2} cells (92).

Although allergen challenges and experimental models suggest the participation of specific mechanisms of inflammation, it should be emphasized that an analysis of the AD skin lesion does not allow simple classification discretely into an IgE-mediated LPR or a T-cell-mediated immune reaction. Thus, in all likelihood, the mononuclear cell infiltrate in the AD skin lesion may reflect a combination of both IgE-dependent mast cell degranulation and T-cell-mediated responses elicited during acute exacerbations. Chronic AD may result from several different cellular mechanisms that serve to perpetuate inflammation.

B. Gastrointestinal Tract and Food Allergy

GALT consists of four lymphoid compartments: Peyer's patches, lymphocytes and plasma cells scattered throughout the lamina propria, mesenteric lymph nodes, and intraepithelial lymphocytes interdigitated between enterocytes (93). Macrophages and dendritic cells transport macromolecules from the intestinal lumen to resident B cells and T cells in lymphoid follicles. Although all Ig isotypes can be synthesized after oral antigen ingestion, the predominant antibody response in the gastrointestinal tract is IgA (94).

IgA antibodies found in intestinal secretions are particularly well suited for mucosal function because of their resistance to enzymatic digestion. Indeed, the generation of these dimeric secretory IgA molecules provides a good example of the specialization of the intestinal mucosal immune system. In this regard, two molecules of monomeric IgA synthesized by intestinal IgA plasma cells are linked by a peptide "J chain." While dimeric IgA is transported across the intestinal mucosal epithelium, epithelial cells covalently link a secretory component to dimeric IgA, thus forming secretory IgA.

Despite the ingestion of enormous amounts of food during a lifetime, only a small percentage of the population develops food allergy. Thus, the gastrointestinal immune system has been designed to tolerate ingested antigens and thus avoid deleterious, e.g., IgE-mediated, immune responses to foods. A number of nonimmunological and immunological mechanisms have been described for protection against mucosal antigens. Nonimmunological factors such as gastric acid and proteolytic enzymes degrade food proteins while normal gut motility and mucous production minimize mucosal contact with potentially antigenic substances. The epithelium also acts as a barrier to prevent significant uptake of large molecules. Local IgA production also prevents antigen uptake.

Despite these various protective mechanisms, intestinal uptake of immunologically intact proteins does occur. Immune mechanisms for the development of oral tolerance, however, remain poorly understood. In experimental animal models, it has been found that oral feeding of protein antigens results in suppression of systemic IgM, IgG, and IgE antibody responses (95). This appears to be the result of $CD8^+$, suppressor T-cell activation. Elimination of these suppressor cells, e.g., using cyclophosphamide, prevents the development of tolerance. Based on the mechanisms discussed in previous sections on the mechanisms of IgE regulation, it is likely that patients who are prone to develop gastrointestinal allergy have an expansion of food antigen–specific T_{H2} T cells that secrete IL-4 and thus induce the synthesis of IgE directed against specific foods.

The production of IgE by gastrointestinal lymphoid tissues can sensitize mast cells locally as well as in distant organs, e.g., the skin and airways. Thereafter, ingestion and intestinal uptake of food allergens can result in the degranulation of mast cells in the gastrointestinal tract to induce local symptoms, e.g., diarrhea or vomiting, or alternatively, circulating food antigen can deposit in a number of tissues to cause clinical symptoms at distant organs (see Table 2). Of note, immunological reactions to foods can also involve mechanisms other than immediate hypersensitivity. Immune complex formation and complement deposition as well as cell-mediated immune reactions to food antigens have been reported to play a role in a variety of food-induced diseases, including eosinophilic gastroenteritis, food-induced colitis, dermatitis herpetiformis, and celiac disease (96,97).

C. Lung and Airway Hyperresponsiveness

The lining of the respiratory tract is continuous with the skin and with the lining of the alimentary tract, from which the lower respiratory tract develops in utero. In contrast to the alimentary tract, ambient air moves frequently and

TABLE 2 Allergen Sensitization of Specific
Target Organs and Their Clinical Syndromes

1. **Skin**
   Urticaria/angioedema
   Atopic dermatitis
2. **Gastrointestinal**
   Food-induced enterocolitis
   GI anaphylaxis
   Allergic eosinophlic gastroenteritis
3. **Respiratory**
   Asthma
   Rhinitis

freely over the respiratory lining, making it particularly susceptible to the environment. Lymphoid tissue within the lung falls into three main categories; lymph nodes, bronchial-associated lymphoid tissue (BALT), and lymphoreticular aggregates. Although present in humans (and mice), BALT is less prominent than in other species.

Most allergens that provoke attacks of asthma enter the body by inhalation. The role of sensitization through the airways, although critical, has not received a great deal of attention. In many of the animal models of airway hyperresponsiveness, subsequent challenge of the airways usually followed a protocol of parenteral sensitization, often using adjuvant to elicit a systemic IgE response (98,99). The response to allergen challenge in humans has been characterized by the appearance of eosinophils and neutrophils in lavage fluid accompanied by lymphocytes with a T_{H2}-like phenotype (reviewed in Ref. 100). A similar pattern of cells is also seen infiltrating bronchial and broncheolar tissues (101). T-cell clones established from bronchial or nasal mucosal biopsy specimens following provocation also primarily exhibit a T_{H2} phenotype capable of inducing IgE synthesis in the presence of autologous peripheral blood B cells and sensitizing antigen (101). These data suggest that inhalation of the clinically relevant allergen can induce activation of specific T cells in the airway mucosa of a phenotype that contributes to IgE synthesis and airway inflammation.

Although the appropriateness of using animal models for studying allergic diseases of the lung can be debated, important insights can be gained. Since adjuvants may induce nonspecific T-cell as well as inflammatory responses and affect several cellular functions, their avoidance is important in dissecting the immune-inflammatory response. To study the local response in the lung, we developed a system to sensitize mice exclusively via the airways, in the absence of adjuvant, and examined the local and systemic consequences of this form of sensitization on IgE production and airway responsiveness (102–108). Mice were exposed to antigen (ovalbumin, ragweed, or the major cat dander allergen, Fel d1) by placing them in a plastic box and using ultrasonic nebulization to ensure the delivery of small particles of antigen in the respirable range. In parallel to the development of the sensitization procedure, we also established the means for assaying specific IgE antibody production and for performing immediate cutaneous skin tests and studying airway responsiveness in vivo and in vitro. In addition, we examined the consequences of local sensitization on the local lymph nodes of the airways and lung, the peribronchial lymph nodes (PBLN).

In BALB/c mice, sensitization via the airways in the absence of adjuvant results in an antibody response that is predominately IgE and to a lesser degree IgG1 and is associated with the development of antigen-specific immediate cutaneous hypersensitivity responses and airway hyperresponsiveness measured in vivo, following intravenous methacholine challenge, or in vitro, monitoring responsiveness of tracheal smooth muscle preparations to electrical field stimulation. The PBLN are enlarged in sensitized animals, consisting of increased numbers of lymphocytes that, when transferred into naïve recipients, result in the development of IgE responses and immediate cutaneous hypersensitivity. Despite circulating IgE levels in the recipient animals equivalent to the primary sensitized animals, airway responsiveness is increased only in recipient animals that receive a single challenge with the relevant antigen via the airways (107).

Further characterization of the relevant cells in PBLN revealed that passive transfer of IgE responsiveness could be achieved with $CD4^+$ cells but not $CD8^+$ T lymphocytes (109). In addition, it appeared that in response to ovalbumin or ragweed sensitization via the airways, T cells expressing different Vß elements of the T-cell receptor are selectively expanded in the PBLN (and spleen). The expansion of these Vß-expressing T-cell subsets also reflected which sensitizing antigen was used; ovalbumin triggered expansion of $Vß8.1^+$ and $Vß8.2^+$, $Vß2^+$ and $Vß14^+$ T cells, whereas ragweed sensitization increased the numbers of $Vß8.2^+$ T cells. The expansion of distinct subsets of T cells was also accompanied by functional differences; following sensitization to ovalbumin, we demonstrated, in vitro and in vivo, the capacity of $Vß8^+$ T cells to provide help for IgE synthesis whereas the $Vß2^+$ T cells from sensitized animals prevented the induction of IgE synthesis (106). Recent studies suggest that at least in part, the results may reflect the cytokine profile of the individual Vß-expressing T-cell subset from sensitized animals.

It thus appears that interesting differences in the immune response emerge depending on the genetic background, the route of sensitization, and the nature of the sensitizing antigen. While sensitization via the airways leads to the preferential development of an IgE response in a susceptible strain (BALB/c mice), sensitization in the same fashion of a nonsusceptible strain (SJL/J mice) triggers an IgG response without any alteration in airway function (103). Of interest, SJL/J mice are depleted of Vß8[+] T cells. Further studies are obviously needed but the data in this model have provided evidence for an association between the development of an IgE response and airway hyper-responsiveness and the sensitization of specific T-cell subsets in the local environment of the airways, which control development of this IgE-specific antibody response.

V. MODIFICATION OF THE ALLERGIC RESPONSE

A. Inhibitory Cytokines

As described above and in Chapter 10, many of the cytokines may have a negative regulatory influence on IgE production, at least in vitro (Table 2). Among these, the best-studied inhibitory cytokine is IFN-γ. In in vitro studies of IgE production by murine and human lymphocytes, IFN-γ was inhibitory (110–113), and in mice, administration of IFN-γ also inhibited IgE production (114). The inhibitory action of IFN-γ is not fully defined, but it reduces IL-4-induced germline ε mRNA by more than 50% and productive ε transcripts by more than 80% (2,3). The therapeutic role of IFN-γ in allergic diseases has, however, yielded inconsistent results. Treatment of severe atopic dermatitis with subcutaneous recombinant IFN-γ showed reduction in skin disease despite a lack of effect on serum IgE levels (115,116). Placebo-controlled trials with IFN-γ showed no clinical improvement in patients with seasonal allergic rhinitis and no changes in serum IgE levels (117). These inconsistent results have been related to the inability to achieve therapeutic levels of IFN-γ at regional lymph nodes.

Since the human trials were limited in terms of examining variables such as route of administration, dosage, and, to some extent, timing of IFN-γ administration and its immunomodulatory effects, we examined some of these issues in the murine model of allergen sensitization described above. The data highlight the differences in effects observed between parenteral and local (nebulized via the airways) delivery of IFN-γ (118). As predicted from other studies, administration of IFN-γ intraperitoneally resulted in a reduction in total serum IgE but failed to interfere with the generation of allergen-specific IgE. In contrast, nebulized IFN-γ had little effect on serum polyclonal IgE production, but markedly decreased allergen-specific IgE, inhibited the development of immediate cutaneous reactivity, and prevented the alteration in airway function observed with sensitization through the airways. As previously shown in a human trial, nebulized IFN-γ is available in the lung and local lymphoid tissue, with little systemic effect. Further, the timing of administration was critical, with maximum benefit observed when IFN-γ was begun prior to allergen exposure.

B. Anticytokine/Anticytokine Receptor

In view of the central role of IL-4 in IgE production, a number of strategies have been used to limit the production of IgE by interfering with the functional activities of this cytokine. These include inhibiting IL-4 synthesis, neutralizing circulating IL-4, and limiting accessibility of IL-4 to its receptor. Because of the widespread (in vitro) effects of IL-4 on T and B lymphocytes, it might have been predicted that neutralization of this cytokine in vivo could suppress all antibody responses, regardless of isotype. However, in in vivo murine studies, administration of a monoclonal anti-IL-4 antibody inhibited B-cell MHC class II expression and completely suppressed IgE antibody production, but had little or no effect on IgG1 antibody responses (119). Similar results were seen following immunization with a protein-alum conjugate, injection of a goat anti-mouse IgD antibody, or a nematode infection (119,120). Although IL-4 was reasonably effective in selectively inhibiting primary and secondary IgE responses, high concentrations of antibody were required, rendering this approach somewhat impractical.

Another approach is to prevent IL-4 interaction with IL-4R receptors on lymphocytes using anti-IL-4 receptor antibody. The results with this approach were very similar to the results with anti-IL-4 antibody, namely blocking of IgE responses almost completely but only a modest and variable effect on the induction of IgG1 responses (121,122).

A third approach has been to use soluble IL-4 receptor molecules (sIL-4R). These sIL-4R effectively bind IL-4 resulting in inhibition of IL-4-dependent, mitogen-stimulated T-cell proliferation, IL-4 induced up-regulation of CD23 on B cells, and in vitro IgE production (123,124). In an allergen-specific system, IgE and IgG1 production were inhibited in the presence of sIL-4R, especially when present during the first three days of culture; delaying addition of sIL-4R beyond day 6 (in 14-day cultures) had no inhibitory effect (125).

Administration of sIL-4R in high doses also inhibited the production of IgE in mice. The effect of treatment with sIL-4R was tested in the murine model of allergen-induced sensitization (126). Mice, sensitized through the airways and treated by intraperitoneal injections of sIL-4R, developed significant suppression of immediate hypersensitivity responses (IgE and IgG1 antibody formation and immediate cutaneous reactivity) and normalized airway responsiveness. When sensitized mice were treated with nebulized sIL-4R, the effects were even more dramatic with complete normalization of airway function.

C. Immunosuppression

Corticosteroids

In in vitro studies of corticosteroid effects on IgE production, conflicting results have been reported, with both inhibition and enhancement being observed (127,128). Some of the controversy may reside in the different preparations of cells used, the nature of the steroid used, and the source of the B cells. As described earlier, together with anti-CD40 antibody, hydrocortisone can provide a second signal for purified B cells, stimulating IgE production (72). Soluble CD23 possesses B-cell growth factor activity and can enhance IgE production. IL-4 is a potent stimulator of CD23 expression and dexamethasone can both inhibit the IL-4-dependent up-regulation of CD23 and reduce the levels of soluble CD23 in culture supernates (129).

The in vivo effects of corticosteroids on IgE synthesis are also inconsistent. In a recent study in which 10 asthmatics were given a 7-day course of prednisone (20 mg b.i.d.), all patients demonstrated a rise in serum IgE levels, and cultures of peripheral blood mononuclear cells in the presence of IL-4 produced increased levels of IgE (130). The data confirmed that the observed rise in IgE production associated with prednisone treatment was not clinically deleterious.

D. Cyclosporin A

Cyclosporin A is known to block the transcription of a number of cytokine genes, including IL-4. In vitro, cyclosporin A inhibited IL-4-dependent IgE production and the number of IgE-producing cells (128). The suppression of immunoglobulin production was restricted to the immunosuppressive compounds, but not a nonimmunosuppressive analog. The suppressive effects of cyclosporin A were related to treatment of the T cells but not the B cells. Recently, cyclosporin A was reported to inhibit CD40-ligand expression and inhibited IL-4-driven, CD40-ligand-dependent IgE isotype switching (131).

REFERENCES

1. Ishizaka T, Ishizaka K. Biology of immunoglobulin E. Prog Allergy 1975; 19:60–121.
2. Coffman RL, Lebman DA, Rothman P. Mechanism of immunoglobulin isotype switching. Adv Immunol 1993; 54:229–270.
3. Gauchat JF, Lebman DA, Coffman RL, Gascan H, de Vries JE. Structure and expression of germline ε transcripts in human B cells induced by interleukin 4 to switch to IgE production. J Exp Med 1990; 172:463–473.
4. Jabara HH, Schneider LC, Shapira SK, Allieri C, Moody CT, Kieff E, Geha RS, Vercelli D. Induction of germline and mature C_ε transcripts in human B cells stimulated with rIL-4 and EBV. J Immunol 1990; 145:3468–3473.

5. Jabara HH, Fu SM, Geha RS, Vercelli D. CD40 and IgE: synergism between anti-CD40 mAb and IL-4 in the induction of IgE synthesis by highly purified human B cells. J Exp Med 1990; 172:1861–1864.

6. Beiber T, de la Salle H, Wollenberg A, Hatkimi J, Chizzonite R, Ring J, Hanan D, de la Salle C. Human epidermal Langerhans cells express the high affinity receptor for immunoglobulin E. J Exp Med 1992; 175:1285–1290.

7. Wang B, Rieger A, Kilgus O, Ochiai K, Maurer D, Fodinger D, Kinet JP, Sting LG. Epidermal Langerhans cells from normal human skin bind monomeric IgE via FcεRI. J Exp Med 1992; 175:1353–1365.

8. Geha RS, Helm B, Gould H. Inhibition of the Prausnitz-Kustner reaction by an immunoglobulin ε-chain fragment synthesized in *E. coli.* Nature 1985; 315:577–578.

9. Helm B, Marsh P, Vercelli D, Padlan E, Gould H, Geha R. The mast cell binding site on human immunoglobulin E. Nature 1988; 331:180–183.

10. Vercelli D, Helm B, Marsh P, Padlan E, Geha RS, Gould H. The B cell binding site on human immunoglobulin E. Nature 1989; 338:649–651.

11. Kinet J-P. The high affinity receptor for immunoglobulin E. Curr Opin Immunol 1990; 2:499–505.

12. Serafin WE, Austen KF. Current concepts: mediators of immediate hypersensitivity reactions. N Engl J Med 1987; 317:30–34.

13. Burd PR, Rogers HW, Gordon JR, Martin CA, Jayaraman S, Wilson SD, Dvorak AM, Galli SJ, Dorf ME. Interleukin 3-dependent and -independent mast cells stimulated with IgE and antigen express multiple cytokines. J Exp Med 1989; 170: 245–257.

14. Galli SJ, Gordon JR, Wershil BK. Cytokine production by mast cells and basophils. Curr Opin Immunol 1991; 3:865–872.

15. Plaut M, Pierce JH, Watson CJ, Hanley-Hyde J, Nordan RP, Paul WE. Mast cell lines produce lymphokines in response to cross-linkage of FcεRI or to calcium ionophores. Nature 339:64–67.

16. Conrad DH, Squire CM, Barlett WC, Dierks SE. Fcε receptors. Curr Opin Immunol 1991; 3:859–864.

17. Yokota A, Kikutani H, Tanaka T, Sato R, Barsumian EL, Suemura M, Kishimoto T. Two species of human Fcε receptor II (FcεRII/CD23): tissue specific and interleukin 4-specific regulation of the gene expression. Cell 1988; 55:611–618.

18. Ikuta K, Takami M, Kim CW, Honjo T, Miyoshi T, Tagaya Y, Kawabe T, Yodoi J. Human lymphocyte Fc receptor for IgE: sequence homology of its cloned cDNA with animal lectins. Proc Natl Acad Sci USA 1987; 84:819–823.

19. Pirron U, Schlunck T, Prinz JC, Rieber EP. IgE-dependent antigen focusing by human B lymphocytes can also be mediated by the low-affinity receptor for IgE. Eur J Immunol 1990; 20:1547–1551.

20. Fuller R, Morris P, Richmond R, Sykes D, Varndell IM, Kemeny DM, Cole PJ, Dollery CT, MacDermot J. Immunoglobulin E-dependent stimulation of human alveolar macrophages: significance in type 1 hypersensitivity. Clin Exp Immunol 1986; 65:416–426.

21. Rouzer CA, Scott WA, Hamill AL, Liu FT, Katz DH, Cohn ZA. Secretion of leukotriene C and other arachidonic acid metabolites by macrophages challenged with immunoglobulin E immune complexes. J Exp Med 1982; 156:1077–1086.

22. Vercelli D, Jabara HH, Arai K, Geha RS. Induction of human IgE synthesis requires interleukin 4 and T-B cell interaction involving the T cell receptor/CD3 complex and MHC class II antigens. J Exp Med 1989; 169:1295–1307.

23. Parronchi P, Tiri A, Macchia D, DeCarli M, Biswas P, Simonelli C, Maggi E, Del-Prete G, Ricci M, Romagnani S. Noncognate contact-dependent B cell activation can promote IL-4 dependent in vitro human IgE synthesis. J Immunol 1990; 144: 2102–2108.

24. Clark EA. CD40: a cytokine receptor in search of a ligand. Tissue Antigens 1990; 36:33–36.

25. Gascan H, Gauchat J-F, Aversa G, Van Viasselaer P, deVries JE. Anti-CD40 monoclonal antibodies or CD4$^+$ T cell clones and IL-4 induce IgG4 and IgE switching in purified human B cells via different signaling pathways. J Immunol 1991; 147:8–13.

26. Ke Z, Clark EA, Saxon A. CD40 stimulation provides an IFN-γ independent and IL-4-dependent differentiation signal directly to human B cells for IgE production. J Immunol 1991; 146:1836.

27. Renz H, Brodie C, Bradley K. Leung DYM, Gelfand EW. Enhancement of IgE production by anti-CD40 antibody in atopic dermatitis. J Allergy Clin Immunol 1994; 93:658–668.

28. Spriggs MK, Armitage RJ, Strockbine L, Clifford KN, Macduff BM, Sato TA, Maliszewski CR, Fanslow WC. Recombinant human CD40 ligand stimulates B cell proliferation and immunoglobulin E secretion. J Exp Med 1992; 176:1543–1550.

29. Graf D, Korthauer U, Mages HW, Senger G, Kroczek RA. Cloning of TRAP, a ligand for CD40 on human T cells. Eur J Immunol 1992; 22:3191–3194.

30. Hollenbaugh D, Grosmaire LS, Kullas CD, Chalupny NJ, Braesch-Andersen S, Noelle RJ, STamenkovic I, Ledbetter JA, Aruffo A. The human T cell antigen gp39, a member of the TNF gene family, is a ligand for the CD40 receptor expression of a soluble form of gp39 with B cell co-stimulatory activity. EMBO J 1992; 11:4313–4321.

31. Armitage RJ, Fanslow WC, Strockbine L, Sato TA, Clifford KN, Macduff BM, Anderson DM, Gimpel SD, Davis-Smith T, Maliszewski CR, Clark EA, Smith CA, Grabstein KH, Cosman D, Spriggs MK. Molecular and biological characterization of a murine ligand for CD40. Nature (Lond) 1992; 357:80–82.

32. Allen RC, Armitage RJ, Conley ME, Rosenblatt H, Jenkins NA, Copeland NG, Bedell MA, Edelhoff S, Disteche CM, Simoneaux DK, Fanslow WC, Belmont J, Spriggs MK. CD40 ligand gene defects responsible for X-linked hyper-IgM syndrome. Science 1993; 259:990–993.

33. Aruffo A, Farrington M, Hollenbaugh D, Li X, Milatovich A, Nonoyama S, Bajorath J, Grosmaire LS, Stenkamp R, Neubauer M, Roberts RL, Noelle RJ, Ledbetter JA, Francke U, Ochs HD. The CD40 ligand, gp39, is defective in activated T cells from patients with X-linked hyper-IgM syndrome. Cell 1993; 72:291–300.

34. Korthauer U, Graf D, Mages HW, Briere F, Padayachee M, Malcolm S, Ugazio AG, Notarangelo LD, Levinsky RJ, Kroczek RA. Defective expression of T-cell CD40 ligand causes X-linked immunodeficiency with hyper IgM. Nature (Lond) 1993; 361:539–541.

35. DiSanto JP, Bonnefoy JY, Gauchat JF, Fischer A, de Saint Basile G. CD40 ligand mutations in X-linked immunodeficiency with hyper-IgM. Nature (Lond) 1993; 361:541–543.

36. Geha RS, Hyslop N, Alami S, Farah F, Schneeberger EE, Rosen FS. Hyper immunoglobulin M immunodeficiency (dysgammaglobulinemia): presence of immunoglobulin M-secreting plasmacytoid cells in peripheral blood and failure of immunoglobulin M-immunoglobulin G switch in B-cell differentiation. J Clin Invest 1979; 64:385–391.

37. Armitage RJ, Macduff BM, Spriggs MK, Fanslow WC. Human B cell proliferation and Ig secretion induced by recombinant CD40 ligand are modulated by soluble cytokines. J Immunol 1993; 150:3671–3680.

38. Fanslow WC, Anderson D, Grabstein KH, Clark EA, Cosman D, Armitage RJ. Soluble forms of CD40 inhibit biological responses of human B cells. J Immunol 1992; 149:655–660.

39. Ren CL, Morio T, Fu SM, Geha RS. Signal transduction via CD40 involves activation of lyn kinase and phosphatidylinositol-3-kinase, and phosphorylation of phospholipase Cγ2. J Exp Med 1994; 179:673–680.

40. Pene J, Rousset F, Briere F, Chretien I, Wildeman J, Bonnefoy JY, deVries JE. Interleukin-5 enhances interleukin-4 induced IgE production by normal human B cells: the role of soluble CD23 antigen. Eur J Immunol 1988; 18:929–935.

41. Vercelli D, Jabara HH, Arai K, Yakota T, Geha RS. Endogenous IL-6 plays an obligatory role in IL-4 induced human IgE synthesis. Eur J Immunol 1989; 19: 1419–1424.

42. Gauchat J-F, Gascan H, de Waal Malefyt R, deVries JE. Regulation of germ-line ε switching in cloned EBV-transformed and malignant human B cell lines by cytokines and CD4$^+$ T cells. J Immunol 1992; 148:2291–2299.

43. Punnonen J, Aversa G, Cocks BG, McKenzie ANJ, Menon S, Zurawski G, de Waal Malefyt R, de Vries JE. Interleukin-13 induces interleukin-4-independent IgG4 and IgE synthesis and CD23 expression by human B cells. Proc Natl Acad Sci USA 1993; 90:3730–3734.

44. McKenzie ANJ, Culpepper JA, de Waal Malefyt R, Briere F, Punnonen J, Aversa G, Sato A, Dang W, Cocks BG, Menon S, de Vries JE, Bancherau J, Zurawski G. Interleukin 13, a novel T cell-derived cytokine that regulates human monocyte and B cell function. Proc Natl Acad Sci USA 1993; 90:3735–3739.

45. Zurawski G, de Vries JE. Interleukin 13, an interleukin 4-like cytokine that acts on monocytes and B cells, but not on T cells. Immunol Today 15:19–26.

46. Mosmann TR, Coffman RL. T_{H1} and T_{H2} cells: different patterns of lymphokine secretion lead to different functional properties. Annu Rev Immunol 1989; 7:145–173.

47. Cher DJ, Mosmann TR. Two types of murine helper T cell clones. 2. Delayed-type hypersensitivity is mediated by T_{H1} clones. J Immunol 1987; 138:3688–3694.

48. Rothman P, Chen Y-Y, Lutzker S, Li SC, Stewart V, Coffman R, Alt FW. Structure and expression of germline immunoglobulin heavy-chain ε transcripts: interleukin-4 plus lipopolysaccharide-directed switching to Cε. Mol Cell Biol 1990; 10:1672–1679.

49. Mosmann TR, Bond MW, Coffman RL, Ohara J, Paul WE. T cell and mast cell lines respond to B cell stimulatory factor-1. Proc Natl Acad Sci USA 1986; 83: 5654–5658.
50. Yamaguchi Y, Suda T, Suda J, Eguchi M, Miura Y, Harada M, Tominada A, Takatsu K. Purified interleukin 5 supports the terminal differentiation and proliferation of murine eosinophilic precursors. J Exp Med 1988; 167:43–56.
51. Cocks BG, de Waal Malefyt R, Galizzi JP, de Vries JE, Aversa G. IL-13 induces proliferation and differentiation of human B cells activated by the CD40 ligand. Int Immunol 1993; 5:657–663.
52. Swain SL, Weinberg AD, English M, Huston G. IL-4 directs the development of T_{H2}-like helper effectors. J Immunol 1990; 145:3796–3806.
53. Del Prete GF, De Carli M, Mastromauro C, Biagiotti R, Macchia D, Falagiana P, Ricci M, Romagnani S. Purified protein derivative of mycobacterium tuberculosis and extretory-secretory antigen(s) of toxocara canis expand in vitro human T cells with stable and opposite (type 1 T helper or type 2 T helper) profile of cytokine production. J Clin Invest 1991; 88:346–350.
54. Parronchi P, Macchia D, Piccinni MP, Biswas P, Simonelli C, Maggi E, Ricci M, Ansari AA, Romagnani S. Allergen- and bacterial antigen-specific T-cell clone established from atopic donors show a different profile of cytokine production. Proc Natl Acad Sci USA 1991; 88:4538–4542.
55. Wierenga EA, Snoek M, deGroot C, Chretien I, Bos JD, Jansen HM, Kapsenberg ML. Evidence for compartmentalization of functional subjects of $CD4^+$ T-lymphocytes in atopic patients. J Immunol 1990; 144:4651–4656.
56. Finkelman FD, Svetic A, Gresser I, Snapper C, Holmes J, Troptta PP, Katona IM, Gause WC. Regulation by interferon-α of immunoglobulin isotype selection and lymphokine production in mice. J Exp Med 1991; 174:1179–1188.
57. Firestein GS, Roeder WD, Laxer JA, Townsend KS, Weaver CT, Hom JT, Linton J, Torbett BE, Glasebrook AL. A new murine $CD4^+$ T cell subset with an unrestricted cytokine profile. J Immunol 1989; 143:518–525.
58. Quinti I, Brozek C, Geha RS, Leung DY. Circulating IgG antibodies to IgE in atopic syndromes. J Allergy Clin Immunol 1986; 77:586–594.
59. Swain SL, McKenzie DT, Weinberg AD, Hancock W. Characterization of T helper 1 and 2 cell subsets in normal mice: helper T cells responsible for IL-4 and IL-5 production are present as precursors that require priming before they develop into lymphokine-secreting cells. J Immunol 1988; 141:3445–3455.
60. Swain SL, Weinberg AD, English M. $CD4^+$ T cell subsets: lymphokine secretion of memory cells and of effector cells which develop from precursors in vitro. J Immunol 1990; 144:1788–1799.
61. Maggi E, Biswas P, Del Prete GF, Parronchi P, Macchia D, Simonelli C, Emmi L, DeCarli M, Tiri A, Ricci M. Accumulation of T_{H2}-like helper T cells in the conjunctiva of patients with vernal conjunctivitis. J Immunol 1991; 146:1169–1174.
62. Robinson DS, Hamid Q, Ying S, Tsicopoulos A, Barkans J, Bentley AM, Corrigan C, Durham SR, Kay AB. Predominant T_{H2}-like bronchoalveolar T-lymphocyte population in atopic asthma. N Engl J Med 1992; 326:298–304.
63. Leung DYM. Immunopathology of atopic dermatitis. Springer Semin Immunopathol 1992; 13:427–440.

64. DeFrance T, Aubry J, Rousset F, Vanbervliet B, Bonnefoy JY, Arai N, Takebe Y, Yokota T, Lee F, Arai K. Human recombinant interleukin-4 induces Fcε receptors (CD23) on B lymphocytes. Proc Natl Acad Sci USA 1987; 165:1459–1467.

65. Vercelli D, Jabara HH, Lee BW, Woodland N, Geha RS, Leung DY. Human recombinant interleukin-4 induces FcεR2/CD23 on normal human monocytes. J Exp Med 1988; 167:1406–1416.

66. Rousset F, Robert J, Andary M, Bonnin JP, Souillet G, Chretien I, Briere F, Pene J, DeVries JE. Shifts in interleukin-4 and interferon-γ production by T cells of patients with elevated serum IgE levels and the modulatory effects of these lymphokines on spontaneous IgE synthesis. J Allergy Clin Immunol 1991; 87:58–69.

67. Vollenweider S, Saurat J-H, Rocken M, Hauser C. Evidence suggestsing involvement of interleukin-4 (IL-4) production in spontaneous in vitro IgE synthesis in patients with atopic dermatitis. J Allergy Clin Immunol 1991; 87:1088–1095.

68. Jujo K, Renz H, Abe J, Gelfand EW, Leung DY. Decreased gamma interferon and increased interleukin-4 production promote IgE synthesis in atopic dermatitis. J Allergy Clin Immunol 1992; 90:323–331.

69. Reinhold U, Pawelec G, Wehrmann W, Herold M, Wernet P, Kreysel HW. Immunoglobulin E and immunoglobulin G subclass distribution in vivo and relationship to in vitro generation of interferon-gamma and neopterin in patients with severe atopic dermatitis. Int Arch Allergy Appl Immunol 1988; 87:120–126.

70. Jabara HHJ, Schneider LC, Shapira SK, Alfieri C, Moody CT, Kieff E, Geha RS, Vercelli D. Induction of germline and mature Cε transcripts in human B cells stimulated with rIL-4 and EBV. J Immunol 1990; 145:3468–3473.

71. Thyphronitis G, Tsokos GC, June CH, Levine AD, Finkelman FD. IgE secretion by Epstein-Barr virus-infected purified human B lymphocytes is stimulated by interleukin 4 and suppressed by interferon-γ. Proc Natl Acad Sci USA 1989; 86: 5580–5584.

72. Jabara HH, Ahern DJ, Vercelli D, Geha RS. Hydrocortisone and IL-4 induce IgE isotype switching human B cells. J Immunol 1991; 147:1557–1560.

73. Wu CY, Sarfati M, Heusser C, Fournier S, Rubio-Trujillo M, Peleman R, Delespesse G. Glucocorticoids increase the synthesis of immunoglobulin E by interleukin 4–stimulated human lymphocytes. J Clin Invest 1991; 87:870–877.

74. Settipane GA, Pudupakkam RK, McGowan JH. Corticosteroid effect on immunoglobulins. J Allergy Clin Immunol 1978; 62:162–166.

75. Guy-Grand D, Griscelli C, Vassali P. The gut-associated lymphoid system: nature and properties of the large dividing cells. Eur J Immunol 1974; 4:435–443.

76. Streilein JW. Lymphocyte traffic, T-cell malignancies and the skin. J Invest Dermatol 1978; 78:167–171.

77. Dolovich J, Hargreave FE, Chalmers R, Shier KJ, Gauldie J, Bienenstock J. Late cutaneous allergic responses in isolated IgE-dependent reactions. J Allergy Clin Immunol 1973; 52:38–46.

78. Solley GO, Gleich GJ, Jordan RE, Schroeter AL. The late phase of the immediate wheal and flare skin reaction: its dependence upon IgE antibodies. J Clin Invest 1976; 58:408–420.

79. Kay AM, Ying S, Varney V, Gaga M, Durham SR, Moqbel R, Wardlaw AJ, Hamid Q. Messenger RNA expression of cytokine gene cluster, interleukin 3 (IL-3), IL-5,

and granulocyte/macrophage colony-stimulating factor, in allergen-induced late-phase cutaneous reactions in atopic subjects. J Exp Med 1991; 173:775–778.

80. Bochner B, Charlesworth E, Lichtenstein L, Derse C, Gillis S, Dinarello C, Schleimer R. Interleukin-1 is released at sites of human cutaneous allergic reactions. J Allergy Clin Immunol 1990; 86:830–839.

81. Cotran RS, Pober JS. Endothelial activation: its role in inflammatory and immune reactions. In: Simionescu N, Simionescu M. Endothelial Cell Biology. New York: Plenum Press, 1988:335–347.

82. Groves RW, Allen MH, Haskard DO, MacDonald DM. Endothelial leukocyte adhesion molecule-1 in acute and chronic eczema. In: Immunological and Pharmacological Aspects of Atopic and Contact Eczema. Basel: Karger, 1991: 85–88.

83. Leung DYM, Cotran RS, Pober JS. Expression of an endothelial leukocyte adhesion molecule (ELAM-1) in elicited late phase allergic skin reactions. J Clin Invest 1991; 87:1805–1809.

84. Bieber T, de la Salle H, Wollenbereg A, Hakimi J, Chizzonite R, Ring J, Hanau D, de la Salle C. Human epidermal Langerhans cells express the high affinity receptor for immunoglobulin E (FcεRI). J Exp Med 1992; 175:1285–1290.

85. Vercelli D, Jabara HH, Lee B, Woodland N, Geha RS, Leung DYM. Human recombinant interleukin-4 induces FcεR$_2$/CD23 on normal human monocytes. J Exp Med 1988; 167:1406–1416.

86. Bieber T, Ring J. In vivo modulation of the high-affinity receptor for IgE (FcεR1) on human epidermal langerhans cells. Int Arch Allergy Immunol 1992; 99:204–207.

87. Beaven M, Metzger H. Signal transduction by Fc receptors: the Fc epsilon RI case. Immunol Today 1993; 14:222–226.

88. Borish L, Mascali J, Rosenwasser L. IgE-dependent cytokinc production by human peripheral blood mononuclear phagocytes. J Immunol 1991; 146:63–67.

89. Rouzer CA, Scott WA, Hamill AL, Liu F-T, Katz DH, Cohn ZA. Secretion of leukotriene C and other arachidonic acid metabolites by macrophages challenged with immunoglobulin E immune complexes. J Exp Med 1982; 156:1077–1086.

90. Quinti I, Brozek C, Geha RS, Leung DYM. Circulating IgG antibodies to IgE in atopic syndromes. J Allergy Clin Immunol 1986; 77:586–594.

91. Mudde GC, Van Reijsen FC, Boland GJ, DeGast GC, Bruijnzeel PLB, Bruijnzeel-Koomen CAFM. Allergen presentation by epidermal Langerhans cells from patients with atopic dermatitis is mediated by IgE. Immunology 1990; 69:335–341.

92. Hauser C, Snapper CM, Ohara J, Paul WE, Katz SI. T helper cells grown with hapten-modified cultured Langerhans cells produce interleukin 4 and stimulate IgE production by B cells. Eur J Immunol 1989; 19:245–251.

93. Patrick MK, Gall DG. Protein intolerance and immunocyte and enterocyte interaction. Pediatr Clin North Am 1988; 35:17–34.

94. Gearhart PJ, Cebra JJ. Differentiated B-lymphocytes: potential to express particular antibody variable and constant regions depends on site of lymphoid tissue and antigen load. J Exp Med 1979; 149:216–227.

95. Tomasi TB. Oral tolerance. Transplantation 1980; 29:353–356.

96. Savilahti E, Verkasalo M. Intestinal cow's milk allergy: pathogenesis and clinical presentation. Clin Rev Allergy 1984; 2:7–23.

97. Strober W, James SP. The immunopathogenesis of gastrointestinal and hepato-biliary diseases. JAMA 1992; 268:2910–2917.

98. Frew AJ, Mogbel R, Azzawi M, Hartnell A, Barkans J, Jeffery PK, Kay AB, Scheper RJ, Varley J, Church MK, Holgate ST. T-lymphocytes and eosinophils in allergen-induced late-phase asthmatic reactions in the guinea pig. Am Rev Respir Dis 1990; 141:407–413.

99. Renzi PM, Olivenstein R, Martin JG. Inflammatory cell populations in the airways and parenchyma after antigen challenge in the rat. Am Rev Respir Dis 1993; 147:967–974.

100. Kay AB. Asthma and inflammation. J. Allergy Clin Immunol 1991; 87:893–910.

101. del Prete GF, de Carli M, D'Elios MM, Maestrelli P, Ricci M, Fabbri L. Romang-nani S. Allergen exposure induces the activation of allergen-specific T_{H2} cells in the airway mucosa of patients with allergic respiratory disorders. Eur J Immunol 1993; 23:1445–1449.

102. Renz H, Smith HR, Henson JE, Ray BS, Irvin CG, Gelfand EW. Aerosolized antigen exposure without adjuvant causes increased IgE production and in-creased airway responsiveness in the mouse. J Allergy Clin Immunol 1992; 89: 1127–1138.

103. Larsen GL, Renz H, Loader JE, Bradley KL, Gelfand EW. Airway response to electrical field stimulation in sensitized inbred mice: passive transfer of increased responsiveness with peribronchial lymph nodes. J Clin Invest 1992; 89:747–752.

104. Saloga J, Renz H, Lack G, Bradley K, Larsen G, Gelfand EW. Development and transfer of immediate cutaneous hypersensitivity in mice exposed to aerosolized antigen. J Clin Invest 1993; 91:133–140.

105. Larsen GL, Fame TM, Renz H, Loader JE, Graves JP, Gelfand EW. Increased catecholine release and M2 muscarinic autoreceptor dysfunction in tracheas from allergen-exposed IgE-immune mice. Am J Physiol (Lung Cell Mol Physiol) 1994; 10:L263–L270.

106. Renz H, Bradley K. Saloga J, Loader J, Larsen GL, Gelfand EW. T cells express-ing specific Vβ elements regulate IgE production and airways responsiveness in vivo. J Exp Med 1993; 177:1175–1180.

107. Saloga J, Renz H, Larsen GL, Gelfand EW. Increased airways responsiveness depends on local challenge with antigen. Am J Respir Crit Care 1994; 149:65–70.

108. Renz H, Saloga J, Bradley KL, Loader JE, Greenstein JL, Larsen G, Gelfand EW. Specific Vβ T cell subsets mediate the immediate hypersensitivity response to ragweed allergen. J Immunol 1993; 151:1907–1917.

109. Renz H, Lack G, Saloga J, Schwinzer R, Bradley K, Loader J, Kupfer A, Larsen GL, Gelfand EW. Inhibition of IgE production and normalization of airways re-sponsiveness by sensitized CD8 T cells in a mouse model of allergen-induced sensitization. J Immunol 1993; 152:351–360.

110. Snapper CM, Paul WE. Interferon-γ and B cell stimulatory factor-1 reciprocally regulate Ig isotype production. Science 1987; 236:944–947.

111. Coffman RL, Carty J. A T cell activity that enhances polyclonal IgE production and its inhibition by interferon-γ. J Immunol 1986; 136:949–954.

112. Pene J, Rousset F, Briere F, Chretien I, Bonnefoy JY, Spits H, Yokota T, Arai N, Arai KI, Banchereau J, De Vries JE. IgE production by normal human lym-

phocytes is induced by interleukin 4 and suppressed by interferons α, γ and pro-staglandin E_2. Proc Natl Acad Sci USA 1988; 85:6880–6884.

113. Chretien E, Pene J, Briere F, De Waal-Malefijt R, Rousset F, De Vries JE. Regulation of human IgE synthesis. I. Human IgE synthesis in vitro is determined by the reciprocal antagonistic effects of interleukin 4 and interferon-γ. Eur J Immunol 1990; 20:243–251.

114. Finkelmann FD, Katoni IM, Mosmann TR, Coffman RL. IFN-γ regulates the isotypes of Ig secreted during in vivo humoral immune responses. J Immunol 1988; 140:1022–1027.

115. Reinhold U, Wehrmann W, Kukel S, Kreysel HW. Recombinant interferon-γ in severe atopic dermatitis. Lancet 1990; 335:1282.

116. Boguniewicz M, Jaffe HS, Izu A, Sullivan MJ, York D, Geha RS, Leung DYM. Recombinant γ-interferon in treatment of patients with atopic dermatitis and elevated IgE levels. Am J Med 1990; 88:365–370.

117. Li JTC, Yunginger JW, Reed CE, Jaffe HS, Nelson DR, Gleich GJ. Lack of suppression of IgE production by recombinant interferon-γ: a controlled trial in patients with allergic rhinitis. J Allergy Clin Immunol 1990; 85:934–940.

118. Lack G, Renz H, Saloga J, Bradley KL, Loader J, Leung DYM, Larsen G, Gelfand EW. Nebulized but not parenteral interferon-γ decreases IgE production and normalizes airways function in a murine model of allergen sensitization. J Immunol 1994; 152:2546–2554.

119. Finkelman FD, Katoni IM, Urban JF Jr, Holmes J, Ohara J, Tung AS, Sample JVG, Paul WE. Interleukin 4 is required to generate and sustain in vivo IgE responses. J Immunol 1988; 141:2335–2341.

120. Finkelman FD. Katoni IM, Urban JF Jr, Snapper CM, Ohara J, Paul WE. Suppression of in vivo polyclonal IgE responses by monoclonal antibody to the lymphokine BSF-1. Proc Natl Acad Sci USA 1986; 83:9675–9678.

121. Beckmann MP, Schooley KA, Gallis B, VandenBos T, Friend D, Alpert AR, Raunio R, Prickett KS, Paker PE, Park LS. Monoclonal antibodies block murine IL-4 receptor function. J Immunol 1990; 144:4212–4217.

122. Finkelman FD, Urban JF Jr, Beckmann MP, Schooley KA, Holmes JM, Katona IM. Regulation of murine in vivo IgG and IgE responses by a monoclonal anti-IL-4 receptor antibody. Int Immunol 1991; 3:599–607.

123. Maliszewski CR, Sato TA, VandenBos T, Waugh S, Darver SK, Slack J, Beckmann MP, Grabstein KH. Cytokine receptors and B cell functions. J Immunol 1990; 144:3028–3033.

124. Sato TA, Widmer MB, Finkelmann FD, Madani H, Jacobs CA, Grabstein KH, Maliszewski CR. Recombinant soluble murine IL-4 receptor can inhibit or enhance IgE responses in vivo. J Immunol 1993; 150:2717–2723.

125. Renz H, Enssle K. Lauffer L, Kurrle R, Gelfand EW. Inhibition of allergen-induced IgE and IgG1 production by soluble IL-4 receptor (sIL-4R). J Allergy Clin Immunol 1994 (submitted).

126. Renz H, Bradley K , Enssle K. Loader J, Larsen GL, Gelfand EW. Prevention of the development of immediate hypersensitivity and airway hyperresponsiveness following in vivo treatment with soluble IL-4 receptor. J Immunol 1994 (submitted).

127. Del Prete GF, Vercelli D, Tiri A, Maggi E, Rossi O, Romangnani S, Ricci M. Effect of in vitro irradiation and cell cycle-inhibitory drugs on the spontaneous human IgE synthesis in vitro. J Allergy Clin Immunol 1987; 79:69–77.

128. Renz H, Mazer BD, Gelfand EW. Differential inhibition of T and B cell function in IL4-dependent IgE production by cyclosporin A and methylprednisolone. J Immunol 1990; 145:3641–3646.

129. Kaufman Paterson RL, Or R, Domenico JM, Delespesse G, Gelfand EW. Regulation of CD23 expression by IL-4 and corticosteroid in human B lymphocytes; altered response following EBV infection. J Immunol 1994; 152:2139–2147.

130. Zieg G, Lack G, Harbeck RJ, Gelfand EW, Leung DYM. In vivo effects of glucocorticoids in IgE production. J Allergy Clin Immunol 1994; 94:222–230.

131. Fuleihan R, Ramesh N, Horner A, Ahern D, Belshaw PJ, Alberg DG, Stamenkovic I, Harmon W, Geha RS. Cyclosporin A inhibits CD40 ligand expression in T lymphocytes. J Clin Invest 1994; 93:1315–1320.

5

Clinical Methods to Study the Immune System in Asthma and Allergy

Bengt Björkstén

University Hospital
Linköping, Sweden
and Tartu University
Estonia

I. INTRODUCTION

A correct diagnosis of asthma and allergy is a prerequisite for all epidemiological and genetic studies of these conditions. Unfortunately, many studies have been performed without employing uniform criteria for diagnosis. In this chapter, reasonably simple methods are discussed that could be considered to define clinically individuals with and without an allergic disease. As discussed in Chapter 1, there are no generally accepted definitions of "asthma" and "hyperreactivity" and this makes comparisons between different studies difficult to perform.

The clinical history of the patient, combined with the demonstration of IgE antibodies to an allergen, is the most important part of the work to confirm a certain allergy. This can be done by skin tests, challenge of various chock organs, and laboratory tests for the demonstration of circulating IgE antibodies.

In addition, some less well documented tests of potential interest in clinical allergology will be briefly discussed.

The basis for documentation of diagnostic efficiency of any method must be standardization of the reagents that are used in the test. This poses a major problem for the diagnosis of asthma and allergy, as only a few of all the relevant allergens are purified (1,2).

The demonstration of IgE antibodies in a chock organ does not prove the presence of clinical disease. It does, however, prove that the individual has encountered the allergen previously and reacted to it. False positive tests are uncommon. Thus, the demonstration of IgE antibodies in the skin or in the circulation is strongly associated either with the presence of allergy or with a history of allergy that the patient has not become clinically tolerant, alternatively that allergy will appear later, usually within the next year (3–5).

The ideal test procedure should yield a positive result in all patients with disease and be negative in all healthy persons. Unfortunately, this is never the case, as no procedure has an accuracy of 100%. The performance of a method is defined by the sensitivity, specificity, positive and negative predictive value, and efficiency. The sensitivity and specificity are given as percentage figures, defined and calculated as shown in Figure 1. Sensitivity indicates the number of true positive results as a percentage of affected individuals. Specificity in-

	Test result:		
Disease	**Positive**	**negative**	
Yes	true positive	false negative	TP +FN
No	false positive	true negative	FP +TN

$$\text{Sensitivity} = \frac{TP}{TP + FN} \qquad \text{Specificity} = \frac{TN}{TN + FP}$$

$$\text{Positive predictive value:} \quad \frac{TP}{TP + FP}$$

$$\text{Negative predictive value:} \quad \frac{TN}{FN + TN}$$

$$\text{Efficiency:} \quad \frac{TP + TN}{TP + FP + TN + FN}$$

FIGURE 1 Definitions of sensitivity, specificity, positive and negative predictive value, and diagnostic efficiency.

dicates the number of true negative in percent of the nonaffected individuals. In Figure 1 are also defined the terms "positive" and "negative predictive values" (affected persons in percent of all test-positive individuals and nonaffected individuals in percent of test-negative individuals, respectively) and "diagnostic efficiency" (correctly classified by the test in percent of all tested).

The clinical value of a diagnostic procedure is decided not only by the sensitivity, specificity, and diagnostic efficiency, as calculated from data obtained in a clinical study. The performance of the test also varies significantly when it is employed in populations with a different prevalence of the disease. This is ex-

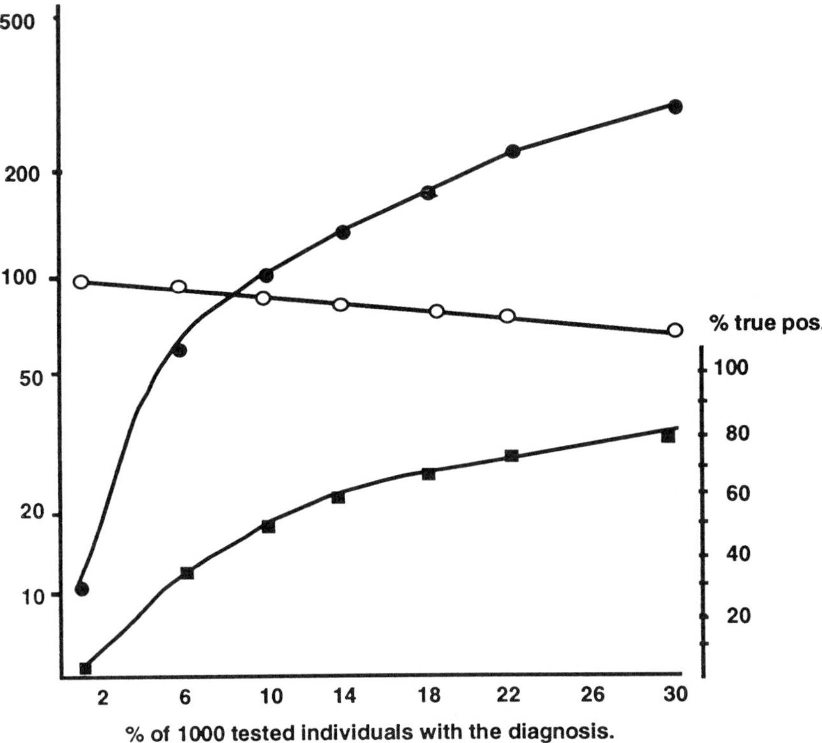

FIGURE 2　The proportion of the true positive test results of all positive results (solid squares) is related to how common the disease is in the tested population. Shown are the consequences for a test with a 95% sensitivity and 90% specificity. When the test is used in a population with few affected individuals, e.g., when screening a general population, the number of false positive tests (open circles) will be higher than the number of true positive tests (solid circles). The reverse is true when the test is used in a population with many affected individuals.

emplified in Figure 2 for a test intended for the diagnosis of allergy to a certain allergen. Assuming a sensitivity of 95% and specificity of 90%, the proportion of true positive tests of all the positive test results will be low if it is used for screening purposes in the general population with a relatively low prevalence of allergy. The test performance will be higher if it is used in patients with a history suggesting allergy to the particular allergen. Thus, the usefulness of a test is heavily influenced by the clinical situation under which it is employed.

For all the reasons discussed above, i.e., lack of generally accepted definitions of disease, technical variations in performing the tests, varying potency of allergens, and varying prevalence of disease owing to different selection criteria, it is difficult to compare the results of different epidemiological studies of asthma and allergy. Great efforts should therefore be taken to define all the parameters and tests that are used in the study. Some means of increasing the reproducibility of the various procedures are discussed in the following sections. Both tests employed in the diagnosis of IgE antibodies and other com-

TABLE 1   In Vivo and In Vitro Tests for the Diagnosis of Asthma and Allergy

Immunity	
Laboratory tests	
S-IgE levels	Confirmed
Allergen-specific IgE antibodies in serum	Confirmed
Basophil degranulation	Confirmed
Allergen-specific IgG antibodies in serum	?
Immune complexes	?
In vivo tests	
Skin tests; prick test and intracutaneous test	Confirmed
Provocation of chock organ; bronchial, nasal, conjunctival, food challenges	Confirmed
Inflammation and hyperreactivity	
Laboratory tests	
Histamine in blood and other body fluids	?
Tryptase in blood and other body fluids	?
Eosinophil cationic protein, eosinophil peroxidase, in blood and other body fluids	?
Quantitation of eosinophils and basophils in blood and other body fluids	Confirmed
In vivo tests	
Histamine and metacholine provocation	Confirmed
Cold air provocation	Confirmed
Exercise provocation	Confirmed
Other	
Bronchial alveolar lavage	Confirmed

ponents of the immune system, as well as methods to assess inflammation and hyperreactivity (Table 1), will be discussed. Some methodological problems in epidemiological studies are discussed in Chapter 7.

II. CLINICAL HISTORY

A carefully obtained clinical history is the hallmark of diagnosis. There are, however, many pitfalls, as the perceptions of symptoms varies among individuals, people forget, many symptoms are unspecific, and the symptoms have a varying etiology. Furthermore, cultural differences may influence the interpretation of symptoms.

Questionnaires are usually employed to assess the clinical history in epidemiological studies. The questionnaires are either answered by the participants of the study or they are used by interviewers for a structured interview. Independent of how they are used, they should be carefully validated. This can be done, e.g., in a pilot study on a representative group of people with and without the disease. The individual responses are then compared with the "true" diagnosis. The pilot study may reveal that some of the questions can be misunderstood, interpreted in different ways, that they do not differentiate between healthy and affected persons, or that different ethnic groups respond differently. The questionnaire is then modified appropriately. A second pilot study may be advisable if major changes are made of the questionnaire.

Generally, questions of previous symptoms or exposure are much less reliable than questions related to current prevalence. As an example, retrospective questions about breast feeding and infant diet are almost worthless, as occasional administration of a food is easily forgotten. This is also true even for pronounced clinical symptoms of disease. In a prospective study comprising 1700 children who were followed from birth to 11 years of age, questionnaires related to symptoms of allergy were answered by the parents when the children were 1 1/2, 4, 7, and 11 years old (6,7). When asked in the latter questionnaire about previous symptoms, the parents of 30% of children who were now healthy, but who had reported symptoms in the previous questionnaires, now stated that their children never had any symptoms.

When a questionnaire is being translated, great care should be taken that the translation is not merely verbally correct but also that the words are interpreted in a similar way in the second language. The translation is preferably checked by a backtranslation into the original language by an independent person. Some terms may not be available in a certain language. For example, several languages do not have a word for "wheezing." If this is the case, a list of possible words describing the symptom can be made and then a representative group of patients with the symptom in question are asked to select the most appropriate term or terms.

III. ALLERGENS

A major limitation in the diagnosis of allergy to defined allergens is the lack
of characterized extracts with a defined potency. This is true for material used
for skin tests, provocations, and laboratory tests. The term "allergen usually
indicates a mixture of compounds from one source, e.g., tree pollen or animal
dander. Many of the proteins in this mixture are "allergenic"; i.e., they may
stimulate an IgE antibody response in a susceptible individual. The term "allergen" could also mean a defined protein, one of many in an extract from an
allergen source.

The general features of many of the clinically important aeroallergens
have been known for some time. The data indicate that structurally, allergens
are indistinguishable from other antigens. Recent studies indicate, however,
that the majority of the clinically important aeroallergens are biochemically
active; e.g., they are enzymes, enzyme inhibitors, or have other regulatory properties (2). In addition, some allergens are glycosylated and/or are structurally
similar to proteins that have evolved to function in the respiratory system.

The amino acid sequences of more than 40 allergens are now known (2).
Only some of them are, however, yet commercially available. The relevance
of the source material from which an extract is produced and the quality of the
allergen extract are critical for all diagnostic work aimed at defining an allergy
to a particular allergen.

When allergy to foods is being tested, fresh food items can be used instead of extracts (8). This can be done by pressing the skin prick test (SPT)
needle into the food item and then into the skin. The "prick-prick" method is
usually more sensitive and reproducible than using commercially available extracts, as no manufacturer has standardized the food allergen extracts. To improve "standardization" of the test material, a batch of the food item is frozen
and stored in small vials that can be thawed as needed.

IV. SKIN TESTS

By skin testing, allergenic material is introduced into the superficial layer of the
skin (1). Providing IgE antibodies, with an idiotype corresponding to the allergen, are attached to skin mast cells, mast cell mediators are released, causing
an early and, under certain circumstances, also a late-phase reaction. The latter
is uncommon in children and it is only seen in about 8% of adults, provided a
concentration suitable for routine use is employed. If very high concentrations
of allergen are used, then the number of late reactions will increase.

Methods for performing skin tests include intradermal, SPT, and scratch
patch tests (1). Scratch patch tests offer no advantage over SPT and they are

technically more difficult to perform. They are even more difficult than the other skin test procedures to standardize.

Intracutaneous tests (ICT) are sometimes used, as they are more sensitive than SPT. They are, however, less specific. Moreover, ICT are potentially dangerous, as systemic reactions can be elicited in highly sensitive individuals. For these reasons ICT should be avoided. If the method is used at all, it should be preceded by a negative SPT.

For practical reasons, the SPT therefore remains the test of choice for demonstrating sensitization in the skin to defined allergens. The test results are unfortunately heavily influenced by many factors that are often difficult to control in epidemiological studies, including the quality and potency of extracts, type of needle, subtle individual variations in test technique, and how the test results are interpreted. Several methods for performing SPT have been suggested. A suitable test procedure has been recommended in a position paper issued by the European Academy of Allergy and Clinical Immunology (EAACI) (1). One drop of an allergen solution is applied on the volar surface of the underarm. The skin is punctured with a needle with a 1-mm tip that is carried through the drop of allergen at 90° angle. The same pressure should be applied every time for 1 sec by the volar surface of the fingertip. The solution is removed by pressing a clean soft tissue against the test position.

After 15 min, the outline of the wheal is encircled with a fine filter-tip pen, not crossing any part of the wheal and not leaving any part of the surrounding erythema inside the circle. The drawing can be transferred to a record sheet by pressing a piece of translucent tape against the test area. This will give an imprint of the wheal diameter on the tape, which is then transferred to the patient record. By this procedure, wheal sizes obtained over time can be compared, as well as wheal sizes between individuals.

In some studies the SPT results are expressed as the size of the flare reaction, rather than of the wheal. The flare is more influenced by other factors than the allergic reaction and it is less reproducible and more difficult to read, compared to the wheal reaction.

There are several methods for estimating the wheal size. The most common method is to express the size as the mean diameter. The longest and the midpoint orthogonal diameters are measured with a transparent ruler and the mean diameter is recorded, by taking the mean value of the two diameters. A more accurate way of defining the size of the wheal is to measure the area of the wheal, e.g., by scanning the area with a scanning program and storing the data directly into a computer.

There are several potential pitfalls when SPT are used in population studies, particularly if the purpose is to compare the prevalence of sensitization in different populations (9). In addition to the methodological aspects already discussed, the SPT results may be influenced by skin texture, as a tough skin is more difficult to puncture. As a consequence, a falsely low prevalence may be obtained in persons exposed to the sun and/or those spending much time outdoors.

Ideally, SPT should be done in duplicate, as single prick tests may easily yield a negative result in moderately sensitive individuals. On the other hand, this limits the number of allergens that can be tested, particularly in children. The question about duplicate or single pricks can to some degree be overcome by assessing the variation (CV) of the different people performing the skin prick tests. This could be done by performing 10–20 histamine pricks in volunteers on three occasions, i.e., before, during, and after the study. This procedure would improve the technical reproducibility of the person performing the tests and also be a control that it is not altered over time. With a reasonably low CV, the individual allergens could then be tested by single pricks. A positive control, histamine dihydrochloride 10 mg/ml (53.4 mmol/L), should always be included in duplicate. To reduce the number of tests, e.g., in young children, a negative control could be excluded as a routine and be employed only in patients showing positive results to all allergens, i.e., in patients who do not have at least one negative prick test.

V. CIRCULATING IgE ANTIBODIES

The search for specific IgE antibodies in serum is an alternative to SPT. The basic problem related to the quality of antigen material is similar to that for extracts used for SPT; i.e., it is acceptable for most pollen allergens, mites, pets, and protein foods like eggs, cow's milk, fish, and peanuts but undocumented for most other foods and most "local" airborne allergens.

The major advantages of the blood tests are that many tests can be done on a single sample, that many samples can be done in one assay, and that the reproducibility can be continuously checked. As a consequence, determination of IgE antibodies is more reliable for comparisons of sensitization in different individuals and populations. The disadvantages are mainly high cost, that the results are not immediately available when the patient is still in the office, that relevant allergens may be missing, and that there may be practical and cultural problems in obtaining blood samples.

There are several commercially available tests for IgE antibodies. Results obtained with different tests cannot automatically be compared because of differences in antigen composition and test performance. The composition may be influenced by the coupling procedures, i.e., how the antigens are attached to the solid phase in the test kit. It may also be affected by the presence of lectins and other compounds that may give nonspecific binding or increased background and by various technical modifications in the laboratory.

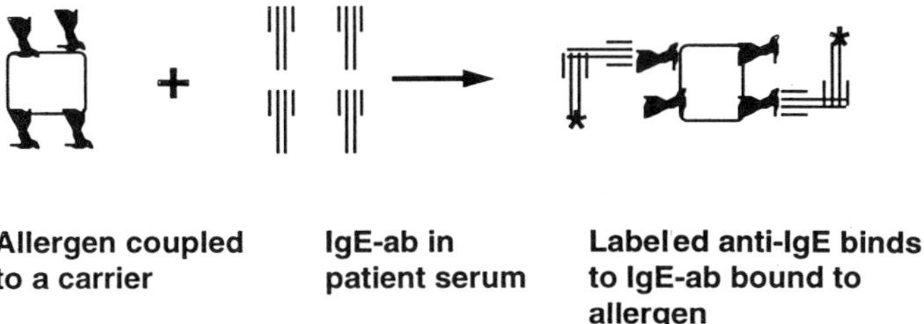

FIGURE 3   Radio allergosorbent test (RAST). The allergen is coupled to a solid surface. The serum sample is added, and after appropriate incubation, the nonattached IgE antibodies are removed by washing. Anti-IgE antibodies labeled with a radioactive tracer are then added and bind to the IgE antibodies. The nonbound anti-IgE are washed away and the remaining radioactivity represents a semiquantitative estimation of the amount of specific IgE antibodies in the patient serum.

Because of inherent problems with the standardization of a mixture of allergens and the variable avidity of the antibodies, IgE antibody determinations are never more than semiquantitative. This is probably not important in clinical situations, as there is no clear relationship between the concentration of IgE antibodies in the circulation and the severity of disease.

The two most common tests are the radioallergosorbent test (RAST) and the enzyme-linked immunosorbent assay (ELISA) (Figs. 3 and 4). All tests

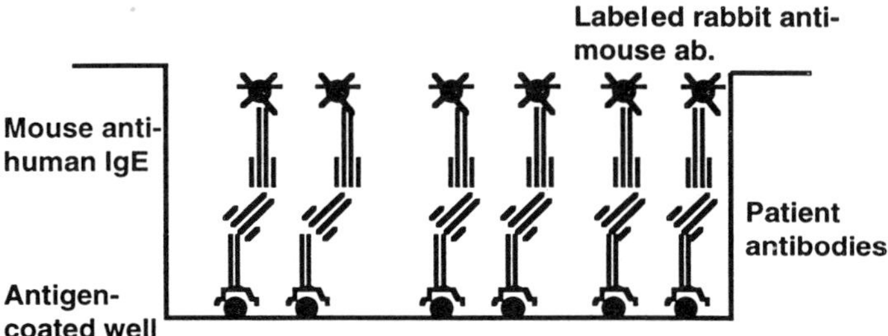

FIGURE 4   Enzyme-linked immunosorbent assay (ELISA). The allergen is bound to the surface of, e.g., a test tube. The principle is then the same as for the RAST, except that the anti-IgE antibodies are labeled with an enzyme. After the incubations, a substrate is added and the resulting color reaction is proportional to the amount of enzyme (bound to the anti-IgE antibodies) remaining in the test tubes.

used to demonstrate IgE antibodies are based on a similar principle. The allergen is bound to a solid phase, e.g., a plastic tube, a well in a microtiter plate, or a cellulose disk. The test sample is added and the antibodies directed against the allergen bind to it. After an appropriate incubation time, the test sample is removed and loosely attached antibodies are washed away. Then, an antibody directed against human IgE is added. This antibody is labeled with a radioactive isotope (radioimmuno assay), an enzyme (enzyme immunoassay), or a light-generating compound (chemiluminescence). The radioactivity and so forth is then determined with the appropriate equipment and the quantity of it is taken as a measure of the amount of antibodies bound to the allergen.

In principle, a determination of circulating IgE antibodies and skin prick tests yield the same information, i.e., that the individual has become sensitized. In Table 2 a comparison is made between the methods.

TABLE 2 Comparison of Different Methods to Detect IgE Antibodies Against Defined Allergens

Skin prick tests
    Advantages
        Rapid
        Cheap
        Fresh foods can be used for testing
    Disadvantages
        Standardization of allergens
        Standardization of method
In vitro tests
    Advantages
        Standardization of method possible
        Simple
    Disadvantages
        Answer not immediately available
        Standardization of allergens
        Expensive
Provocation tests
    Advantages
        Biologically relevant
    Disadvantages
        Time-consuming
        Potentially dangerous

VI. OTHER LABORATORY TESTS

A. Basophil Degranulation

Basophil or leukocyte degranulation tests are used by some laboratories, although the use is mainly limited to certain countries (10). The test procedure is derived from the observation that peripheral blood leukocytes from allergic individuals degranulate in vitro in the presence of antigen. The test is performed by mixing heparinized blood or separated washed leukocytes with an extract in plastic tubes. The mixture is then incubated for a defined time period, usually 30 min. The basophilic cells are counted after appropriate staining and the counts are compared in tubes with and without allergen present. If there is degranulation of basophils in the tubes containing the allergen, then the numbers of identified cells will be lower than in the control tubes. A reduction of more than 20% in the number of basophils is regarded as a positive result. Alternatively, degranulation can be assessed by measuring liberated histamine.

The test depends on the presence of IgE antibodies that are bound to the basophils. In theory, it would offer an advantage over conventional IgE assays, since it would detect only antibodies that are cell-associated. The test does not, however, offer any appreciable advantage over other methods to demonstrate IgE antibodies against allergens. From a clinical point of view it is at best comparable with in vitro determinations of IgE antibodies, e.g., RAST and ELISA, but only under carefully controlled conditions. The test is highly susceptible to the environmental conditions and requires viable cells from the patients.

B. Lymphocytes

Different subpopulations of lymphocytes can be identified and quantitated based on the presence of different CD antigens on their surface. This is done by incubating the cells with monoclonal antibodies directed against the various antigens. The antibodies are labeled with a fluorescing agent that stains the cell surface. The cells can then be identified in the microscope, or in a fluorescent antibody cell sorter (FACS). Deviations in the CD profiles have been observed in atopic individuals in several studies (c.f. Chapter 10), although not consistently. Determination of the various surface markers on lymphocytes remains a research tool, however, as normal values in different age groups are lacking for most of them, the clinical significance of the determinations is unknown, and the tests are expensive.

Reduced suppressor cell function in atopic individuals has been confirmed employing several different methods (11). This appears to be a primary defect, as indicated by the fact that it can be demonstrated in clinically healthy children who later in life develop asthma and other allergic manifestations.

Results obtained in different laboratories cannot be compared, however, as the functional assays are poorly standardized. Furthermore, they are relatively complicated and time-consuming to perform and are therefore not suited for population studies.

C. Eosinophils

Elevated eosinophil counts have long been known to be associated with allergic manifestations. Total numbers of blood eosinophils are counted on stained samples of capillary blood. Values over 4×10^8 per liter are regarded as moderate, and over 800×10^8 as pronounced eosinophilia (12,13). Eosinophilia is strongly associated with allergic disease in the absence of parasitosis.

A relation between eosinophilia and allergic disease is also true for eosinophils in secretions (13). Thus, the cytology in smears of nasal secretions from a patient with allergic rhinitis is often dominated by eosinophils, in contrast to the dominating presence of neutrophil granulocytes in nasal secretions of nonallergic origin.

D. Mast Cells and Basophils

Metachromatically staining cells, i.e., mast cells and basophil leukocytes, are pivotal cells in the allergic inflammation. After appropriate stimulation they degranulate and release numerous potent mediators, notably histamine, tryptase, and compounds that are chemotactic for eosinophils, monocytes, and neutrophils. Normally, the number of basophils in the blood is low, comprising less than 1% of all the white blood cells. In patients with an ongoing allergic manifestation, however, the number may be increased.

There is a considerable overlap in cell counts between healthy and allergic individuals and both the sensitivity and specificity are rather poor. Therefore, the clinical use of quantitation of metachromatically staining cells and their products (see below) is undefined and the tests remain research tools.

E. Mediators of Inflammation

Various inflammatory mediators are released from mast cells and basophils by mechanisms other than IgE. A direct analysis of such products locally or in the circulation would therefore conceivably be of great clinical use. Of the potential test compounds, however, only determination of histamine has been shown to be of clinical value, and then only under special circumstances (14).

When mast cells and basophils are activated during an allergic inflammatory reaction, their granular constituents are released. There are now commercially available tests for quantitation of two of the compounds, i.e., histamine and tryptase. Histamine is rapidly degraded and the half-time in secretions and the circulation is only a few minutes. The metabolite methyl histamine is more stable and can be determined in urine samples. The levels are influenced by the diet and may be increased after consumption of histamine- and histidine-containing foods (15). To relate the levels of histamine and methyl histamine to a possible ongoing allergic inflammatory reaction, the patient's diet has to be standardized (10).

The levels of tryptase in the circulation are very low and the presently commercially available assay is not sensitive enough to detect subtle changes caused by an inflammatory reaction. It therefore remains a research tool, e.g., to detect tryptase in nasal secretions as an indicator of a local reaction in the nose (16,17).

In recent years, immunoassays have become commercially available by which the levels of two dominating eosinophil enzymes can be determined, i.e., eosinophil cationic protein (ECP) and eosinophil peroxidase (EPX). The test procedure is similar to that described for IgE tests. Several clinical studies indicate that the serum levels are elevated in patients with an ongoing allergic inflammation, e.g., in active asthma (18–21). After appropriate treatment the levels appear to decrease. Elevated levels of the two enzymes have also been observed in secretions, e.g., nasal secretions and bronchial lavage fluid. Unfortunately, only a few studies have been published so far. In all these studies merely differences between groups of patients were compared. In none of them was test performance, as defined in Figure 1, analyzed in relation to the clinical condition, however. The precise clinical usefulness of ECP and EPX determinations therefore has yet to be defined.

F. Interleukins

Very recently, it has become possible to measure by radioimmunoassays (RIA) the very low levels of interleukins that are present in secretions and the circulation. Some of them, including IL-3, IL-4, and IFN-γ, are of particular interest in asthma and allergy. The sensitive methods that have been developed also allow the analysis of cytokine production in vitro by blood cells from atopic and healthy individuals. It has been established that the levels of IL-4 are higher and of IFN-γ lower in atopic and nonatopic individuals (22). This is also true at least for IL-4 in healthy infants who later develop allergy as compared to babies who remain healthy (23). The interleukin assays provide valuable tools for research but their clinical role has yet to be determined.

Receptor analysis has also recently become possible, although the clinical relevance of such determinations is not established. The T-cell surface antigen CD23 is identical with the low-affinity receptor for the epsilon chain on the IgE molecule, Fcϵ. This receptor is present on many cells and also in the serum. It appears to have immune regulatory properties but the precise role has yet to be defined.

G. Non-IgE Immunoglobulins

Non-IgE antibodies directed against allergens are common findings in healthy, as well as atopic, individuals. There are several methods to detect these IgG, IgG subclass, IgM, and IgA antibodies (24). As the levels of IgG antibodies are 100–1000 times higher than for IgE, less sensitive assays can be employed, however. There is also less risk for the interference of antibodies of other isotypes directed against the allergen.

Antibodies of the IgG isotype appear to be part of the normal immune response and their role in the pathogenesis of asthma and allergy is unknown. Thus, the clinical significance of determinations of other antibodies than IgE remains to be determined. They may possibly be part of a defense mechanism against allergic reactions. This is most likely true for secretory IgA antibodies that are present in the mucosal membranes and secretions.

Determination of antibodies of different IgG subclasses, particularly IgG4, has been suggested to be useful in the diagnosis of allergies, particularly food allergy (25). It is true that elevated levels are common in some patients, but since they are also frequently encountered in nonallergic individuals, these antibodies are most likely part of a general immune response to antigens that the individual is exposed to for long periods.

Even if the clinical significance of non-IgE antibodies against allergens is limited, such antibodies are of interest in genetic studies, e.g., in the search for immune response genes in family and population studies. One method employed for determination of IgG antibodies against allergens is a competitive double-antibody radioimmunoassay (DARIA) (26).

H. Immune Complexes

There are several studies in which immune complexes containing allergen and antibodies of various isotypes, including IgG, IgM, IgA, and IgE, have been demonstrated in the circulation. None of the studies, however, has shown a clear correlation between the laboratory findings and clinical disease. It is equally possible that such immune complexes play a protective role in the defense against allergy, or that they are part of the normal immune regulation.

Antibodies directed against IgE have received renewed interest recently. IgG anti-IgE antibodies have been suggested to play a role in the regulation of IgE antibody formation (27). Elevated levels of anti-IgE antibodies in cord blood have also been reported to be associated with a reduced incidence of allergic manifestations in early childhood (28). As for other immune complexes, there are several types of IgG anti-IgE antibodies, with different compositïon and directed against different epitopes. It is reasonable to assume that they would also have different biological activities. For these reasons, the determination of such antibodies remains a research tool of unknown significance.

VII. PROVOCATION TESTS

A. Conjunctival Provocation Test (CPT)

The CPT is the most easily performed provocation test and it is regarded as safe. There are no reported systemic reactions after CPT. Continuously higher concentrations of an allergen solution are administered into the lower conjunctival sac at 10-min intervals (29,30). A positive reaction is defined as redness of more than 50% of the conjunctiva and itching. Usually the test is done with increasing doses into one eye, and the second eye can then be tested with another allergen. The interpretation is somewhat subjective, but it has been shown to be reproducible within one dilution step. Using half-10 log increments in allergen concentration, 10-fold differences in sensitivity to the allergen are thus identified.

B. Nasal Provocation Test (NPT)

Nasal lavage involves the instillation of a liquid into the nasal cavity and the subsequent recovery of that liquid admixed with a sample of nasal secretions. The methods of instillation vary but all seem reasonably reproducible and well tolerated (16,31). With proper handling of recovered lavage fluid, multiple mediators, marker substances, and cells can be evaluated, thus offering means to study the local inflammation.

C. Bronchial Provocation (BPT) and Other Lung Function Tests

Inhalation challenge tests are being used in research studies as well as in clinical practice. From clinical and epidemiological studies it appears that airway responsiveness measurements provide valuable information about airways disease. The relationships between various clinical symptoms of asthma and hyperreactivity, on one hand, and the various lung function tests, on the other, have not been established, however. This is partly due to the fact that there is no clear definition of "asthma." In epidemiological studies there are statistically significant correlations between the presence of hyperreactivity as measured by lung function tests and the presence of clinical symptoms. This is not always true for the individual patient, however, as patients with a disabling asthma may have an almost normal lung function when tested and a person with a pronounced hyperreactivity in a histamine challenge may deny having any problems. Several aspects of the methods to assess lung function in asthma are also discussed in Chapter 12.

Bronchial provocations can be performed with pharmacological agents, hypo- and hypertonic solutions, physical stimuli, and allergens (Table 1). They should never be done without proper training of the involved personnel, as the patient may develop a strong bronchoconstriction needing immediate treatment. A detailed description of the various methods used, including preparation of solutions, suitable equipment, administration, safety aspects, and interpretation of the results, has recently been published by the European Working Party (32). Pharmacological agents used for the assessment of bronchial reactivity include histamine and metacholine. Usually, four to six doses are administered over 1–2 hr and the lung function is determined before each dose. A fall in $FEV_1 > 15\%$ over the baseline value is usually taken as a positive reaction.

Exercise provocation and challenge with cold/dry air have the advantage of being more clinically relevant than provocation tests using pharmacological agents or high concentrations of allergens. Exercise tests are reasonably easy to perform, even in large epidemiological studies. To confirm that the patient has actually been adequately challenged, the pulse rate should be tested immediately after the exercise. For challenges with cold/dry air special equipment is needed. These tests are therefore less suitable for epidemiological studies.

Daily measurements of peak flow can be done with simple and inexpensive equipment in epidemiological studies (33,34). Both maximal values and diurnal variations can be taken as indicators of hyperreactivity. There are, however, no epidemiological studies in which the relationships between the various tests and clinical symptoms have been clearly defined. Therefore, no test can yet be recommended as clearly superior to the other methods.

Allergen provocations are rarely done for clinical purposes and their use is limited to certain research problems. The main reasons for this are that the tests are time-consuming, expensive, and potentially dangerous. Furthermore, their clinical relevance may be questioned, as the doses are much higher than those that the individual is exposed to under natural conditions.

D. Food Challenge

Elimination diets can be used in patients with chronic symptoms. The patient is first asked to keep a daily record of his symptoms for 2 weeks (basic registration of symptoms) (8). The elimination diet is given for another 2 weeks. If there is not a clear improvement within 2 weeks, it is unlikely that food allergy is the cause of the patient's complaints. In patients who report clinical improvement, the diet period is followed by an open challenge or a double-blind, placebo-controlled food challenge (DBPCFC). A negative open challenge excludes food allergy, whereas a positive challenge should be confirmed by DBPCFC, except in obvious cases.

A positive DBPCFC is the only conclusive evidence of an adverse reaction to food, provided it is performed properly. It does not reveal, however, the mechanism underlying the reaction. There are several procedures for performing oral provocations, as summarized in a position paper by the European

Academy of Allergy and Clinical Immunology (8). The DBPCFC should be performed in a hospital setting where emergency care is immediately available. Negative results in DBPCFC should be followed by an open meal provocation with normally processed food.

VIII. CONCLUSIONS

None of the clinical methods that are used to study the immune system in allergic patients are perfect. At best, the methods to demonstrate the presence of IgE antibodies are semiquantitative. All share a common problem, in that only a few of the allergens that are used for the detection of antibodies are available in a standardized form. For epidemiological studies, the determination of IgE antibodies in serum would be the method of choice. Unfortunately, however, it is not always feasible to draw blood samples from large population samples. Furthermore, the tests are expensive. Skin prick tests are difficult to standardize and great care should be taken to check the variations in test performance between individuals, as well as for the same individual over time.

Provocation tests would in principle be the gold standard used to confirm or exclude the presence of a clinically relevant allergy or hyperreactivity. None of the lung function tests are, however, generally accepted as a measure of asthma, or even of hyperreactivity, and the relation to clinical symptoms has not been documented in large studies for any of them. Provocation tests are also time-consuming and relatively expensive.

Whatever methods are used to study the immune system and inflammatory reactions in asthma and allergy, the methodology should be described in detail to allow comparisons between different studies.

REFERENCES

1. Dreborg S, Frew A. Position paper: allergen standardization and skin tests. Allergy 1993; 48(Suppl)14:49–82.
2. Stewart G, Thompson P, McWilliams A. Biochemical properties of aeroallergens: contributory factors in allergic sensitization? Pediatr Allergy Immunol 1993; 4:163–172.
3. Hattevig G, Kjellman B, Björkstén B, Johansson SGO. The prevalence of allergy and IgE antibodies to inhalant allergens in Swedish school children. Acta Paediatr Scand 1987; 76:349–355.
4. Hattevig G, Kjellman B, Björkstén B. Appearance of IgE antibodies to ingested and inhaled allergens during first 12 years of life in atopic and non-atopic children. Pediatr Allergy Immunol 1993; 4:182–189.
5. van Asperen PP, Kemp AS. The natural history of IgE sensitization and atopic disease in early childhood. Acta Paediatr Scand 1989; 78:239–245.
6. Croner S, Kjellman N-IM. Natural history of bronchial asthma in childhood—a prospective study from birth to 14 years of age. Allergy 1992; 47:150–157.

7. Croner S, Kjellman N-IM. Development of atopic disease in relation to family history and cord blood IgE levels: eleven-year follow-up in 1654 children. Pediatr Allergy Immunol 1990; 1:14–20.

8. Bruijnzeel-Koomen L, Ortolani C, Aas K, Bindslev-Jensen C, Björkstén B, et al. Position paper of the European Academy of Allergy and Clinical Immunology on adverse reactions to food. Allergy 1995; 50:623–635.

9. Haahtela T. Skin tests used for epidemiological studies. Allergy 1993; 48(Suppl 14): 76–80.

10. Nolte H. The clinical utility of basophil histamine release. Allergy Proc 1993; 14: 251–254.

11. Björkstén B, Kjellman N-IM. Immunological abnormalities in atopic infants. Allergologie 1989; 12(Suppl):176–179.

12. Foucard T. A follow-up study of children with asthmatoid bronchitis. II. Serum IgE and eosinophil counts in relation to clinical course. Acta Paediatr Scand 1974; 63:129–139.

13. Borres MP. Metachromatic cells and eosinophils in atopic children: a prospective study. Pediatr Allergy Immunol 1991; 2(Suppl)1:1–24.

14. Norgaard A, Skov P, Bindslev-Jensen C. Egg and milk allergy in adults: comparison between fresh foods and commercial extracts in skin prick test and histamine release from basophils. Clin Exp Allergy 1992; 22:940–945.

15. Sampson H, Broadbent K, Bernhisel-Broadbent J. Spontaneous release of histamine from basophils and histamine-releasing factor in patients with atopic dermatitis and food hypersensitivity. N Engl J Med 1989; 321:228–232.

16. Nacleiro R, Togias A, Flowers B, et al. Nasal lavage: a technique for elucidating the pathophysiology of allergic rhinitis. In: Mygind N. Pipkorn U, Dahl R, eds. Rhinitis and Asthma. Copenhagen: Munksgaard, 1990:213–221.

17. Naclerio RM. Effects of antihistamines on inflammatory mediators. Ann Allergy 1993; 71:292–295.

18. Venge P. Serum measurements of eosinophil cationic protein (ECP) in bronchial asthma. Clin Exp Allergy 1993; 2:3–7.

19. Venge P. The eosinophil granulocyte in allergic inflammation. Pediatr Allergy Immunol 1993; 4(Suppl 4):19–24.

20. Zimmerman B, Enander I, Zimmerman R, Ahlstedt S. Asthma in children less than 5 years of age: eosinophils and serum levels of the eosinophil proteins ECP and EPX in relation to atopy and symptoms. Clin Exp Allergy 1994; 24:149–155.

21. Zimmerman B, Lanner A, Enander I, Zimmerman RS, Peterson CG, Ahlstedt S. Total blood eosinophils, serum eosinophil cationic protein and eosinophil protein X in childhood asthma: relation to disease status and therapy. Clin Exp Allergy 1993; 23:564–570.

22. Romangnani S. Human TH1 and TH2 subsets: Regulation of differentiation and role in protection and immunopathology. Int Arch Allergy Immunol 1992; 98:279–285.

23. Borres M, Einarsson R, Björkstén B. Serum levels of interleukin-4, soluble CD23 and IFN-gamma in relation to the development of allergic disease during the first 18 months of life. Clin Exper Allergy 1995; 25:543–548.

24. Hvatum M, Scott H, Brandtzaeg P. Pitfalls in determining IgG and IgG subclass antibodies to food antigens. J Immunol Methods 1992; 148:77–85.
25. Björkstén B. In vitro diagnostic methods in the evaluation of food hypersensitivity. In: Metcalfe D, Sampson H, eds. Adverse Reactions to Foods and Food Additives. Cambridge, MA: Blackwell Scientific Publications, 1991:67–80.
26. Ghosh B, Rafnar T, Perry MP, et al. Immunologic and molecular characterization of Amb p V allergens from *Ambrosia psilostachya* (Western ragweed) pollen. J Immunol 1994; 152:2882–2889.
27. Stadler BM. Anti-IgE autoantibodies: a possible specific feedback on the cytokine network in allergy? Eur Cytokine Netw 1992; 3:437–441.
28. Vassella C, Odelram H, Kjellman N-I, Borres M, Vanto T, Björkstén B. High anti-IgE levels at birth are associated with a reduced allergy incidence in early childhood: a prospective study. Clin Exp Allergy 1994; 24:771–777.
29. Rimås M, Gustafsson P, Kjellman N-I, Björkstén B. Conjunctival provocation test: high clinical reproducibility but little temperature change. Allergy 1992; 47:324–326.
30. Möller C, Björkstén B, Nilsson G, Dreborg S. The precision of the conjunctival provocation test. Allergy 1984; 39:37–41.
31. Pipkorn U. Pharmacological influence of antiallergic medication on in vivo allergen testing. Allergy 1988; 43:81–86.
32. Sterk P, Fabbri L, Quanjer P, et al. Airway responsiveness: standardized challenge testing with pharmacological, physical and sensitizing stimuli in adults. Eur Respir J 1993; 6(Suppl 16):53–83.
33. Bråbäck L, Breborowicz A, Dreborg S, Knutsson A, Pieklik H, Björkstén B. Atopic sensitization and respiratory symptoms among Polish and Swedish schoolchildren. Clin Exp Allergy 1994; 24:826–835.
34. Riikjärv MA, Julge K, Vasar M, Bråbäck L, Knutsson A, Björkstén B. The prevalence of atopic sensitization and respiratory symptoms among Estonian schoolchildren. Clin Exp Allergy 1995; 25:1198–1204.

6

Genetic Studies of Asthma and Allergy
Statistical Methods

Newton E. Morton
University of Southampton
Southampton, Hampshire, England

I. INTRODUCTION

Statistical analysis of familial traits is one aspect of genetic epidemiology, the science that deals with etiology, distribution, and control of disease in relatives and with inherited causes of disease in populations (1). Its initial focus was on confirming a major locus inferred from examination of pedigrees (2). Then emphasis shifted to complex inheritance, in which recurrence risks are variable among families of a given mating type (3). This history was recapitulated when DNA markers made the mapping of disease loci dramatically successful, even when indistinguishable phenotypes were produced by different genes in different families (4). However, the search for linkage often fails in two limiting cases of complex inheritance: when the number of genes with large effects is great but each is rare (as for nonspecific mental retardation and deafness) and when several common genes interact to produce affection (as for schizophrenia and type II diabetes). Asthma and atopy presumably belong to the latter class, which is currently the focus of much research but few triumphs. Not surprisingly, there is considerable disagreement about goals and methods, and the opinions expressed herein may soon have to be revised. Beginning with the observation that asthma and atopy are multivariate, I will consider the consequences of treating them as quantitative or qualitative, the impact of ascertainment through probands, strategies for gene mapping, and possibilities for combining different studies by meta-analysis.

II. MULTIVARIATE TRAITS

A. Principal Component Regression

Atopy is a condition characterized by a persistent and heritable immunoglobulin E (IgE) response to protein allergens. *Asthma* is a disorder characterized by wheezing and bronchial hyperresponsiveness, for which atopy is the major cause. As defined, the two traits are correlated and multivariate, including total and specific IgE titers, skin prick tests, medical history, and provocation tests of bronchial reactivity. How should the several components be characterized and combined?

Bronchial response to inhalation challenge gives a dose-response curve that may be summarized by area under the curve and other statistics, and it is not self-evident how to choose the best one. We have taken the view that total IgE, despite its environmental triggers, is the best single criterion to characterize bronchial response. We let $Y = \log$ IgE be a dependent variable and X_i be the ith principal component of statistics taken during the challenge or subsequently computed. Then stepwise regression gives $a + \Sigma_i b_i X_i$ as the measure of bronchial reactivity. This is turn may be used to characterize wheezing, which consists of responses to a questionnaire and a symptom video. Other components (circulating IgE to defined antigens, skin prick testing, eczema, hay fever, and migraine) are best characterized like bronchial reactivity by total IgE. In our work so far we have not used specific IgEs (RAST).

We have applied this procedure to a sample of 131 random families selected through at least three children without regard to atopy or asthma (Table 1). The resultant traits are quantitative, with high values indicative of atopy and atopic asthma. Their intercorrelations are dominated by total IgE, and the principal component defining atopy correlates almost perfectly with that variable (Table 2).

This use of principal components is reminiscent of the way in which psychometricians have defined IQ. Binet used age of children as we have used total IgE, selecting questionnaire items that correlated highly with age. Later workers grouped items into homogeneous sets and defined a general factor g (analogous to atopy) and specific factors for spatial, verbal, and other abilities (corresponding to wheeze, hay fever, etc.). Principal component regression

TABLE 1 Definition of Indices

Index	Symbol	Dependent variable	Independent variables
log IgE	IGE	IGE	—
Bronchial reactivity	BR	IGE	Doubling dilutions of histamine/bronchodilator challenge
Skin prick	SP	IGE	12 common allergens and controls (diameter product)
Hay fever	HF	IGE	Questionnaire (includes medication, desensitization)
Eczema	EZ	IGE	Questionnaire (includes medication)
Migraine	MG	IGE	Questionnaire
Wheeze	WZ	BR	Questionnaire (includes symptoms, medication, asthma) and video (5 episodes, 15 questions)
Atopy	AY	—	First principal component of above 7 indices
Asthma	AS	—	First principal component of WZ and BR
Situation	S	AY, AS	Age, sex
Environment	I	AY, AS	Smoking, smoke exposure, house dust, pets

TABLE 2 Trait Correlations

	IGE	BR	SP	WZ	EZ	HF	MG	AY
Log IGE	1.00	0.39	0.54	0.39	0.28	0.30	0.13	0.98
Bronchial reactivity		1.00	0.38	0.63	0.14	0.27	0.09	0.49
Skin prick			1.00	0.45	0.19	0.43	0.07	0.67
Wheeze				1.00	0.23	0.34	0.03	0.49
Eczema					1.00	0.13	0.09	0.30
Hay fever						1.00	−0.09	0.38
Migraine							1.00	0.13
Atopy								1.00

became feasible with advances in computers. Its function is to summarize information in interrelated items of data.

B. Alternative Multivariate Procedures

Although principal component analysis works well, it is not unique. Each multivariate method has certain optimal properties that may be irrelevant to genetic analysis. Some investigators prefer definitions that do not depend on the data. These are mostly of two types: Boolean union (A *and/or* B) and Boolean intersection (A *and* B), where A and B are arbitrary dichotomies. For example, Cookson et al. (5) designated individuals atopic by Boolean union if they satisfied at least one of the following criteria: (1) a wheal response 2 mm > negative control to any one or more of the allergens tested; (2) a positive RAST (> 0.35 RU) to any of the allergens tested; (3) an elevated total serum IgE > 100 units of adults and > 1 standard deviation above an age-related geometrical mean in children. Shirakawa et al. (6) required that *all* three criteria be met (Boolean intersection). These definitions are subjective, they force a dichotomy on quantitative data, and they lead to frequencies that are unrelated to any supported genetic model.

Goldin et al. (7) have shown ingeniously how a small number of quantitative traits may be combined to optimize fit to a monogenic model. However, all analysis that allows for two or more genetic mechanisms has shown that a monogenic model for atopy or asthma does not fit family data. Another alternative would be to maximize heritability, the proportion of the variance that is genetic. However, there is no reason to suppose that the genetic basis of such a selection index (a linear combination that maximizes heritability) would be simple. Dispute about the most appropriate definition of multivariate traits is bound to continue until they have been reduced to effects of known loci.

III. QUANTITATIVE TRAITS

A. Principal Components

When multiple variables are reduced to a single quantitative trait Y by the first principal component or other linear function $Y = a + \Sigma bX$, the genetic model specifies that genotypes act cumulatively and in the simplest case additively. This monotonicity means that reduction of the quantitative trait to a dichotomy of normal versus affected must lose genetic information. On the other hand, quantitative traits introduce distributional assumptions that affect tests of significance and can be confounded with genetic mechanisms. For example, kurtosis can make polygenic inheritance give spurious evidence for a major locus in segregation analysis. This illustrates a general principle in statistics, that the most efficient methods make the most assumptions, but even the least efficient ones are not assumption-free. Any violation of assumptions is a potential source of error that should be recognized and, if possible, avoided.

B. Commingling

The effect of major genes on a quantitative trait is to cause a commingling (admixture) of two or more distributions. Estimates and tests of hypotheses are straightforward if these distributions are normal with the same variance. MacLean et al. (8) introduced a power transform to remove skewness so that $n - 1$ skewed distributions could be distinguished by a likelihood test from n normal distributions on the hypothesis of uniform variance (homoscedasticity). A likelihood test compares the probability of the data under two hypotheses. Commingling is consistent with (but does not imply) a major gene. Four other causes are biased ascertainment, mixtures of populations, multiple measures of the same variable in principal component analysis, and failure of homeostasis beyond a threshold with larger values initiating progressive pathology that forms a separate population. Graphical or statistical comparison of the observed and expected cumulative distributions provides a supplementary test of goodness of fit. Consistency of the genetic parameters in commingling and segregation analysis strengthens a major gene hypothesis (Table 3). There is evidence of commingling for total IgE, but its biological interpretation is uncertain (9).

TABLE 3 Parameters in Commingling Analysis

p	The power transform to eliminate skewness, conditional on commingling of normal homoscedastic distributions
q	Frequency of gene G'
t	Displacement of G'G'
d	Dominance of G'
u	Mean of the commingled distribution
v	Variance of the commingled distribution
F	Coefficient of inbreeding

Genotype	Density[a]	Frequency
GG	$N(z, \sigma^2)$	$(1 - q)^2 + q(1 - q)\,F$
GG'	$N(z + dt, \sigma^2)$	$2q(1 - q)(1 - F)$
G'G'	$N(z + t, \sigma^2)$	$q^2 + q(1 - q)\,F$

[a]The symbol $N(M, \sigma^2)$ denotes a normal distribution with mean M and variance σ^2. In this case the mean takes values z, $z + dt$, and $z + t$ for the three genotypes defined by alleles G, G', where z is a constant that can be eliminated by substitution in the population mean.

C. Path Analysis

In path analysis a correlation matrix is fitted to a causal model. Correlations between pairs of relatives give estimates and tests of hypotheses about variance proportions due to genes and family environment (10). This is contrary to the reductionism that pervades modern science, so path analysis is usually incidental to other studies and therefore based on nuclear families. More unusual relationships (twins, adoptions, etc.) tend to introduce small samples and biased ascertainment. Normality, additivity, and random sampling are assumed, although there has been some progress by adjusting nonprobands for relationship to the proband. Full use of nuclear families requires a fairly good estimate of the environment. Despite clear evidence that smoking and allergen exposure promote atopy and asthma, the correlation with the environmental index is often too small to give good resolution of genetic heritability and family environment (cultural heritability). Systematic underestimation of cultural heritability is avoided by treating the environment as a latent (unmeasured) variable that is estimated by its index if the number of observed correlations is at least as great as the number of parameters to be estimated. The object of the analysis is to eliminate models that fit poorly (Table 4). A model that fits familial correlations is undoubtedly oversimplified, but it beats any model that does not fit. For atopy defined as total IgE, Gerrard et al. (9) obtained a parsimonious model that agrees well with segregation analysis (Table 5).

Sandford et al. (11) favour FCER1B on chromosome 11q12 as the major locus for atopy, with imprinting in males. This region is homologous to mouse chromosome 19, on which imprinting has not been observed. Familial correlations provide more direct evidence (Table 6). Contrary to their hypothesis, the father-child correlation exceeds (nonsignificantly) the mother-child correlation and shows no evidence of imprinting. Had the opposite been true, not

TABLE 4   Parameters in Path Analysis

h	Effect of genotype on phenotype (square root of heritability)
c	Effect of indexed environment on phenotype (square root of cultural heritability)
f_F	Effect of father's indexed environment on child's indexed environment
f_M	Effect of mother's indexed environment on child's indexed environment
u	Correlation between parental indexed environments
b	Effect of nontransmitted common sibship environment on child's indexed environment
i	Effect of indexed environment on index

TABLE 5 Variance Components for Atopy

| | Variance component ±SE from: | |
	Path analysis	Segregation analysis
Source		
Heritability	0.425 ± 0.058	0.485 ± 0.078
Indexed environment	0.070 ± 0.026	0.024 ± 0.030
Residual	0.505 ± 0.059	0.491 ± 0.082

Source: After Ref. 9.

only imprinting but a maternal effect would have to be considered (12). The intermediate sib-sib correlation argues against any nutritional or other intrauterine effect that persists in successive births (13). These conclusions are of sufficient interest to continue study of familial correlations (not yet extended to asthma) as a by-product of studies with greater resolution.

D. Segregation

1. Single-Locus Models

Classic segregation analysis assumed a single locus with Mendelian segregation frequencies ($\frac{1}{4}$, $\frac{1}{2}$, $\frac{3}{4}$) specific for each mating type (3). This was adequate to confirm or refute monogenic inheritance with high penetrance (not necessarily the same locus in different families). However, it is inappropriate for complex inheritance, in which no locus may be sufficient for affection and different genotypes may act in different families.

The next development was extension to pedigrees by Elston and Stewart (14), a landmark in genetic computation. However, an equally important aspect was its use of population parameters (gene frequencies, dominance, etc.) that were not mating-type-specific. This was satisfactory to test for monogenic inheritance with high penetrance, but it provided no distinction between the

TABLE 6 Familial Correlations

Source	Correlation (*r*)	Sample size (*n*)
Father-child	0.313	220
Mother-child	0.222	230
Sib-sib	0.264	317

Source: After Ref. 9.

general single-locus model and more complex inheritance. The transmission frequencies (taus) that were a feature of this model are Mendelian for both a major locus and polygenes (15,16), and their only value is to detect obliquely some failures of assumptions, usually with respect to ascertainment or distribution. Single-locus models have no utility for atopy and asthma as currently defined.

2. The Mixed Model

To address such problems, Morton (17) suggested a mixed model that includes a major locus and polygenes. This was implemented by Morton and MacLean (18) for nuclear families and extended by Lalouel and Morton (19) to ascertainment through affected relatives called *pointers* of which there could be up to three per family (pointers to father, mother, and/or the children). Selection through multiplex (two or more) affected or multiplex probands was provided as special cases. The cost of allowing for rather general types of ascertainment was to lose some of the information in large pedigrees, for which ascertainment corrections are still controversial and not available in any computer program.

Special attention was given in the mixed model to quantitative traits because of their informativeness. The additive model for effects of genes and environment led naturally to representation of affection by truncation of commingled normal distributions with all values beyond the threshold taken as affected. Affection status need not be defined under complete selection (random families) but is essential under incomplete selection (through a proband). We therefore introduced liability classes denoted by a liability indicator 1, 2, . . . 9 for situational variables like age, sex, or birth order that alter risk but can be defined independent of phenotype (and even if the phenotype is unknown). For example, liability class 1 might be males aged 0–9. The mixed model achieved parsimony by expressing penetrance through displacements t for the homozygote at risk and dt for the heterozygote, assumed constant for each liability class, which therefore was completely characterized by a truncation threshold. As many as 3×9 penetrances are described by only two parameters and nine morbid risks. In this way we were able to avoid arbitrary assumptions about penetrance in the normal homozygote and genotype-specific age-of-onset distributions, letting the data speak for themselves. This model has stood the test of time, although it could be violated by genetic heterogeneity (for example, a genotype with high lifetime penetrance but exceptionally late onset).

Applied to quantitative traits, there have been three difficulties with the mixed model as programmed in POINTER (20). First, it assumes that genetic liability g, the continuous latent variable underlying both the quantitative trait and affection, is more highly correlated with the former: i.e., the quantitative trait $y = g + e$, but liability for affection is $y + w$, where e and w were nonheritable, normally distributed errors with variances Ve and Vw, respectively. Therefore, affection status is ignored for an individual whose quantitative value y is known. However, sometimes affection is based on critical evidence, whereas the quantitative trait is measured only once with significant error. Then a better model for liability would be $g + w$, where $Vw < Ve$. More complicated attempts at bivariate analysis have been made (21) but are not in general use.

A second problem is that segregation analysis of a quantitative trait is exquisitely sensitive to distributional assumptions. Skewness of a polygenic trait can simulate a major locus. Even if skewness is removed by transformation, residual kurtosis can still simulate a major locus. Leptokurtosis tends to cause sporadic outliers that favor a recessive model ($d = 0$), but are easily recognized on careful study of families that support a mixed model against a polygenic alternative. Unfortunately, this aspect of the POINTER program is so generally neglected that it has been deleted from the "portable" version. Platykurtosis is more insidious, since spurious evidence for a major locus is distributed thinly over many families. The conservative choice is to normalize the quantitative trait (e.g., by a rank transform) and do analysis conditional on parental mating types, or to use a method that does not assume normality. Studies that fail to do this or even to examine critical families generate an unacceptable frequency of spurious major loci as type I errors (16).

Atopy, whether measured by total IgE or in a more complicated way, is skewed, and the power transform used for commingling analysis does not induce normality within genotype. This may account for the diversity of results when POINTER was applied, with claims of recessive, codominant, and polygenic inheritance. This work was done before the seriousness of distributional assumptions was fully recognized and should be reexamined by more robust methods. However, there is a consensus that the data do not fit a single-locus model.

A third problem with the mixed model and its successors is the frequent assumption that a model can be accepted if Mendelian transmission probabilities are not rejected. Unfortunately, this is not the case, since they do not distinguish a major locus from additive oligogenes or polygenes (15,16). Conversely, rejection of Mendelian values does not exclude a major locus, unless all other assumptions (ascertainment, distribution, etc.) are satisfied. No biological meaning has yet been attached to the unconfirmed claim of non-Mendelian transmission for breast cancer (22), and the programming of transmission probabilities in POINTER fails a critical test (23), but see Dizier et al. (24) for an obscure counterargument.

3. Oligogenic Models

The mixed model is formulated in terms of two alleles but has some ability to detect multiple allelism through local maxima (25). It assumes an infinitely large number of additive modifiers. A model with few modifier loci is called oligogenic. Of the oligogenic models the two-allele, two-locus model has been most frequently used, primarily to test the "major locus" for linkage to a marker on the assumption that the "modifier locus" can describe residual genetic factors adequately, but formal comparison with the mixed model has not been made. Computing time is similar for the two models, and errors in numerical integration at high values of polygenic heritability are avoided in oligogenic models. Nearly all experience has been with an ordered polychotomy defined on percentiles to minimize distributional assumptions (see Section IV.A).

4. Regressive Models

Bonney (26) has introduced four classes of regressive models incorporating a major locus and residual correlations with family members. The correlation structure assumed for A, B, and C models corresponds to no genetic mechanism, whereas the class D model is equivalent to the mixed model for a quantitative variable (27). An advantage of the regressive approach is that it can be applied to pedigrees. A disadvantage is that ascertainment correction is rudimentary. All the distributional cautions of the mixed model apply with equal force to regressive models (perhaps with greater force because of the more complex pedigree structure). They were neglected in a recent application to "basal IgE," defined as total IgE adjusted for atopy, like death adjusted for cardiac arrest (28). The recessive model favored in that study contradicts a dominant gene with paternal imprinting claimed by the same group (29).

E. Linkage

1. Multiple Pairwise Tests (Lods)

Given a prior genetic model, perhaps determined by segregation analysis, the evidence on linkage to a particular marker in a sample S may be summarized by the logarithm of the odds (lod), $Z(\theta) = \log_{10}[f(S;\theta)/f(S;^{1}/_{2})]$ where θ is a recombination frequency (30). In practice, two modifications are made: recombination is sex-specific, giving θ_f, θ_m for females and males, respectively (do not confuse the subscripts with *f*athers and *m*others), and we are especially interested in maximum likelihood values $\hat{\theta}$. If the null hypothesis is true (i.e., if recombination equals $^{1}/_{2}$ and the function $f(S;\theta)$ is correctly specified), a value of $Z > \log A$ for any $A > 1$ will be observed with frequency less than $1/A$ (31,32), and this holds for $\hat{\theta}$ as for any other value of θ (33). For random markers, A is usually taken to be 1000 to protect against type I errors. For markers known to be on the same chromosome (syntenic), a smaller value of A is appropriate. Double intercrosses with dominance or involving fewer than three alleles confound male and female recombination. This is typically a small part of the data and the joint lod $Z(\hat{\theta}_m, \hat{\theta}_f)$ can be factored as $Z(\hat{\theta}_m) + Z(\hat{\theta}_f)$.

Information about sample size that is lost when $\hat{\theta} = \frac{1}{2}$ and $Z(\hat{\theta}) = 0$ can be recovered on the assumption of a distribution (usually taken to be binomial as for backcrosses of known phase) if the lod is reported for $\theta < \frac{1}{2}$ (34).

It has been found that good linkage maps can be constructed by treating lods for different markers as if independent (35). Moreover, typing errors can be filtered and interference allowed for (36) even in maps of several hundred loci. The significance levels are not exact because the lods for linked markers really are not independent, but there is usually good agreement between nominal chi-square and its degrees of freedom. Although errors attributable to multiple pairwise analysis are rare and may be more than outweighed by errors in multilocus analysis without error filtration or a realistic level of interference, many investigators feel that confirmation by other methods is necessary, especially if the significance is borderline. Of course, in that case the need for more data is even more pressing.

2. Multipoint Tests

The LINKAGE program was the first practical implementation of multipoint tests, in which several markers are considered simultaneously without the intermediary of pairwise lods (37). Computations are so slow that the number of markers considered for disease mapping must be small. The CRIMAP program is much faster but is applicable only to codominant loci (P. Green, personal communication). Segregation parameters cannot be meaningfully estimated in the absence of any defined sampling design and appropriate correction. All $2N$ gametes defined by N heterozygous loci can be described by multipoint-feasible interference functions that unfortunately lack statistical support and genetic credibility. The liability index can be used wrongly to stratify the data into groups with different gene frequencies, although the calculations assume constant gene frequencies for a single locus. Because of these constraints, multipoint analysis is rarely used to detect linkage, more commonly to support pairwise or other evidence. Multipoint analysis has been successful with monogenic disease but has given misleading results with complex inheritance. The reasons for these errors are only partly understood (38). Any violation of the null hypothesis (including distributional assumptions for a quantitative trait) can distort the linkage test, but usually not grossly. Unconscious bias in classifying the phenotype is always possible unless markers and phenotypes are scored blindly.

3. Sib Pairs

Haseman and Elston (39) introduced a sib pair test based on a quantitative phenotype and the probability of identity by descent (ibd), assumed to be known and not estimated from gene frequencies. For example, at a given locus sibs may have 0, 1, 2 alleles ibd, whereas unilineal relatives can have only 0 or

1 alleles ibd. Classified in this way relatives are pairwise independent, but treating the $n(n - 1)/2$ pairs of n relatives as independent makes the significance test unreliable even in large samples. The phenotype enters as the quadratic form $(Y_i - Y_j)^2$, where Y_i is the phenotype of the ith sib ($i \neq j$). The SIBPAL program performs this analysis. Quadratic forms do not have a normal distribution, but the central limit theorem makes a normalizing transformation unnecessary in large samples. Almost nothing is known about the power of this approach compared with more parametric alternatives, especially mixed and oligogenic models. Relative power presumably depends on the unknown mechanisms in complex inheritance, with a parametric approach favored only when it is good approximation.

Power of any linkage test depends on frequency, effect, mode of ascertainment, and recombination rate. The classic Haseman-Elston test is appropriate for small common effects, but may well not have high power against rare alleles with large effects. Perhaps they would be detected better by rejecting small values of $(Y_1 - Y_2)^2$ and doing a normalizing rank transform on the remainder. However, this makes the test more sensitive to sporadic outliers. There is simply not enough experience with sib pairs and parametric alternatives to justify more than conjecture. We need observation, not computer simulations under models that may well be irrelevant to the disease of interest.

There has been virtually no experience with less efficient methods that use identity by state (ibs). They are gene-frequency-dependent and therefore much less informative unless there is a rare founder allele (a monophylon). Multiple pairwise independence fails for identity by state and weighting of different alleles and pedigree structures is arbitrary, so the reliability of ibs methods is in doubt even in large samples (40).

F. Combined Segregation and Linkage

Having failed to justify parametric analysis of linkage under an unsupported segregation model, it is reasonable to develop combined analysis. The segregation component requires conditioning on the mode of ascertainment, and a realistic model must incorporate more than one mechanism. To my knowledge, there is no general and public computer program available for quantitative data under the mixed, two-locus, or regressive models. Morton et al. (41) have suggested that the distributional assumptions required for quantitative data are restrictive and have introduced ordered polychotomies as an alternative approach (see Section IV.A).

Positional cloning through noncandidate loci ("reverse genetics") has been rather unsuccessful in complex inheritance and cannot be used for exclusion mapping since the mode of inheritance is unknown. Close linkage to a moderately polymorphic marker is more easily detected than moderate linkage to a highly polymorphic marker (42). Therefore, candidate loci (including in-terleukins and immunoglobulins and their receptors) are favored for linkage studies of atopy and asthma.

G. Allelic Association

Alleles predisposing to a particular disease may be identified by case-control studies in which the controls are drawn from the same population as the cases. Owing to the anthropological bias toward small isolated populations thought to be representative of primitive man, little is known about variation of gene frequencies within national populations of postindustrial countries, and this has been a source of much forensic argument (43). Within a regional popula-tion, often centered on a metropolis, it appears sufficient to match case-control pairs for major ethnic groups, but avoiding deliberate divergence (for example, cases from inpatients, but controls from laboratory personnel). The adequacy of national gene frequencies as regional controls remains to be determined and should be distrusted if only because of technical variation in measuring fragment lengths. There are statistical methods of kinship bioassay to deter-mine population structure within and among samples (44). Whereas structural loci show unique and sometimes striking variation among ethnic groups sug-gesting divergent selection, variation among loci is below the level of detection within ethnic groups, suggesting uniform selection pressures. This is likely to be true a fortiori for nonexpressed loci.

Falk and Rubinstein (45) have proposed intrafamily controls: i.e., the alleles not transmitted from tested parents to a proband child. However, with domi-nance, untested parents, or other uncertainties this gives biased frequencies.

Allelic association has been most frequently studied for the ABO blood groups, especially for diseases requiring surgery and therefore blood typing and for the HLA system because of its protean effects on immune response (46). Candidate loci for cardiovascular and other diseases are beginning to give consistent results. Failure to replicate a reputed association may be due to four causes: either the first report was a type I error, perhaps caused by inappro-priate controls, or the association is restricted to a subgroup of cases, or power to detect the association is low, or the marker does not have a pleiotropic effect but is in linkage disequilibrium with a more potent allele, and that disequili-brium differs among populations. Many examples of the latter phenomenon are known for the HLA system. Consistency of an allelic association among popu-lations argues against linkage disequilibrium and in favor of pleiotropic effects.

Whatever the complexity of allelic association, it is usually detectable only over distances less than 1% crossing over (1 cM) because even that small systematic pressure dominates selection and drift. However, a unique founder of a disease cluster creates linkage disequilibrium that for some generations may be detectable in an isolate even over distances greater than 1 cM: this is the basis for autozygosity mapping through inbred probands (47,48). Cases of other etiology weaken this test. Both atopy and asthma are too common to make autozygosity mapping feasible except perhaps for a distinctive, rare, monogenic form that could easily be mapped by conventional methods.

Since allelic association is constrained to small distances between disease and marker, there is a clear advantage to candidate loci whose alleles may have pleiotropic effects or be in disequilibrium with closely linked homologous loci or regulatory sequences. Positional cloning through noncandidate markers ("reverse genetics") has less power to detect allelic association.

In a case-control study in which individuals are independent, an appropriate analysis is by stepwise multiple regression of quantitative value on binary variables representing alleles. Unless the model were specified a priori, it would be reasonable to use the Bonferroni correction, multiplying the significance level by the number of variables in stepwise regression. When controls (or more commonly cases) are interrelated, the extra source of variation must be allowed for. One approach is to incorporate allelic association into combined segregation and linkage analysis as coupling frequencies where the gene frequency at a linked disease locus is $q = \Sigma c_i p_i$ and c_i is the coupling frequency of the ith marker allele with frequency p_i: i.e., c_i is the probability that a haplotype carrying allele i also carries the linked disease allele. George and Elston (49) have proposed a method that uses kinship between pairs of relatives and stays within the framework of relatively nonparametric association tests.

Pairwise independence is lost if kinship at the marker locus is uncertain. Confirmation in other samples remains the best way to establish the significance and magnitude of allelic association supported by kinship or combined segregation and linkage analysis.

Extension to haplotypes requires inference of coupling, either by transmission from parents or in probability. The possible number of haplotypes can be large and ways to reduce the number of independent variables have been sought. Cladistic analysis fits haplotypes to a phylogenic tree and assumes that disease susceptibility appeared at one bifurcation and was propaged in descendant clads (50). There is no provision for an evolutionary network produced by recombination or admixture, nor for multiple origins of a single haplotype. The utility of cladistic analysis for haplotype association is therefore sub judice.

IV. QUALITATIVE TRAITS

A. Segregation

Quantitative traits may be reduced to a polychotomy, which in the extreme case is a simple dichotomy between normal and affected. This loses some genetic information unless there is a clear antimode between genotypes, the loss increasing with distributional overlap. Commingling analysis cannot be applied to a polychotomy, and path analysis has seen little use (51).

There are three reasons to consider qualitative traits. First, many diseases cannot yet be represented as extreme values of a continuous metric. Second, reducing a quantitative trait to an ordered polychotomy escapes the assumptions of normality and uniform variance (homoscedasticity) for all genotypes, replacing them by the weaker assumption of ordered risk in relatives (41). Third, affection status must be defined under incomplete selection, so that bias may be removed by conditioning on the event or measure of ascertainment (see Section V). Under complete selection there is no need to define affection: all individuals may be taken as normal with the polychotomy representing a scale of *diathesis* from lowest to highest risk in relatives.

Under incomplete selection diathesis is retained for normals. Affection may be ordered by *severity* that includes information supplementary to liability class: for example, age of onset among affected individuals with onset substantially before the cohort in which they were last observed, by which their liability class is defined. The population frequencies of diathesis and severity classes must be specified. Among a finite number of alternative frequency vectors, the one that maximizes the likelihood is preferred.

The mixed model of a major locus with polygenes allows for a dichotomy of normal versus affected, in addition to progenitors of unknown phenotype. More general polychotomies are not yet accommodated in the mixed model.

The two-locus model has been extended to severity and diathesis. Locus-specific scaling parameters (S, S_m for severity and B, B_m for diathesis) allow the model to describe interaction of rare and common genes to produce both a disease and a preclinical trait, which less general models force into a common allele (e.g., 52). The general two-allele, two-locus model has 10 parameters: four scaling and six segregation parameters representing dominance at both loci (d, d_m), displacements (t, t_m), and gene frequencies (q, q_m). There may be local maxima and convergence is delicate, but tests of restricted models are easier. Useful polychotomies are ordered so that if there are n classes the jth is associated with a higher (or lower) risk in relatives than the $(j-1)^{\text{st}}$ class for all $j = 1, \ldots, n$ (53). Probit and logistic models are applicable to such situations: they are equivalent in practice. The probit model corresponds more closely to an underlying continuity that has been truncated to form a polychotomy. Both are included in the COMDS program (41).

We have used the two-locus model to test and exclude single-locus inheritance for atopy. We conjecture that the same result would be obtained with other methods and with asthma if the number of classes is not too small. Departures from single-locus inheritance are hardest to detect when the underlying continuum is truncated into the dichotomy of normal versus affected.

Regressive models for polychotomies do not correspond to any genetic mechanism, unlike the quantitative case where the class D regressive model is equivalent to the mixed model (54). Polychotomies with n classes are represented by $n - 1$ design variables and are therefore not strictly ordered in the statistical sense (53,55). In regressive models the matrix inversion that is implicit with quantitative data has no genetic interpretation with polychotomies. There has been little comparative study of oligogenic and regressive models. Both can be used to test single genes, but adequacy of their representation of complex inheritance remains in doubt for linkage analysis and risk prediction.

The effect of situational variables like age and sex can be controlled for quantitative traits by covariance analysis, but affection status requires that population morbid risk be entered through a liability indicator. In the absence of genotype-specific mortality, the morbid risk equals cumulative incidence to the class midpoint. The morbid risk is less than cumulative incidence if there is genotype-specific mortality. No modification of morbid risk is sufficient to represent the resultant gene frequency decline with age.

Genotype-specific mortality is not allowed for in any current method of segregation analysis. This is inconsequential for atopy but perhaps not for asthma. The effect of neglecting this factor will not be understood until life table methods are introduced into segregation analysis.

In COMDS the diathesis and severity classes are assumed for mathematical simplicity to be independent of liability class, which is rarely true unless affection status is defined on the same covariance-adjusted quantitative trait used for severity and diathesis, so there is a single liability class. Otherwise only affected individuals atypical of their liability class should be scored as severe.

B. Combined Segregation and Linkage

Segregation analysis assumes that gene frequency is constant for all liability classes, and violation by genotype-specific mortality is cause for concern. The LINKAGE computer program allows the investigator to *define* "liability classes" that have unique gene frequencies: for example, an intermediate phenotype may be treated incorrectly as a liability class, although the *calculations* assume constant gene frequency as in segregation analysis. LINKAGE does not allow for incomplete ascertainment, cannot fit a genetic model, and is commonly applied under untested assumptions.

This has not been a serious problem with monogenic disorders, but there is no evidence justifying its use under complex inheritance. The current choice is between combined segregation and linkage analysis with a computer program like COMDS or a "nonparametric" approach through pairs of affected relatives, neglecting information provided by severity and diathesis (Section IV.C). It is not clear which is more powerful and the advantage may depend on the unknown mode of inheritance. The COMDS program allows simultaneous analysis of segregation and linkage with up to nine ordered classes of diathesis and severity, or a total of 18 possible classes. A false model inflates estimates of recombination and to some unknown degree reduces power.

To my knowledge the mixed and regressive models do not yet provide combined segregation and linkage analysis.

C. Sib Pairs

Affected pairs of relatives discard all information in severity and diathesis. Methods that use identity by descent may be unreliable in small samples. For example, R sibs concordant for a parental allele have probability $(^1/_2)^{R-1}$ on the null hypothesis of no linkage but are assigned probability $(^1/_2)^{R(R-1)/2}$ when all possible pairs are made. Pairwise independence does assure a valid test in the limit for large samples if the other assumptions (correct assignment of identity by descent and no typing or parentage errors) are satisfied. Simulation provides a useful check on significance. Identity by state is not pairwise independent and so is less reliable even if gene frequencies are accurate. There is active development of affected pair theory in the hope that it can be more powerful than a false parametric model for some undefined class of complex inheritance.

D. Allelic Association

Multiple logistic analysis replaces linear regression when a quantitative trait is dichotomized, and chi-square replaces the F test. All other considerations for a quantitative trait apply, except that normality of the dependent variable is not assumed. Information in diathesis and severity is lost.

V. ASCERTAINMENT

Every genetic analysis assumes that families are selected in a particular way. A false ascertainment model biases estimates of genetic parameters and can lead to wrong inference.

Complete ascertainment implies no selection of sibships through their phenotypes. Selection of parental phenotypes may be allowed for by conditioning the likelihood on them: this *conditional* probability of children given parents is contrasted with *joint* likelihood of parents *and* children. Selection through phenotypes of relatives outside the nuclear families may in simple cases be allowed for by *pointers*, taken as the closest relative through whom the family was ascertained. A nuclear family may have up to three pointers, to the mother, father, and set of children. Two or more probands with the same relationship to the nuclear family pose a problem, as do more complex sampling schemes through multiplex (two or more) affected. Analysis can be made more realistic if the ascertainment details are specified precisely, as they rarely are.

Ascertainment falls into two classes. In *ascertainment event* models the family is conditioned on the exact event that led to its selection. For example, an unusual concentration of cases in part A of a pedigree might lead to its extension to a set of relatives B, and then $P[(A+B)|A]$ would be appropriate (26). This allows the ascertainment event A to be atypically severe, provided severity is included in the analysis.

The only ascertainment event that has seen much use is the case where A is a single proband (56). This was called the proband method by Weinberg (2) and, unfortunately, the sib method by Fisher (57). If two probands occasionally occur in the same pedigree, say A and A', an unbiased but approximate solution is to replicate the family to give $P[(A+B \mid A)]$ and $P(A'+B) \mid A')$. This is the general proband method of Weinberg (2). At high levels of ascertainment this could lead to inflated sample sizes and excessive type I errors unless the effect of replication on chi-square were allowed for.

Maximum likelihood leads to *ascertainment measure* models in which each family is counted only once, however many probands it contains, and probabilities are conditional on the measure of the set of ascertained families. In the simplest case, with a constant segregation frequency p and ascertainment probability Π, the probability of ascertaining a family with r affected sibs is $1 - (1 - \Pi)^r$, and the measure of the set of ascertained families is $1 - (1 - p\Pi)^s$, with obvious generalization to more complex cases. There has been criticism of this binomial model, but no more realistic one has been proposed. Models in r^α give sensible results for $\alpha = 0$ (truncate selection) and $\alpha = 1$ (single selection), but do not rest on any sampling scheme (58). Ewens and Schute (59) proposed an "ascertainment-assumption-free method" for which all of the limited genetic information comes from linkage or the distribution of parental mating types.

Ascertainment measure models avoid replication of families, but they assume that probands are drawn at random from affected within a given liability class. Ascertainment event models are preferred when this is not true but severity is incorporated in the analysis.

To summarize, ascertainment bias is a complicated and controversial subject. The investigator who plans a study of atopy and/or asthma may be sure that if his sampling scheme violates all known ascertainment models, his results will be questionable. A practical solution is to sample families at random (primarily for segregation analysis) and by multiplex selection of families with two or more affected (primarily for linkage analysis). This can be achieved by asking each proband, "Do you have a brother or sister who is similarly affected?" and selecting all pedigrees in which the response is positive. Then the proband's children are sampled under complete selection (but conditional likelihood) and the proband's sibship under multiplex selection (joint likelihood).

Affection is best defined on the sampling scheme. No definition is required for random samples when diathesis or a quantitative trait is used. If the probands are asthma patients, the investigator should not define affection on atopy unless he is prepared to use ascertainment events with severity and/or diathesis classes, in the knowledge that few methods of analysis provide these refinements.

VI. LINKAGE STRATEGY

The object of linkage analysis is to localize a disease gene preparatory to cloning and sequencing. In the final stages of localization, linkage fails to order markers correctly. Then gametic disequilibrium (60) and physical methods are useful to continue positional cloning in the absence of a candidate locus. Identification of a candidate locus within the region may lead to structure-function cloning by recognizing DNA sequences in which a mutation for disease susceptibility has occurred.

Linkage to random markers chosen solely on the basis of polymorphism and location has been amazingly successful for monogenic disorders. With complex inheritance candidate loci may be more successful because exclusion mapping is not feasible when inheritance is complex, the genetic basis is unclear, and a noncandidate marker sweeps only a small radius. On the other hand, a large proportion of cDNAs code for previously unrecognized loci or even multigene families, or there may be no tightly linked hypervariable region. Therefore, the candidate locus strategy cannot be exhaustive. The relative merits of random and candidate loci to map disease genes are controversial. A mixed strategy includes all polymorphic candidate loci, a close hypervariable locus as a surrogate for nonpolymorphic candidates, and random polymorphisms in regions without a candidate locus. The density of markers required to detect linkage is determined by the unknown mode of inheritance and may, in an unfavorable case, be exorbitant.

Sequential analysis gives substantial saving over fixed-sample methods (30). Ideally each family would be entered into the analysis for a particular marker as soon as it has been tested. More conveniently, but with some loss of efficiency, a set of families may be entered (61). In either event we dispense with further tests on that marker when there is no evidence of linkage, but test other markers in the region when there is sufficient evidence of linkage.

VII. INTERACTION

Epidemiologists find that factor interaction can be represented by simple additive and multiplicative models, usually of first order. Most geneticists agree with Sewall Wright (62) that possibly "additivity of loci and semidominance is the rule for most of the loci that are concerned and that deviations from these depend on only a few major loci."

Against this view are a number of observations suggesting greater complexity, such as interactive microphenic effects and genes that increase variance with no main effect. None of these is well established, and their significance depends on false assumptions of a normal distribution and independence of relatives. An extreme position is that interactions are so complex as to demand novel models of indeterminacy (63).

The genetic determination of atopy and asthma is too uncertain to abandon simplicity, but there is evidence for at least two interactions: allergen exposure provokes an extravagant response in atopic individuals, and HLA-determined specificity is most apparent among individuals who are not extremely atopic (64). DR2 is associated with allergy to Amb a V without asthma, but DR2 favors allergy to Amb a V with asthma. Genetic analysis should explore interaction, but be cautious about acceptance without strong confirmation.

VIII. META-ANALYSIS

In a strict sense meta-analysis is the quantitative study of published results relating to a particular problem, leading to conclusions about heterogeneity and overall significance (65). There is insufficient agreement about definitions, genetic models, and statistics to apply this to atopy or asthma. However, quantitative study of results obtained by different collaborators could be useful.

Principal component analysis is one way to derive similar metrics for atopy and asthma in different studies. Alternatively, total IgE appears from our results to convey most of the information. There is little reason to adopt an arbitrary dichotomy (5) when the data can speak for themselves to give a quantitative trait.

There should be no attempt to force agreement on genetic models until experience has been gained. Whatever the model, it should give a statistic that can be presented as a lod score (or alternatively as a χ^2 or other large-sample statistic). This gives both a pooled estimate and test of heterogeneity among samples.

Another test is appropriate to heterogeneity within samples. If Z_i is the lod for the ith family on some genetic hypothesis that specifies a single major locus, then $L_i = \alpha 10^z + 1 - \alpha$ is the likelihood ratio if the major locus is completely linked in a proportion α of families and unlinked in the remainder. Tests on α and recombination are sensitive to this type of heterogeneity among families, which is almost the rule for monogenic disorders and may well play a role in complex inheritance. Other metrics than lods are less closely related to likelihood.

Candidate loci may show allelic association with either common or rare alleles. Genetics provides examples of disease associated with some rare alleles that may be hard to detect because of the large number of candidates and the small number of families informative for any one of them. Perhaps a test on rare alleles collectively would be useful. Unexpected associations should be cross-validated in an independent sample. The possibility for pooling collaborative studies is enhanced if fragments are determined with an error of less than 1 bp, or ideally sequenced.

IX. ENVOI

More than 300 disease loci have been mapped by positional or structure/function cloning and the number is increasing explosively (4). It was inevitable that the search be extended to complex inheritance, where results have so far been modest. To what extent is this inherent in multifactorial traits or simply a result of inadequate methods and little experience? The next few years will tell. Atopy and asthma can reasonably be represented by quantitative traits or ordered polychotomies, and there are many candidate loci in immunological pathways that are beginning to be clear.

There have been several advances in complex inheritance while this chapter was in press. Logistic regression with asthma as the dependent variable is replacing total IgE to define severity and diathesis, but arbitrary Boolean definition has not been abandoned. Risch and Zhang (66) have demonstrated the power of extremely discordant sib pairs to detect linkage, effectively destroying the Haseman-Elston test that does not discriminate between concordant pairs in different parts of the distribution. The advantages of lods over procedures that depend on means and variances (67) have abolished the distinction between identity by descent and identity in state, since the latter is merely a function of the former: failure to use parental information makes for greater dependence on gene frequencies but does not constitute a different method. Among nonparametric methods the most powerful expresses lods in terms of a single parameter β (68) that applies equally well to relatives other than sibs, to a quantitative trait or ordered polychotomy (which in the simplest case could be pairs of affected), and to sequential trials, meta-analysis, and multipoint mapping (69). The "transmission disequilibrium" test (70) is a special case of the β model limited to fully informative sib pairs. Finally, success of linkage studies on type 1 diabetes (IDDM) and other diseases of complex inheritance (71–73) justifies optimism that genes for atopy and asthma can be mapped with available statistical methods.

Sewall Wright (62) defined *leading factors* as genes with the largest effect on a continuous trait, which could be resolved from the polygenic background by genetic analysis. A leading factor need not be *megaphenic* (i.e., have a large effect relative to the phenotype standard deviation). The time seems ripe for a serious effort to characterize leading factors in atopy and asthma. If in the process we determine which genetic analyses are most useful for that purpose, the results will have implications for other diseases of complex inheritance.

REFERENCES

1. Morton NE. Genetic epidemiology. Annu Rev Genet 1993; 27:521–536.
2. Weinberg W. Methode und Fehlerquellen der Untersuchung auf Mendelschen Zahlen beim Menschen. Arch Rass Ges Biol 1912; 9:165–174.
3. Morton NE. Genetic tests under incomplete ascertainment. Am J Hum Genet 1959; 11:1–16.
4. Cooper ND, Schmidtke J. Molecular genetic approaches to the analysis and diagnosis of human inherited disease: an overview. Ann Med 1992; 24:29–42.
5. Cookson WOCM, Sharp PA, Faux JA, Hopkin JM. Linkage between immunoglobulin E responses underlying asthma and rhinitis and chromosome 11q. Lancet 1989; 1:1292–1295.
6. Shirakawa T, Morimoto K, Furuyama J, Yamamoto M, Takai S. Linkage between IgE responses underlying asthma and rhinitis (atopy) and chromosome 11q in Japanese families. Cytogenet Cell Genet 1991; 58:1970.
7. Goldin LR, Elston RC, Graham JB, Miller CH. Genetic analysis of von Willebrand's disease in two large pedigrees: a multivariate approach. Am J Med Genet 1980; 6:279–293.
8. MacLean CJ, Morton NE, Elston RC, Yee S. Skewness in commingled distributions. Biometrics 1976; 32:695–699.
9. Gerrard JW, Rao DC, Morton NE. A genetic study of immunoglobulin E. Am J Hum Genet 1978; 30:46–58.
10. Rao DC, McGue M, Wette R, Glueck CJ. Path analysis in genetic epidemiology. In: Chakravarti A, ed. Human Population Genetics. New York: Van Nostrand Reinhold, 1984:35–82.
11. Sandford AJ, Shirakawa T, Moffatt MF, Daniels SE, Ra C, Faux JA, Young RP, Nakamura Y, Lathrop GM, Cookson WOCM, Hopkin JM. Localisation of atopy and ß subunit of high-affinity IgE receptor (FceRI) on chromosome 11q. Lancet 1993; 341:332–334.
12. Billewicz WZ, McGregor A, Roberts DF, Wilson RJM. Family studies in immunoglobulin levels. Clin Exp Immunol 1974; 16:13–22.
13. Barker DJP, Martyn CN. The maternal and fetal origins of cardiovascular disease. J Epidemiol Commun Health 1992; 46:8–11.
14. Elston RC, Stewart J. A general model for the genetic analysis of pedigree data. Hum Hered 1971; 21:523–542.
15. Elston RC. Likelihood models in human quantitative genetics. In: Sing CF, Skolnick M, eds. The Genetic Analysis of Common Diseases; Applications to Predictive Factors in Coronary Heart Disease. New York: Alan R Liss, 1979:391–450.
16. Go RCP, Elston RC, Kaplan EB. Efficiency and robustness of pedigree segregation analysis. Am J Hum Genet 1978; 30:28–37.

17. Morton NE. The detection of major genes under additive continuous variation. Am J Hum Genet 1967; 19:23–34.
18. Morton NE, MacLean CJ. Analysis of family resemblance. III. Complex segregation of quantitative traits. Am J Hum Genet 1974; 26:489–503.
19. Lalouel JM, Morton NE. Complex segregation analysis with pointers. Hum Hered 1981; 31:12–21.
20. Lalouel JM. Segregation analysis of familial data: the mixed model. In: Morton NE, Rao DC, Lalouel JM, eds. Methods in Genetic Epidemiology. Basel: Karger, 1983:75–91.
21. Lalouel JM, Le Mignon L, Simon M, Fauchet R, Bourel, Rao DC, Morton NE. A combined qualitative (disease) and quantitative (serum iron) genetic analysis of idiopathic hemochomatosis. Am J Hum Genet 1985; 37:700–718.
22. Andrieu N, Demenais F, Martinez M. Genetic analysis of human breast cancer: implications for family study designs. Genet Epidemiol 1988; 5:225–233.
23. Iselius L, Littler M, Morton NE. Transmission of breast cancer—a controversy resolved. Clin Genet 1992; 41:211–217.
24. Dizier MH, Bonaiti-Pellie C, Clerget-Darpoux F. POINTER correctly estimates the transmission probabilities under the general transmission model in the case of incomplete selection. Am J Hum Genet 1992; 51:1449–1450.
25. Iselius L, Evans DAP, Eze LC, Tweedie MCK, Bullen MF, Wren PJJ. Complex segregation analysis for a three allele locus: experience from an analysis of acid phosphatase activity. Genet Epidemiol 1989; 6:619–624.
26. Bonney GE. On the statistical determination of major gene mechanisms in continuous human traits: regressive models. Am J Med Genet 1984; 18:731–749.
27. Demenais FM, Bonney GE. Equivalence of the mixed and regressive models for genetic analysis. 1. Continuous traits. Genet Epidemiol 1989; 6:597–617.
28. Dizier MH, Hill M, James A, Faux J, Ryan G, le Souef P, Musk AW, Lathrop M, Demenais F, Cookson W. Genetic control of basal IgE after accounting for specific atopy. Genet Epidemiol 1993; 10:333–334.
29. Cookson WOCM, Young RP, Sandford AJ, Moffatt MF, Skirakawa T, Sharp PA, Faux JA, Julier C, Le Souef PN, Nakamura Y, Lathrop GM, Hopkin JM. Maternal inheritance of atopic IgE responsiveness on chromosome 11q. Lancet 1992; 340: 381–384.
30. Morton NE. Sequential tests for the detection of linkage. Am J Hum Genet 1955; 7:277–318.
31. Wald A. Sequential Analysis. New York: Wiley, 1947.
32. Haldane JBS, Smith CAB. A new estimate of the linkage between the genes for colour-blindness and haemophilia in man. Ann Eugen 1947; 14:10–31.
33. Collins A, Morton NE. Significance of maximal lods. Ann Hum Genet 1991; 55: 39–41.
34. Morton NE, Andrews V. MAP, an expert system for multiple pairwise linkage analysis. Ann Hum Genet 1989; 53:263–269.
35. Lawrence S, Collins A, Keats BJ, Hulten M, Morton NE. Integration of gene maps: chromosome 21. Proc Natl Acad Sci USA 1993; 90:7210–7214.
36. Shields DC, Collins A, Buetow KH, Morton NE. Error filtration, interference and the human linkage map. Proc Natl Acad Sci USA 1991; 88:6501–6505.

37. Lathrop GM, Lalouel JM, Julier C, Ott J. Strategies for multilocus linkage analysis in humans. Proc Natl Acad Sci USA 1984; 81:3443–3446.

38. Risch N. Genetic linkage and complex diseases, with special reference to psychiatric disorders. Genet Epidemiol 1990; 7:3–46.

39. Haseman JK, Elston RC. The investigation of linkage between a quantitative trait and marker locus. Behav Genet 1972; 2:1–19.

40. Bishop DT, Williamson JA. The power of identity-by-state methods for linkage analysis. Am J Hum Genet 1990; 46:254–265.

41. Morton NE, Shields DC, Collins A. Genetic epidemiology of complex phenotypes. Ann Hum Genet 1991; 55:301–314.

42. Terwilliger JD, Dang Y, Ott J. On the relative importance of marker heterozygosity and intermarker distance in gene mapping. Genomics 1992; 13:951–956.

43. Morton NE. DNA in court. Eur J Hum Genet 1993; 1:172–178.

44. Morton NE. Genetic structure of forensic populations. Proc Natl Acad Sci USA 1992; 89:2556–2560.

45. Falk C, Rubinstein P. Haplotype relative risks: an easy reliable way to construct a proper control sample for risk calculations. Ann Hum Genet 1987; 51:227–233.

46. Tiwari JL, Terasaki PL. HLA and Disease Associations. New York: Springer-Verlag, 1985.

47. Smith CAB. The detection of linkage in human genetics. J Roy Statist Soc B 1953; 15:153–192.

48. Lander ES, Botstein D. Homozygosity mapping: a way to map human recessive traits with the DNA of inbred children. Science 1987; 236:1567–1570.

49. George VT, Elston RC. Biostatistical methods for the familial study of cancer. In: Lynch, Hirayama, eds. Genetic Epidemology of Cancer, Boca Raton, FL: CRC Press, 1989.

50. Templeton AR, Sing CF, Kessling A, Humphries S. A cladistic analysis of phenotype associations with haplotypes inferred from restriction endonuclease mapping. 2. The analysis of natural populations. Genetics 1988; 120:1145–1154.

51. Rao DC, Morton NE, Gottesman II, Lew R. Path analysis of qualitative data on pairs of relatives: application to schizophrenia. Hum Hered 1981; 31:325–333.

52. Skolnick MH, Cannon-Albright LA, Goldgar DE, Ward JH, Marshall CJ, Schumann GB, Hogle H, McWhirter WP, Wright EC, Tran TD, Bishop DT, Kushner JP, Eyre HJ. Inheritance of proliferative breast disease in breast cancer kindreds. Science 1990; 250:1715–1720.

53. Agresti A. Categorical Data Analysis. New York: Wiley, 1990.

54. Demenais FM, Laing AE, Bonney GE. Numerical comparison of the formulations of the logistic regressive models with the mixed model in segregation analysis of discrete traits. Genet Epidemiol 1992; 9:419–435.

55. Bonney GE. Regressive logistic models for familial disease and other binary traits. Biometrics 1986; 42:611–625.

56. Cannings C, Thompson EA. Ascertainment in the sequential sampling of pedigrees. Clin Genet 1977; 12:225–236.

57. Fisher RA. The effects of methods of ascertainment upon the estimation of frequencies. Ann Eugen 1934; 6:13–25.

58. Stene J. Choice of ascertainment model. II. Ann Hum Genet 1979; 42:493–505.

59. Ewens WJ, Schute NCE. A resolution of the ascertainment sampling problem. I. Theory. Theor Pop Biol 1986; 30:388–412.
60. Morton NE, Wu D. Alternative bioassays of kinship between loci. Am J Hum Genet 1988; 42:173–177.
61. Elston RC. Designs for the global search of the human genome by linkage analysis. Proc Sixteenth International Biometric Conference, Hamilton, New Zealand, 1993.
62. Wright S. Evolution and the Genetics of Populations. I. Genetic and Biometric Foundations. Chicago: University of Chicago Press, 1968:417.
63. Sing CF, Hanis C. Genetics of Cellular, Individual, Family and Population Variability. New York: Oxford University Press, 1993.
64. Blumenthal M, Marcus-Bagley D, Awdeh Z, Johnson B, et al. HLA-DR2, [HLA-B7, SC31, DR2] and [HLA-B8, SC01, DR3] haplotypes distinguish subjects with asthma from those with rhinitis only in ragweed pollen allergy. Immunology 1992; 148:411–416.
65. Marriott FHC. A Dictionary of Statistical Terms, 5th ed. Singapore: Longman, 1990.
66. Risch N, Zhang H. Extreme discordant sib pairs for mapping quantitative terst loci in humans. Science 1995; 268:1584–1589.
67. Morton NE. Lods past and present. Gentics 1995; 140:7–12.
68. Morton NE. Lods for linkage in complex inheritance. Proc Natl Acad Sci USA 1996 (in press).
69. Krugylak L, Lander ES. Complete multipoint sib-pair analysis of qualitative and quantitative traits. Am J Hum Genet 1995; 57:439–454.
70. Spielman RS, McGinnis RE, Ewens WJ. Transmission test for linkage disequilibrium: the insulin gene region and insulin-dependent diabetes mellitus (IDDM). Am J Hum Genet 1993; 52:506–516.
71. Todd JA. Genetic analysis of type 1 diabetes using whole genome approaches. Proc Natl Acad Sci USA 1995; 92:8560–8565.
72. Lander ES, Schork NH. Genetic dissection of complex traits. Science 1994; 265: 2037–2048.
73. Weeks DE, Lathrop GM. Polygenic disease: methods for mapping complex disease traits. Trends in Genet 1995; 11:513–519.

7

The Epidemiology of Asthma
Risk Factors, Rates, and Trends

Kevin B. Weiss

Rush Presbyterian St. Luke's Medical Center
Chicago, Illinois

Peter J. Gergen

National Institute of Allergy and Infectious Diseases
National Institutes of Health
Bethesda, Maryland

I. INTRODUCTION

Recent trends in the epidemiology of asthma morbidity and mortality have led to an increasing interest to understand the factors associated with asthma and atopic diseases (1–6). This chapter will review some of the key aspects of the changing epidemiology of this syndrome and, where feasible, compare international trends.

The principal epidemiological model that reflects causation of disease is built around an understanding of the interactions among the host, the disease-causing agent, and the environment. For example, the host would reflect the individual at risk for the disease and would include such facets as genetic

"

inheritance, immune status, atopic disposition, and so forth. The agents are those biological and nonbiological objects that upon exposure to the at-risk individual may cause the disease. The environment incorporates both physical and nonphysical (e.g., social) placement of the host and agent in close enough proximity for the critical exposure to occur and the disease to originate. To understand asthma and atopic disease epidemiology, we should separate out which factors "cause" the condition as contrasted with those that "enhance or promote" the effect of the causative factors related to either the host, agent, or environment. The key role of conditions encountered in early childhood for the development of atopy will be discussed in Chapters 8 and 10.

A. A Working Definition of Asthma

Asthma is better thought of as a syndrome rather than a disease (7), and a clear biological marker that defines this disease is not available. More specifically, the epidemiological definition of asthma remains controversial (8). There are, however, several key aspects to the epidemiological definition of asthma upon which there is general agreement. The prevalence of asthma can be recorded in three different ways: (1) point prevalence—asthma at the time of the survey; (2) lifetime prevalence—asthma at any time during an individual's life; (3) period prevalence—asthma within a certain defined period, usually the last 12 months. Period prevalence, active symptoms during the last 12 months, is mostly generally accepted (9). An epidemiological definition is not equivalent to a medical diagnosis. An epidemiological definition can, however, include a medical diagnosis as one component.

Two methods are commonly used to identify self-report of asthma in epidemiological studies: first, self-report of a diagnosis of asthma (with or without physician confirmation); alternatively, self-report of certain symptoms such as wheeze; second, the presence of bronchial reactivity on challenge. Problems exist with both methods. For example, some of the specific problems related to relying only on diagnosed asthma include the following: much disease in the population is underdiagnosed (10–12); overlap occurs in the diagnosis of chronic bronchitis and asthma among children (13); bias may occur in the assignment of the diagnosis of asthma; e.g., in adults over 40 years of age with similar symptom patterns, women tend to be given the diagnosis of asthma more often than men (14). Also, the presence of parenteral illness or symptoms influences the over- or underreporting of symptoms (15–17).

Although wheeze tends to be the predominant symptom of asthma, some individuals only have a cough as a manifestation of their disease and thus are not included in studies focusing exclusively on wheezing (18–20). Alternatively, studies comparing bronchial reactivity with the diagnosis by symptoms of asthma have found a large degree of overlap between these two diagnostic measures; however, these measures also act somewhat independently (21–24).

B. The Frequency of Asthma in the Population: Incidence and Prevalence

There are few studies of the actual incidence of asthma. These studies demonstrate that the incidence of asthma varies with age. For all age groups, the incidence of asthma has been estimated to vary between 2.65 and 4/1,000 per year (14,25). The highest incidence appears to be among children under 5 years of age (14,25,26).

Disease prevalence is a measure of both incidence and duration of illness. Most of the studies of prevalence reflect data based on self-reported diagnosis or symptoms. Therefore, until recently many of the international studies reporting asthma prevalence have been culturally dependent and related to a population's access to medical care. Asthma prevalence is highly dependent on the definition. For example, data from the National Health and Nutrition Examination Survey (NHANES) and the National Health Interview Survey (NHIS) that monitor the health of the U.S. population suggest asthma prevalence can range from 3 to 10.5% depending on how the question to determine prevalence is phrased.

Due to the problems with using a self-report of diagnosis, it may be more useful to examine the prevalence of symptoms of wheeze, breathlessness, or cough rather than the syndrome labeled "asthma" (27). There are more than 100 published studies on asthma prevalence worldwide, which have been summarized in several reviews (28–30). Additional studies continue to be reported (31–36). While it is difficult to draw detailed inferences about the worldwide prevalence of asthma, one broad conclusion can be extracted from this wealth of data. Rates for "nonindustrialized countries" tend to be lower than those for industrialized societies.

Some of the difficulties in interpreting transnational comparisons in prevalence can be reduced by limiting examination to studies that employed the same methodologies. One prevalence study employed this technique to evaluated asthma prevalence in children between New Zealand and Wales. The results of this study suggested that children in New Zealand were more likely to have asthma, history of wheeze, or positive exercise provocation tests than children from Wales (37). This study provides some of the most direct evidence that the variation in asthma prevalence across populations is real.

II. EXAMINING THE NATURAL HISTORY OF ASTHMA

The asthma epidemiological literature provides some insights into the natural history of this condition, including age of onset, frequency and intensity of relapse and remission, and some information on major asthma morbidity as measured by hospitalization and mortality.

Asthma has been noted to begin in two periods during life, childhood and adulthood (14). Childhood asthma tends to begin before the age of 5 and occurs more frequently in boys than girls, with the male:female ratio approaching 2 (38–40). Childhood asthma is usually associated with atopy (c.f. Chapter 8). This is much less common for asthma in adults. Girls tend to equal or exceed the male prevalence of asthma during adolescence and the sex difference is equivocal in adulthood (12,14,41). The implications of the age of onset of asthma are controversial: early onset having a worse outcome (39,42), early onset having a better outcome (43), or no association between onset and outcome (44).

As is true for the severity of any chronic disease, asthma severity is difficult to quantify. Asthma severity is most often defined by its "physiological severity" (45): the number of attacks or certain types of symptoms per unit time, chronic versus intermittent usage of certain types of medications. Asthma severity should also be viewed in terms of "burden of illness": the impact of the disease on the functioning of the family (45).

A number of risk factors have been identified for asthma severity. Atopy has been related to increased asthma severity among children (46,47), but not among adults (48). The relationship of bronchial reactivity to severity is unclear: in studies using hospitalized patients a close relationship was found (49, 50) while in community studies the relationship was much weaker (26).

Cohort studies of persons with asthma suggest that childhood asthma symptoms abate in approximately one-half of asthmatics by their 20s or 30s (39,51–54). In an Australian cohort followed from age 7 years to 28 years, approximately 55% of children with wheezing onset before age 7 years were wheeze-free at 21 and 28 years (55,56). The majority of those who continued to wheeze became less severe. Prognosis at 21 years was not as good as prognosis at 14 years for participants in this study. Other predictors of the duration of asthma include: atopy, allergen-skin-test reactivity, allergic rhinitis, and eczema (39,44,54–57).

Often for epidemiological purposes the population asthma severity is measured in terms of hospitalization or mortality rates. Any discussion of asthma mortality should be prefaced with the knowledge that asthma deaths are rare. For many countries, asthma is attributed to less than a few hundred deaths annually and is measured in rates per 100,000 population. However, the literature in this area abounds and focuses on the belief that these rare events are important case studies as death from this disease is preventable. Asthma mortality rates are obtained via a country's vital records system.

There are limitations of vital records—and particularly international comparative studies—of asthma mortality. Some of these limitations include: the decreasing accuracy of a reported diagnosis of asthma with age of decedent (58–60); the diagnostic reclassification related to revisions in the International

Classification of Diseases (ICD) (61); the degree to which death certificate are validated by autopsy findings (62); and skill at preparing and understanding of death certification.

In spite of the limitations of vital records data, much has been learned about international asthma mortality rates. Most notable is the large variation in asthma mortality by country. During the period 1985–1987, asthma mortality rates varied from a high of 9 per 100,000 in West Germany to a low of 1.5 per 100,000 in Hong Kong for persons all ages (61). Vital records–based studies have found asthma mortality associated with age, race/ethnicity, and poverty on a population level (12,63–66). Age-specific seasonal variations in asthma deaths have also been noted (67,68).

Follow-back studies of individuals dying from asthma have identified a wide variety of risk factors at the individual level that create a profile of the asthmatic who may be at a high risk from dying: a history of severe disease, lack of access to care, suboptimal pharmacotherapy, depression, family disturbances (69–74), rapid onset of fatal attack (75), and allergy to *Alternaria* (76). Perhaps most controversial of these risk factors is the possible association of inhaled beta-agonists use and subsequent mortality (77–82). The debate on this specific issue, to some extent, has persisted over two decades (78,82–84).

III. EXAMINING SOME OF THE EPIDEMIOLOGICAL RISK FACTORS FOR ASTHMA

The epidemiological study of risk factors for asthma, at both the host and environmental level, can point to potential areas for further clinical, cellular, and molecular studies. As discussed in greater detail in Chapter 8, the influence of various environmental risk factors may vary with age, infants and young children being particularly susceptible. This complicates the epidemiological analysis of asthma.

A. Genetics of Asthma

An in-depth review of the epidemiological evidence related to asthma and atopic disease will be the focus of other chapters. However, some observations are key to our understanding of these conditions.

Asthma is well known to cluster in families (85–87). Also, asthma prevalence among siblings tends to increase if the number of parents with asthma increased (86,88). Studies of twins have attempted to separate the issues of heredity and environment. Edfors-Lubs (89) studied 7000 Swedish twin pairs and found a symptoms concordance of 19% for monozygotic twins versus 4.8% for dizygotic twins. Duffy et al. (90) studied 3808 pairs of Australian twins and found approximately a 60% estimated heritability for asthma. In a reanalysis of Edfors-Lubs' data, Duffy reported a similar level of heritability.

From information from these and other studies, a number of genetic mechanisms have been proposed: dominant, recessive, or a polygenic system with incomplete penetrance (86,88,89). Sibbald et al. (85) hypothesized that the tendencies for asthma and atopy are inherited independently, but the presence of atopy enhances the genetic susceptibility to asthma. These and other possible mechanisms will be the focus of other chapters.

A recent study of lung transplantations found that asthmatic lungs transplanted to nonasthmatics "continued" to have asthma, while nonasthmatic lungs transplanted into asthmatics had not developed asthma up to 3 years after transplantation (91).

B. Migrant Studies

Migrant studies provide some additional insight into the nature of asthma. As discussed in Chapter 8, the children of migrants have been reported to acquire the prevalence of asthma in the area to which the parents move. Tokelauan children (aged 0–14 years) living in New Zealand develop asthma at a higher rate than Tokelauan children living in Tokelau, even if they were not born in New Zealand (92). Further studies of New Zealand children found no differences in bronchial hyperresponsiveness or reported symptoms between children born in New Zealand and those born elsewhere and now living in New Zealand (93). In England, Smith et al. (94) reported that Negro children born in England had asthma at rates as high as or higher than those of other native-born English children, while Negro children born outside England but now living in England had lower rates. In contrast, Asians living in England reported a low rate regardless of their place of birth. Positive skin test reactions to mite were common in all asthmatics regardless of their place of birth (95).

C. Atopy

Allergy is recognized as playing an important role in asthma. Asthmatics tend to be more atopic (allergen skin test reactivity, hay fever, asthma) than nonasthmatics (38,96). Eczema has been reported to be associated with both the development and persistence of asthma (39,54,97).

One classification scheme includes risks such as the potential involvement of atopy with asthma by the age of asthma onset; onset before age 30 was allergic, while onset after age 40 was nonallergic (98). As shown in Figure 1, studies demonstrate that asthma at any age increases with increasing IgE levels or skin test reactivity (99–102). However, asthma has been reported not to be related to skin test reactivity in nonsmoking adults over 25 years of age if they did not also have allergic rhinitis.

Exposure to a number of individual allergens appears to correlate well with asthma morbidity. Of various allergens, exposure to dust mite seems to

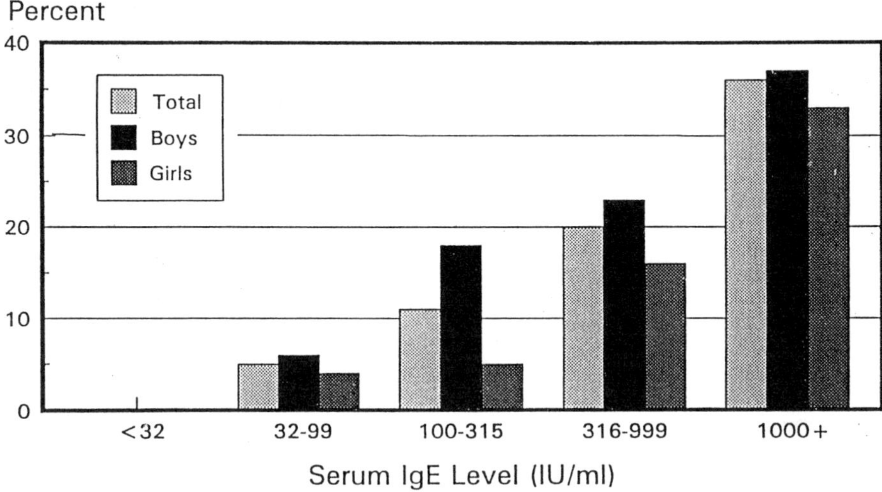

FIGURE 1   Relation between serum total IgE and current asthma in 11-year-old New Zealand children. (From Ref. 100.)

be a strong agent in the development of asthmatic symptoms (74,103–106). In addition, dust mite has been identified as being important etiologically in asthma sensitization (107), and early life exposure has been associated with earlier onset of asthma. The mold *Alternaria* has been implicated in fatal and near-fatal asthmatic attacks (76). Cockroach, cat, and pollens (ragweed and rye grass) have also been reported to be etiologically important agents in asthma (108–111).

D. Birth Factors

As perinatal care has improved, there has also been increased survival of premature infants and an increase in the pulmonary problems associated with premature lung. The role prematurity and premature lung problems play in either the development or severity of asthma has come under increased study.

Survivors of neonatal lung disease, especially its sequelae of bronchopulmonary dysplasia, have been reported to have increased levels of airway obstruction, hyperinflation, and bronchial reactivity in childhood (112). Low birth weight has been associated with decreased flow rates in childhood (113) and in persons with asthma (114). In another study at 7 years of age, infants whose birth weight was under 2000 g had more problems with cough but not wheezing as compared to age-matched schoolmates (115).

One study demonstrated that a family history of asthma, but not other allergies, was identified as a predictor of which children with respiratory distress syndrome of prematurity were likely to develop bronchopulmonary dysplasia (116). This finding was not supported in another study (117). Survivors of neonatal lung disease, especially its sequela bronchopulmonary dysplasia, have been reported to have increased levels of airway obstruction, hyperinflation, and bronchial reactivity in childhood (112,116). Others have reported that low birth weight and prematurity, regardless of neonatal respiratory disease, is associated with decreased flow rates and airway conductance in childhood (113,118). In a follow-up at 7 years of age infants whose birth weight was under 2000 g had more problems with cough but not wheezing as compared to age-matched schoolmates (115). Over a 9-month period, there was no difference between the groups in the number of school days lost due to respiratory symptoms.

Other, less clear, birth factors have been correlated with the occurrence of asthma. For example, a relative deficiency of asthma has been reported among second-born children (119). Also, more asthmatics have been reported to be born in the months of August to January (120) and May to October than in other months (121).

E. Breast Feeding

In spite of the finding that breast feeding protects against wheezing illness in the first months of life (122–125), the role of breast feeding in preventing asthma is controversial. This is discussed in Chapter 8.

F. Smoking

Smoking is a well-recognized respiratory irritant. Children whose parents smoke have been reported to have more problems with wheezing, lower respiratory infections, and asthma than children of parents who do not smoke, especially in the first year of life (126–129). This effect remains even after controlling for other possible risk factors (124). Maternal smoking has consistently been reported to be an important risk factor for childhood asthma morbidity (130). This is probably due to the greater exposure of the children to maternal than paternal smoke. The effect of maternal smoking may be seen even if the moth-er only smoked during pregnancy and quit before delivery, suggesting a congenital effect (131).

Tobacco smoke has been implicated in the development of asthma among children with atopic dermatitis (97), and with the earlier onset of asthma among U.S. children (132), but not in New Zealand (40). Also, tobacco smoke increases the severity of asthma (132,133). Several studies have reported that adolescent asthmatics smoke at a level equal to or higher than that of the general population (38,134,135).

G. Geographical Variation in Disease

Asthma has been reported more frequently in urban areas as compared to rural areas among children (39,136,137) and adolescents (138), but not adults (41).

Also, there appears to be small geographical variation in asthma prevalence. For example, within England and the United States, the prevalence of asthma is reported to be lower in the northern areas as compared to the southern areas (38,139,140), whereas in Sweden and Finland, the prevalence of asthma is reported to be higher in the northern parts of the country as compared to the southern (141).

H. Home Dampness and Molds

Home dampness and the presence of molds in the home have been reported to be associated with an increased prevalence of respiratory symptoms including asthma and wheeze (142–144). It has been suggested that this association may in part be explained by a tendency of parents from homes with visible molds to overreport symptoms (144). This overreporting of symptoms has not been found by others (142). As previously reported, presence of an exposure to the mold *Alternaria* has been reported to be highly correlated with asthma morbidity.

I. Outdoor Pollution

The role of air pollution in either the expression or severity of asthma is still unclear. Obtaining accurate measurements of outdoor pollution is difficult; work from New York has shown that a single monitor does not reflect the experience of a large metropolitan area or even the area surrounding it (145, 146). Another major limitation of epidemiological studies on the effects of air pollution is the difficulty in measuring individual exposure. A confounding factor can be the close relation of weather conditions to levels of various pollutants. Other possible reasons for the diverging results in various studies are discussed in Chapter 8.

The findings on asthma morbidity and pollution are mixed. Asthma has been reported to be increased in polluted areas as compared to nonpolluted areas in Israel (147). In Los Angeles increased asthma morbidity has been associated with high oxidant and particulate pollution (148), nitric oxide, coefficient of haze, hydrocarbons, and airborne allergen counts (149). In contrast, other studies in New Zealand (150) and the United States (151) have found that hospital admissions for asthma were unrelated to pollution levels. A recent study by Dockery et al. (152) suggested that while respiratory mortality seems to be associated with high levels of pollution, asthma mortality per se is not.

There are a number of individual pollutants that may be causing specific environmental effects related to asthma morbidity. An increase in fine particulate pollution has been shown to be associated with increased hospitalizations for asthma and bronchitis in a localized area (153). Sulfur dioxide causes bronchoconstriction and asthma-like symptoms, even at low levels, with chronic exposure (154,155). Nitrogen dioxide, associated with gas stoves, has been implicated as a cause of respiratory disease and has an inconsistent effect on pulmonary function (156). Ozone has been shown to increase bronchial reactivity (154). Airborne acidity has been associated with daily symptoms among moderate to severe asthmatics (157). Exposure to multiple pollutants may have important synergistic effects; e.g., ozone has been shown to potentiate the asthmatic response to sulfur dioxide (158). Acute allergen exposure has been demonstrated to cause community epidemics of asthma morbidity. For example, an epidemic of asthma was caused by soybean dust being blown into nearby neighborhoods during the process of ship loading (159).

J. Race/Poverty

Asthma has been reported to vary by racial groups across the world. In the United States, blacks, at any age, have been reported to have more asthma than whites (38,41). Puerto Rican children living in the New York City area have been reported to have some of the highest rates of asthma in the United States, while Mexican-American children in the Southwest have some of the lowest (160). The rate of hospitalizations (3,161) and mortality (162,163) is also higher among blacks than whites.

Poverty plays a role in these differences. Three studies now suggest that small geographical variations in asthma hospitalization rates are highly correlated with poverty status of the population (65,66,164). Similar increases in asthma morbidity and mortality among groups living in poverty are found in other parts of the world. In New Zealand, Maoris and Pacific Island Polynesians have higher rates of hospitalization (165,166) and mortality than other New Zealanders. The higher rates of hospitalizations among Polynesians appear to be due to different drug management at discharge from hospital and in the community—the Polynesians were less likely to be on prophylactic therapy (167,168).

The reasons for these differences in asthma morbidity by race/ethnicity are not clear.

K. Seasonal, Climatic, and Altitude Effects on Morbidity

Seasonal variations in morbidity and mortality of asthma have been reported. In general, the fall and winter demonstrate the highest rates of morbidity and mortality (169). Variation by day of the week for asthma emergency room (ER) visits have also been reported (170). Changes in temperature, pollen levels, and fungal spore counts have been reported to be associated with asthma ER visits (171–173).

The reasons for these seasonal or climatic changes are poorly understood. For example, asthma hospitalization has been associated with rainfall, low barometric pressure, and counts of colored basidiospores and green algae (174). Asthma is also reported to be less prevalent at higher altitudes (175, 176); a decreased concentration of dust mite at higher altitudes is hypothesized to be responsible for this decrease (177,178). Asthma mortality, however, has been reported not to vary with altitude in the United States (179).

L. Infection

Viral infections are well recognized to be precipitants of asthma attacks (180–184). Bacterial infections do not seem to be important triggers of asthma (179, 185). However, sinusitis, regardless of etiology, is felt to make asthma difficult to control until it is adequately treated (186).

Croup and lower respiratory tract infections, such as bronchiolitis and pneumonia, have been reported to be associated with the later development of asthma (134,187,188). These studies illustrate several important difficulties in interpreting epidemiological studies of this nature: recall bias, and the tendency to study only the most severe patients, e.g., hospitalized patients.

While one report has implicated viral infections in the development of allergenic sensitization (189), other studies have failed to confirm this finding (107,190). Sensitization to the viral agent has been shown to play a role in wheezing illness as production of viral-specific IgE has been found to be associated with the clinical manifestation of wheezy illness for both respiratory syncytial virus (191) and parainfluenza viruses (192).

IV. RECENT EPIDEMIOLOGICAL TRENDS IN ASTHMA

Epidemiological data, duplicated over time, provides a means of identifying secular trends in disease incidence, prevalence, morbidity, and mortality. In many countries, trends in asthma morbidity and mortality have been closely studied, and the changing epidemiology of asthma has been the subject of much discussion (193–196). The following sections present an overview of this literature.

A. Cautions About Trend Comparisons

To obtain a broad epidemiological perspective on trends, it is useful to compare international data on trends in asthma morbidity and mortality. However, due to the many differences in survey and population surveillance methods, interpretations in comparative data should be viewed with caution.

Changes in Diagnostic Coding and Accuracy of Death Certificates

It is customary to present epidemiological data on asthma ambulatory care, hospitalization, and mortality using recorded diagnostic information. These data are abstracted using an international diagnostic classification scheme, the International Classification of Diseases (ICD) codes. Unlike most previous revisions, the coding change of asthma between the eighth and ninth revisions of the ICD in 1979 had an important effect on the diagnosis of asthma. Under the eighth revision, "bronchitis with mention of asthma" was coded as "bronchitis." Under the ninth revision, asthma coexistent with bronchitis was recorded as "asthma." Overall there is an estimated 30% increase in deaths attributed to asthma between ICD-8 and ICD-9. However, for persons aged less than 45 years, the effect is estimated to be less than 5%. The potential implications of this coding change will be highlighted below.

The accuracy of the coding of asthma on death certificates has been of great concern. Studies from New Zealand (59), Britain (58), and the United States (60) have reported that the accuracy of the coding is dependent on the age of the decedent. Under age 35, the coding is virtually 100% accurate; by age 70, the accuracy approaches 50%. As a result, most of the reported literature on asthma mortality focuses on the younger age range.

B. Trends in Incidence

There is little data on trends in incidence. One recent study has examined the trends in the asthma incidence in a study of the Rochester, Minnesota population between 1964 and 1983. In this population, the annual age- and sex-adjusted incidence of definite plus probable asthma increased from 1.8 to 2.8 per 1000. This increase was found only in children aged 1–14 years (197).

C. Recent Trends in Asthma Prevalence

There is evidence that asthma prevalence is increasing in a number of countries and populations.

Data on self-reported* asthma from the U.S. National Health Interview Survey (NHIS) demonstrate an increase in prevalence during the 1980s; how-

---

*For children data are parental-reported.

ever, the increases are largest in younger age groups, persons under 18 years. Results from the special child health supplements to the NHIS, conducted in 1981 and 1988, show the asthma prevalence for children aged under 18 years has increased 39%, from 3.2 to 4.3 per 100 population between 1981 and 1988 (198,199).

In Sweden, the prevalence of asthma increased 47% (from 1.9 to 2.8 per 100 population) among 18-year-old military conscripts between 1971 and 1981 (138). In Finland, the recorded asthma prevalence increased fivefold (from 0.29 to 1.79 per 100 population) among 19-year-old military conscripts, between 1966 and 1989 (200). Two surveys 26 years apart (1964 and 1990) of Melbourne, Australia schoolchildren 7 years of age found reported ever asthma increased 141% (from 19.1 to 46 per 100 population) (201). Shaw et al. reported an increase in asthma prevalence for a rural adolescent population in New Zealand (202).

Not all the international data on trends of asthma prevalence demonstrate an increase. For example, another study of Finnish children and adolescents demonstrated no change in prevalence during a more recent, albeit shorter, time period, 1980–1986 (141). Conflicting data also exist in the trends in asthma prevalence in England. Burney et al. (2) examined the reported prevalence of asthma or bronchitis in the last 12 months and ever wheeze over a 13-year period (1973–1986) among children 4–12 years of age. The asthma prevalence increased 138% among boys and 378% among girls. Persistent wheeze increased 74% among boys and 117% among girls. A different conclusion was reached by Anderson (203), after comparing results of prevalence studies of asthma conducted in the United Kingdom between 1964 and 1986: ". . . prevalence of wheezing over the last year or which was described as 'current' or 'recent' show[s] little evidence of a trend. . . ." However, in spite of these differences, there appears to be an increase in prevalence of "diagnosed" asthma over the recent decade.

V. RECENT TRENDS IN MEDICAL CARE UTILIZATION

Asthma-related ambulatory care visit rates in the United States increased from 2.71 to 2.85 visits per 100 population between 1975 and 1990 (204). This increase appears to be limited to two age-specific groups, persons 15–44 years of age and those 65 years and older. Similarly, general practice visit rates for asthma in England suggest general increases for the period 1971 and 1981 across all age groups and both genders (205).

Asthma hospitalization rates among children have been reported to be increasing for children in several countries. U.S. asthma hospitalization rates increased during the 1970s and leveled off during the 1980s for all but a few age groups (203). Only two notable age-specific trends were noted: a modest decline during the 1980s for persons 45–64 years old, and a notable increase in hospitalization for children under 15 years, a persistent 25-year trend. During the 1980s, the increase in U.S. asthma hospitalization rates for children appeared to be limited to children under 5 years. Limited data suggest that the severity of asthma in U.S. children who were hospitalized for asthma may have increased during the 1980s (161,206). The rate of hospitalizations for children under 18 years with severe respiratory failure leading to intubation or cardiopulmonary arrest increased from 0.11 to 0.50% between 1979 and 1987. In contrast, during the same time period, the length of stay for asthma decreased 0.5 days (which is less than for hospitalizations in general) (161). Other data report a general decrease in U.S. asthma severity (207).

As shown in Figure 2, between 1957 and 1984, hospitalization rates in England and Wales demonstrated an increase in rates that was primarily limited to younger persons, aged 0–4 years and 5–14 years (5). In New Zealand, asthma hospitalizations increased approximately 4.5-fold among the 0–13-year-old children between 1974 and 1989 (208). Since the 1960s, asthma hospitalizations among children 0–14 years old increased 10-fold in New Zealand, eightfold in Queensland, Australia, sixfold in England and Wales, fourfold in Canada, threefold in the United States, and threefold in Tasmania, Australia (209).

VI. TRENDS IN ASTHMA MORTALITY

As shown in Figure 3, asthma mortality rates for persons 5–34 years old have increased since 1980 in the United States, England and Wales, and Japan.

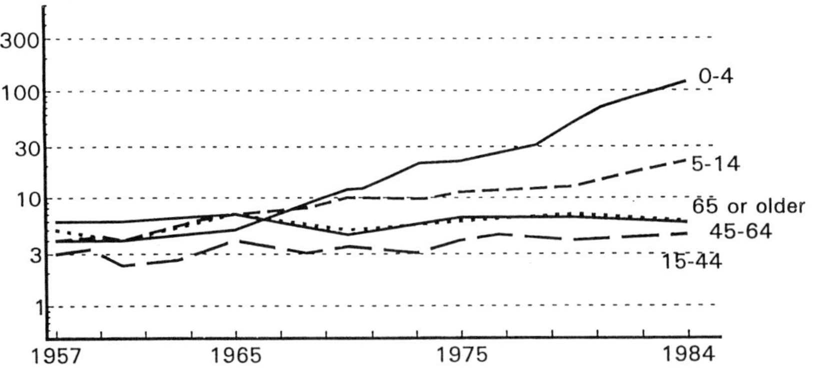

FIGURE 2 Age-specific annual hospital discharge rates for asthma in England and Wales, for males 1957–1984. (From Ref. 205.)

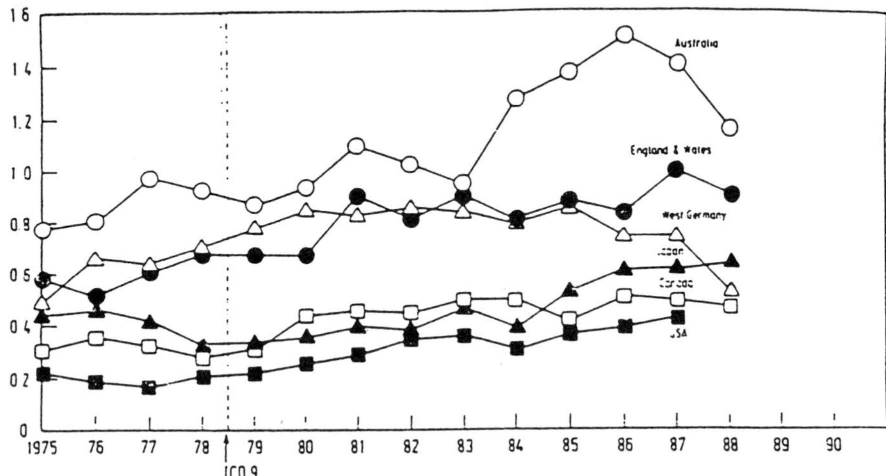

FIGURE 3   Mortality from asthma (rate per 100,000) in 5- to 34-year-old subjects in Australia, England and Wales, West Germany, Japan, Canada, and the United States. (Adapted from Ref. 100.)

During this same period, asthma mortality in Australia demonstrated an increase followed by a decrease, and rates in West Germany declined (61,210). U.S. asthma mortality during the early portion of this century was stable. There was, however, a dramatic increase during the late 1940s and early 1950s, followed by a steady decrease until the late 1970s. Since 1978, the rates appear to be increasing. It is curious that trends for the 5–34-year age group did not demonstrate a dramatic increase in the 1950s. During the 1980s, U.S. asthma mortality within the 5–34-year age range was similar between genders and across each 10-year age group.

A. Comparing the Trends in Prevalence, Medical Care Utilization, and Mortality During the 1980s

The trends in asthma prevalence, medical care utilization, and mortality, when presented individually, suggest general increases. However, when viewed together, these trends tell a rather perplexing story. The age- and country-specific trends in prevalence, hospitalization, and mortality appear different, making any simple explanation of the causes of these changes highly implausible. For example, the most apparent increases in U.S. prevalence rates are for children and adolescents under 18 years, notably children aged 5–17 years. The increases in U.S. hospitalization rates appear to be restricted to persons under 5 years. U.S. mortality seems to be increasing for persons of all ages.

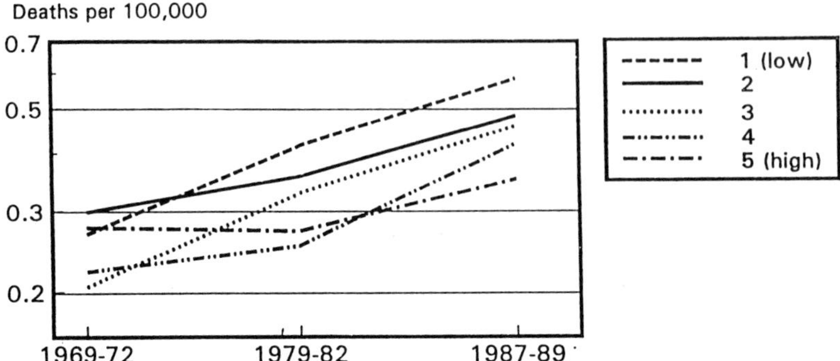

FIGURE 4   U.S. asthma mortality among 5–34-year-old population, county rates by quintile of median income, multiyear averages. (From Ref. 204.)

B. Effect of Race and Socioeconomic Status on Asthma Morbidity and Mortality

There is very little data on epidemiological trends in asthma morbidity by race and socioeconomic status. Data from U.S. surveillance of these trends suggest the differences in rates between whites and nonwhites have remained consistent or increased for asthma prevalence and hospitalization and for mortality, being consistently higher in blacks than whites. There is evidence, however, that over the past two decades a trend toward a strong relationship between U.S. asthma mortality rates and poverty has emerged (see Fig. 4) (204).

VII. PLAUSIBLE EXPLANATIONS FOR THESE RECENT TRENDS

Perhaps the most important question concerning these trends is: are they real changes in population morbidity or are they an artifact of the way we diagnose, record, or analyze the health of the nation? Some of these recent trends may be artifacts introduced by changes in the process of monitoring asthma morbidity, including: changes in diagnostic recognition and accuracy, diagnostic transfer, and the ICD revisions.

A. Changes in Diagnostic Recognition and Accuracy

It is conceivable that some or most of the changes in prevalence are related to a change in the diagnostic recognition of asthma by either the general population or the health care providers. Prevalence is generally "self-reported." During the past 10–15 years, there has been an international effort to increase both physician and public awareness of the signs and symptoms of asthma. Therefore, an increasing asthma awareness could have led to an elevated number of reports without a true increase in the disease burden in the population, as much asthma is undiagnosed (10). It is less likely that diagnostic recognition would have been an important factor in either hospitalization or mortality trends. No new diagnostic technology has appeared that would have improved the recognition of asthma. For asthma mortality, the autopsy rate for children and young adults in the United States is relatively high and has changed very little (163), suggesting that at least for the U.S. trends in mortality, there has been little change in the diagnostic accuracy of this outcome as well.

B. Changes in Diagnostic Transfer

An increase could occur if there was a change in the way another disease was classified so that the disease was now being classified as asthma. This issue of diagnostic transfer—also called diagnostic fashion—has, in fact, been a central concern in recent asthma trends. It has been proposed that the diagnosis of asthma is being substituted for bronchitis, and that this substitution is artificially inflating the estimates of asthma (2,196,211).

C. Effects of the ICD Revision

Change in ICD coding can create a dramatic 1-year increase in both hospitalization (212) and mortality data (3,163,213). Although, coding reclassification probably did have some impact on rates, there is strong evidence that this coding change is not primarily responsible for the recent increases.

Therefore, although some of these recent increases in asthma prevalence, morbidity, and mortality may have been artifacts of changes in diagnostic practices or changes in the health surveillance systems, it seems as though that some true increase in the burden of this illness is occurring.

VIII. CHANGES IN RISK FACTORS AS POSSIBLE LINKS TO RECENT ASTHMA TRENDS

It may be asserted that plausible explanations for the recent trends may be reflected on recent trends in some of the previously noted risk factors for asthma morbidity.

A. Changes in Rates of Prematurity

As previously noted, prematurity with attendant premature lung may be associated with increased asthma symptoms. More low-birth-weight infants are surviving. For example, during the period 1971–1982, U.S. perinatal mortality rates decreased for all birth weights for both blacks and whites (214). Are the increased numbers of surviving premature babies driving up the asthma rates? This is an intriguing possibility that deserves much more study.

B. Changes in the Outdoor Environment

There is very little data on international trends in outdoor air quality. However, during the decade of the 1980s, the trends in U.S. air pollution have uniformly improved (215). From 1981 to 1990 air concentrations of the following pollutants decreased: sulfur dioxide, carbon monoxide, nitrogen dioxide, ozone, and total suspended particles. Small particles, less than $10\,\mu$m (PM-10), are more important for respiratory disease, but have been monitored only since 1989. Thus, nationwide, no evidence exists that supports the role of outdoor pollution levels as the primary factor driving the changes in the epidemiological patterns of asthma morbidity.

C. Changes in the Indoor Environment

Between 1965 and 1985 the age-adjusted prevalence of current smoking in the United States decreased from 52 to 33% for men and from 34 to 28% for women (216). In the past, black women have had a higher prevalence of smoking than white women (122), but late in the 1980s black women were smoking less than white women (217). However, the prevalence of smoking in the United States increased from 40% in 1974 to 44% in 1985 among women aged 20–24 years with a high-school education or less, although by 1987 the rate had dropped to 37.6% in this group (218).

Do changes in smoking play a role in the changing morbidity and mortality of asthma? Smoking probably plays a role, but from the data now available it is not possible to indict smoking as the driving force for the observed increases in asthma. Morbidity and mortality data are not collected by education status of the mother; therefore, the effect of increased smoking among less well educated women cannot be assessed. However, the black-white difference in level of asthma morbidity and mortality may be partially explainable by racial differences in smoking.

Other individual allergens, mostly indoor, are important epidemiologically in eliciting asthma. Could there be increasing exposures to these other indoor allergens? One indirect piece of evidence that there might be changes in indoor exposures relates to the changes in housing conditions over time. For example, the past few decades have brought about important changes in the U.S. housing market. The percentage of new homes with central heating and air-conditioning increased dramatically during the past two decades (219). However, during this period the percent of gas-fueled, forced-air heating remained essentially constant, and the percent of homes with gas ranges used for cooking decreased (220). During the past decade there have been a number of other changes in both residential and work indoor environments, such as increased insulation and wall-to-wall carpeting, that would appear to have an impact on indoor air quality.

It therefore appears that there are a number of possible indoor air pollutants that may affect asthma prevalence and morbidity. However, few studies explicitly examine trends in indoor quality.

D. Changes in Socioeconomic Status

It has also been noted that socioeconomic status (SES) appears to have a modest effect on asthma prevalence (221,222) and a large effect on the small-area geographical variations in both hospitalization and mortality rates (65, 66,164,223). Evidence from the United States suggest that changes in SES may be consistent with the recent epidemiological trends in asthma.

Recent efforts to understand the relationship between asthma and SES in the United States have been focused on the inner city (224). During the past decade, children increasingly have been likely to be raised in families with only one parent and limited financial resources (225). In 1987, nearly 50% of black children and 42% of Hispanic children under 6 were poor versus 10% of white children (226). Forty-six percent of all poor children in the United States lived in the central cities (227), and during the 12-year period 1975–1987, the proportion of poor children living in areas of the central cities where 20% of the population or more are poor rose from 54 to 61% (227).

E. Changes in the Medical Care Environment

During the past decade there have been dramatic changes in health care worldwide. It is difficult, if not impossible, to examine most of these changes as they relate to the trends in asthma morbidity. At least one factor, pharmacotherapy, frequents the asthma literature as a possible link to morbidity. Therefore, the following discussion of possible changes in the health care system will be limited to a discussion of this factor.

Changing Pharmacotherapy

In the past two decades dramatic changes have occurred in the use of medications to control asthma symptoms (228,229). These pharmacoepidemiological trends reflect both increases in total use and the distribution of use among different classes of drugs. Data from the U.S. National Prescription Audit reported an increase in prescriptions of antiasthma drugs (oral and inhaled bronchodilator and inhaled anti-inflammatory drugs) by approximately 9.5% per annum between 1981 and 1985. Sustained-release theophylline formulations increased 138% during this period, while other formulations of this drug decreased (228). During 1980–1986, prescriptions for inhaled sympathomimetics (metered-dose inhalers, MDI) for the State of Michigan Medicaid population increased at a rate of 22% per annum (229).

During the past decade there has been a dramatic increase in the use of MDIs as a principal pharmacotherapeutic agent for asthma symptom control worldwide. Also, methylxanthine use has shifted from immediate- to sustained-release preparations. This change may be an important trend in relation to recent trends in asthma morbidity. MDIs have been at the center of controversy twice during the two decades. It has been proposed that a high-dose inhaler (isoproterenol 0.2 mg/puff) was responsible for an increase in deaths in England during the late 1960s (77,230). More recently, it has been claimed that another MDI that is currently not used in the United States, fenoterol, is causing excess morbidity (79,231). One study has proposed that the regular versus the occasional use of these MDIs may be correlated with risk of morbidity (82). Furthermore, results from a large pharmacoepidemiological study in Canada suggest that frequent use of MDIs along with theophylline and oral steroids can serve as an important epidemiology marker of death and near-death for asthma (80). A recent meta-analysis of beta-agonist use and asthma mortality has suggested a weak association between these two factors (232). The recent and dramatic changes in asthma drug therapy, when viewed in the context of the recent increases in asthma mortality, suggest that further studies are needed to examine whether these two trends represent a causal or coincident occurrence.

IX. SUMMARY

During the past decade our understanding of asthma morbidity has been aided through the epidemiological literature. Through this literature, atopy has emerged as perhaps the most important predisposing factor related to disease onset, while smoking, viral infections, atopy, pollution, health care delivery, and poverty play a role in morbidity and mortality.

There is a growing epidemiological literature to suggest that asthma prevalence and its associated morbidity are increasing. The patterns of this increase by age, race/ethnicity, socioeconomic status, and geographical region are highly variable. Therefore, a simple change in risk factor—whether host, agent, or environment—cannot explain the complex and multiple trends. Yet, a few insights into plausible explanations for the recent epidemiological trends seem to be supported by some evidence. Perhaps the most plausible explanation for at least some of the recent changes may relate to factors related to changes in surveillance methods or population (physician and patient) knowledge and understanding of this disease. The nature of the data on asthma prevalence, self-reported, is very susceptible to enhanced diagnostic recognition. During the past decade, the public and medical community has been exposed to the important message that an unexplained wheeze or chronic cough may be asthma, particularly in children. However, it is not apparent that diagnostic recognition can account for all the recent changes.

If these epidemiological changes are real and not artifact, then several possible explanations seem to emerge. First, much of asthma appears to be atopic, and it is unlikely that the recent increase in prevalence or morbidity can be explained by a genetic change in the host. Another possibility would be changes in either the agents (such as dust mites, cockroach, cat, etc.) or exposure to the agents (such as changing indoor environments). The critical importance of the primary immune response, leading to either tolerance or sensitization (Chapter 10), has some epidemiological support (Chapter 8). Whether artifact or real, the environmental changes are quite dynamic and should be further studied until they are more fully understood.

REFERENCES

1. Asthma—United States, 1980–1987. MMWR 1990; 39:493–496.
2. Burney PG, Chinn S, Rona RJ. Has the prevalence of asthma increased in children? Evidence from the national study of health and growth 1973–86. Br Med J 1990; 300:1306–1310.
3. Evans R, Mullally DI, Wilson RW, Gergen PJ, et al. National trends in the morbidity and mortality of asthma in the US: prevalence, hospitalization and death from asthma over two decades: 1965–1984. Chest 1987; 91:65S–74S.
4. Mitchell EA. Increasing prevalence of asthma in children. NZ Med J 1983; 96:463–464.
5. Mitchell EA, Jackson RT. Recent trends in asthma mortality, morbidity, and management in New Zealand. J Asthma 1989; 26:349–354.
6. Sly RM. Mortality from asthma. J Allergy Clin Immunol 1989; 84:421–434.
7. Gross NJ. What is this thing called love?—Or, defining asthma. Am Rev Respir Dis 1980; 121:203–204 (editorial).
8. Woolcock AJ. Epidemiologic methods for measure prevalence of asthma. Chest 1987; 91:89s–92s.
9. Anderson HR. Is the prevalence of asthma changing? Arch Dis Child 1989; 64:172–175.
10. Speight ANP, Lee DA, Hey EN. Underdiagnosis and undertreatment of asthma in childhood. Br Med J 1983; 286:1253–1256.
11. Banerjee DK, Lee GS, Malik SK, Daly S. Underdiagnosis of asthma in the elderly. Br J Dis Chest 1987; 81:23–29.
12. Burrows B, Lebowitz MD, Barbee RA, Cline MG. Findings before diagnoses of asthma among the elderly in a longitudinal study of a general population sample. J Allergy Clin Immunol 1991; 88:870–877.
13. Taussig LM, Smith SM, Blumenfeld R. Chronic bronchitis in childhood: what is it? Pediatrics 1981; 67:1–5.

14. Dodge RR, Burrows B. The prevalence and incidence of asthma and asthma-like symptoms in a general population sample. Am Rev Respir Dis 1980; 122:567–575.
15. Ware JH, Dockery DW, Spiro AIII, Speizer FE, Gerris BGJ. Passive smoking, gas cooking, and respiratory health of children living in six cities. Am Rev Respir Dis 1984; 129:366–374.
16. Lebowitz MD, Burrows B. Respiratory symptoms related to smoking habits of family adults. Chest 1976; 69:48–50.
17. Bland JM, Bewley BR, Banks MH. Cigarette smoking and children's respiratory symptoms: validity of the questionnaire method. Rev Epidemiol Sante Publ 1979; 27:69–76.
18. Cloutier MM, Loughlin GM. Chronic cough in children: a manifestation of airway hyperreactivity. Pediatrics 1981; 67:6–12.
19. Corrao WM, Braman SS, Irwin RS. Chronic cough as the sole presenting manifestation of bronchial asthma. N Engl J Med 1979; 300:633–637.
20. Johnson D, Osborn LM. Cough variant asthma: a review of the clinical literature. J Asthma 1991; 28:85–90.
21. Pattemore PK, Asher MI, Harrison AC, Mitchell EA, Rea HH, Stewart AW. The interrelationship among bronchial hyperresponsiveness, the diagnosis of asthma, and asthma symptoms. Am Rev Respir Dis 1990; 142:549–554.
22. Sears MR, Jones DT, Holdaway MD, et al. Prevalence of bronchial reactivity to inhaled methacholine in New Zealand children. Thorax 1986; 41:283–289.
23. Peat JK, Britton WJ, Salome CM, Woolcock AJ. Bronchial hyperresponsiveness in two populations of Australian school-children: the relationship between asthma and skin reactivity. Int J Epidemiol 1986; 15:202–209.
24. Cockcroft DW, Murdock KY, Berscheid BA, Gore BP. Sensitivity and specificity of histaminc PC20 determination in a random selection of young college students. J Allergy Clin Immunol 1992; 89:23–30.
25. Broder I, Higgins MW, Mathews KP, Keller JB. Epidemiology of asthma and allergic rhinitis in a total community, Tecumseh, Michigan. IV. Natural history. J Allergy Clin Immunol 1974; 54:100–101.
26. McWhorter WP, Polis MA, Kaslow RA. Occurrence, predictors, and consequences of adult asthma in NHANES I and follow-up survey. Am Rev Respir Dis 1989; 139:721–724.
27. Woolcock AJ. Epidemiologic methods for measuring prevalence of asthma. Chest 1987; 91:89S–92S.
28. Cookson JB. Prevalence rates of asthma in developing countries and their comparison with those in Europe and North America. Chest 1987; 91:97S–103S.
29. Carrasco E. Epidemiologic aspects of asthma in Latin America. Chest 1987; 91: 93S–97S.
30. Chaulet P. Asthma and chronic bronchitis in Africa: evidence from epidemiologic studies. Chest 1989; 96:334S–339S.
31. Woolcock AJ, Peat JK, Keena V, et al. Asthma and chronic airflow limitation in the highlands of Papau New Guinea: low prevalence of asthma in the Asaro Valley. Eur Respir J 1989; 2:822–827.
32. Al Frayh AR. Asthma patterns in Saudi Arabian children. J Roy Soc Health 1990; 110:98–110.

33. Schuhl JF, Alves da Silva, I, Toletti M, Telaine A, Prudente I, Hogado D. The prevalence of asthma in schoolchildren in Montevideo (Uruguay). Allergol Immunopathol 1989; 17:15–19.

34. Holmgren D, Åberg N, Lindberg U, Engström I. Childhood asthma in a rural community. Allergy 1989; 44:256–259.

35. Paoletti P, Carmignani G, Viegi G, et al. Prevalence of asthma and asthma symptoms in a general population sample of North Italy. Eur Respir J 1989; 2:527S–531S.

36. Goren AI, Hellman S. Prevalence of respiratory symptoms and diseases in school children living in a polluted and in a low polluted area in Israel. Environ Res 1988; 45:28–37.

37. Barry DM, Burr ML, Limb ES. Prevalence of asthma among 12 year old children in New Zealand and South Wales: a comparative survey. Thorax 1991; 46:405–409.

38. Gergen PJ, Mullally DI, Evans RIII. National Survey of Prevalence of Asthma among Children in the United States, 1976 to 1980. Pediatrics 1988; 81:1–7.

39. Åberg N, Engström I. Natural history of allergic disease in children. Acta Paediatr Scand 1990; 79:206–211.

40. Horwood LJ, Fergusson DM, Hons BA, Shannon FT. Social and familial factors in the development of early childhood asthma. Pediatrics 1985; 75:859–868.

41. Turkeltaub PC, Gergen PJ. Prevalence of upper and lower respiratory conditions in the U.S. population by social and environmental factors: data from the second National Health and Nutrition Examination Survey, 1976–80 (NHANES II). Ann Allergy 1991; 67:147–154.

42. Williams H, McNicol KN. Prevalence, natural history, and relationship of wheezy bronchitis and asthma in children: an epidemiological study. Br Med J 1969; 4:321–325.

43. Foucard T, Sjöberg O. A prospective 12-year follow-up study of children with wheezy bronchitis. Acta Paediatr Scand 1984; 73:577–583.

44. Park ES, Golding J, Carswell F, Stewart-Brown S. Preschool wheezing and prognosis at 10. Arch Dis Child 1986; 61:642–646.

45. Stein REK, Gortmaker SL, Perrin EC, et al. Severity of illness: concepts and measurements. Lancet 1987; 2:1506–1509.

46. McNichol KN, Williams HE. Spectrum of asthma in children. II. Allergic components. Br Med J 1973; 4:12–16.

47. Zimmerman B, Feanny S, Reisman J, et al. Allergy in asthma. I. The dose relationship of allergy to severity of childhood asthma. J Allergy Clin Immunol 1988; 81:63–70.

48. Inouye T, Tarlo S, Broder I, et al. Severity of asthma in skin test–negative and skin test–positive patients. J Allergy Clin Immunol 1985; 75:313–319.

49. Juniper EF, Frith PA, Hargreave FE. Airway responsiveness to histamine and methacholine: relationship to minimum treatment to control symptoms of asthma. Thorax 1981; 36:575–579.

50. Bleecker ER. Airways reactivity and asthma: significance and treatment. J Allergy Clin Immunol 1985; 75:21–24.

51. Buffum WP, Settipane GA. Prognosis of asthma in childhood. Am J Dis Child 1966; 112:214–217.

52. Gerritsen J, Koeter GH, Postma DA, Schouten JP, Knol K. Prognosis of asthma from childhood to adulthood. Am Rev Respir Dis 1989; 140:1325–1330.

53. Blair H. Natural history of childhood asthma. Arch Dis Child 1977; 52:613–619.

54. Jonsson JA, Boe J, Berlin E. The long-term prognosis of childhood asthma in a predominantly rural Swedish county. Acta Paediatr Scand 1987; 76:950–954.

55. Martin AJ, McLennan LA, Landau LI, Phelan PD. The natural history of childhood asthma to adult life. Br Med J 1980; 280:1397–1400.

56. Kelly WJW, Hudson I, Phelan PD, Pain MCF, Olinsky A. Childhood asthma in adult life: a further study at 28 years of age. Br Med J 1987; 294:1059–1062.

57. Martin AJ, Landau LI, Phelan PD. Predicting the course of asthma in children. Aust Paediatr J 1982; 18:84–87.

58. Accuracy of death certificates in bronchial asthma: accuracy of certification procedures during the confidential inquiry by the British Thoracic Association. Thorax 1984; 39:505–509.

59. Sears MR, Rea HH, De Boer G, et al. Accuracy of certification of deaths due to asthma: a national study. Am J Epidemiol 1986; 124:1004–1011.

60. Barger LW, Vollmer WM, Felt RW, Buist AS. Further investigations into the recent increase in asthma death rates: a review of 41 asthma deaths in Oregon in 1982. Ann Allergy 1988; 60:31–39.

61. Sears MR. Worldwide trends in asthma mortality. Bull Int Union Tuberc Lung Dis 1991; 66:79–83.

62. Sly RM. Mortality from asthma, 1979–1984. J Allergy Clin Immunol 1988; 82:705–717.

63. Sly RM. Increases in death from asthma. Ann Allergy 1984; 53:20–25.

64. Sears MR. International trends in asthma mortality. Allergy Proc 1991; 12:155–158.

65. Carr W, Zeitel L, Weiss K. Variations in asthma hospitalizations and deaths in New York City. Am J Public Health 1992; 82:59–65.

66. Marder D, Targonski P, Orris P, Persky V, Addington W. Effect of racial and socioeconomic factors on asthma mortality in Chicago. Chest 1992; 101:426S–429S.

67. Khot A, Burn R. Seasonal variation and time trends of deaths from asthma in England and Wales 1960–1982. Br Med J 1984; 289:233–234.

68. Weiss KB. Seasonal trends in US asthma hospitalizations and mortality. JAMA 1990; 263:2323–2328.

69. Strunk RC, Mrazek DA, Wolfson-Furhmann GS, LaBrecque JF. Physiologic and psychological characteristics associated with deaths due to asthma in childhood: a case-controlled study. JAMA 1985; 254:1193–1198.

70. Fraser PM, Speizer FE, Waters SD, Doll R, Mann NM. The circumstances proceeding death from asthma in young people in 1968 to 1969. Br J Dis Chest 1971; 65:71–84.

71. Sears MR, Rea HH, Beaglehole R, et al. Asthma mortality in New Zealand: a two year national study. NZ Med J 1985; 98:271–275.

72. Hunt LW, Mair JE, LaPlante JM, et al. Causes of death in a population with asthma. Am Rev Respir Dis 1989; 139:A486.
73. Miller BD, Strunk RC. Circumstances surrounding the deaths of children due to asthma. Am J Dis Child 1989; 143:1294–1299.
74. Birkhead G, Attaway NJ, Strunk RC, Townsend MC, Teutsch S. Investigation of a cluster of deaths of adolescents from asthma: evidence implicating inadequate treatment and poor patient adherence with medications. J Allergy Clin Immunol 1989; 84:484–491.
75. Campbell S, Hood I, Ryan D, Biedrzycki L, Mirchandani H. Death as a result of asthma in Wayne County Medical Examiner Cases, 1975–1987. J Forens Sci 1990; 35:356–364.
76. O'Hollaren MT, Yunginger JW, Offord KP, et al. Exposure to an aeroallergen as a possible precipitating factor in respiratory arrest in young patients with asthma. N Engl J Med 1991; 324:359–363.
77. Speizer FE, Doll R, Heaf P, Strang LB. Investigation into use of drugs preceding death from asthma. Br Med J 1968; 1:339–343.
78. Gandevia B. Pressurized sympathomimetic aerosols and their lack of relationship to asthma mortality in Australia. Med J Aust 1973; 1:273–277.
79. Rae HH, Scragg R, Jackson R, Beaglehole R, Fenwick J, Sutherland DC. A case-control study of deaths from asthma. Thorax 1986; 41:833–839.
80. Spitzer WO, Suissa S, Ernst P, et al. The use of beta agonist and the risk of death and near death from asthma. N Engl J Med 1992; 326:501–506.
81. Grainger J, Woodman K, Pearce N, et al. Prescribed fenoterol and death from asthma in New Zealand, 1981–7: a further case-control study. Thorax 1991; 46: 105–111.
82. Sears MR, Taylor DR, Print CG, et al. Regular inhaled beta-agonist treatment in bronchial asthma. Lancet 1990; 336:1391–1396.
83. Stolley PD, Schinnar R. Association between asthma mortality and isoproterenol aerosols: a review. Prev Med 1978; 7:519–538.
84. Esdaile JM, Feinstein AR, Horwitz RI. A reappraisal of the United Kingdom epidemic of fatal asthma: can general mortality data implicate a therapeutic agent? Arch Intern Med 1987; 147:543–549.
85. Sibbald B, Horn MEC, Brain EA, Gregg I. Genetic factors in childhood asthma. Thorax 1980; 35:671–674.
86. Van Arsdel PPJ, Motulsky AG. Frequency and hereditability of asthma and allergic rhinitis in college students. Acta Genet 1959; 9:101–114.
87. Sibbald B, Turner-Warwick M. Factors influencing the prevalence of asthma among first degree relatives of extrinsic and intrinsic asthmatics. Thorax 1979; 34: 332–337.
88. Kjellman N-IM. Atopic disease in seven-year-old children: incidence in relation to family history. Acta Paediatr Scand 1977; 66:465–471.
89. Edfors-Lubs M-L. Allergy in 7,000 twin pairs. Acta Allergol 1971; 26:249–285.
90. Duffy DL, Martin NG, Battistutta D, Hopper JL, Mathews JD. Genetics of asthma and hay fever in Australian twins. Am Rev Respir Dis 1990; 142:1351–1358.
91. Corrin PA, Dark JH. Aetiology of asthma: lessons from lung transplantation. Lancet 1993; 341:1369–1371.

92. Waite DA, Eyles EF, Tonkin SL, O'Donnell TV. Asthma prevalence in Tokelauan children in two environments. Clin Allergy 1980; 10:71–75.

93. Pattemore PK, Asher MI, Charrison A, Mitchell EA, Rae HH, Stewart AW. Ethnic differences in prevalence of asthma symptoms and bronchial hyperresponsiveness in New Zealand schoolchildren. Thorax 1989; 44:168–176.

94. Smith JM, Harding LK, Cumming G. The changing prevalence of asthma in school children. Clin Allergy 1971; 1:57–61.

95. Smith JM. Skin tests and atopic allergy in children. Clin Allergy 1973; 3:269–275.

96. Kalliel JN, Goldstein BM, Braman SS, Settipane GA. High frequency of atopic asthma in a pulmonary clinic population. Chest 1989; 96:1336–1340.

97. Murray AB, Morrison BJ. It is children with atopic dermatitis who develop asthma more frequently if the mother smokes. J Allergy Clin Immunol 1990; 86:732–739.

98. Rackemann FM. A working classification of asthma. Am J Med 1947; 3:601–606.

99. Hopp RJ, Townley RG, Biven RE, Bewtra AK, Nair NM. The presence of airway reactivity before the development of asthma. Am Rev Respir Dis 1990; 141:2–8.

100. Sears MR, Burrows B, Flannery EM, Herbison GP, Hewitt CJ, Holdaway MD. Relation between airway responsiveness and serum IgE in children with asthma and in apparently normal children. N Engl J Med 1991; 325:1067–1071.

101. Burrows B, martinez FD, Halonen M, Barbee RA, Cline MG. Association of asthma with serum IgE levels and skin-test reactivity to allergens. N Engl J Med 1989; 320:271–277.

102. Gergen PJ, Turkeltaub PC. The association of allergen skin test reactivity and respiratory disease among whites in the U.S. population: data from the second National Health and Nutrition Examination Survey 1976 to 1980. Arch Intern Med 1991; 151:487–492.

103. Van Bever HP, Stevens WJ. Suppression of the late asthmatic reaction by hyposensitization in asthmatic children allergic to house dust mite (*Dermatophagoides pteronyssinus*). Clin Exp Allergy 1989; 19:399–404.

104. Platts-Mills TAE, Mitchell EB, Nock P, Tovery ER, Moszoro H, Wilkins SR. Reduction of bronchial hyperreactivity during prolonged allergen avoidance. Lancet 1982; 2:675–678.

105. Murray AB, Ferguson AC, Morrison BJ. Diagnosis of house dust mite allergy in asthmatic children: what constitutes a positive history? J Allergy Clin Immunol 1983; 71:21–28.

106. Horst M, Hejjaoui A, Horst V, Michel F-B, Bousquet J. Double-blind, placebo-controlled rush immunotherapy with a standardized alternaria extract. J Allergy Clin Immunol 1990; 85:460–472.

107. Sporik R, Holgate ST, Platts-Mills TAE, Cogswell JJ. Exposure to house-dust mite allergen (Der p I) and the development of asthma in childhood. N Engl J Med 1990; 323:502–507.

108. Kang B, Chang JL. Allergenic impact of inhaled arthropod material. Clin Rev Allergy 1985; 3:363–375.

109. Van Metre TE, Marsh DG, Adkinson NFJ, et al. Dose of cat (*Felis domesticus*) allergen 1 (Fel d 1) that induces asthma. J Allergy Clin Immunol 1986; 78:62–75.

110. Sears MR, Herbison GP, Holdaway MD, Hewitt CJ, Flannery EM, Silva PA. The relative risks of sensitivity to grass pollen, house dust mite and cat dander in the development of childhood asthma. Clin Exp Allergy 1989; 19:419–424.
111. Pollart SM, Chapman MD, Fiocco GP, Rose G, Platts-Mills TAE. Epidemiology of acute asthma: IgE antibodies to common inhalant allergens as a risk factor for emergency room visits. J Allergy Clin Immunol 1989; 83:875–882.
112. Bader D, Ramos AD, Lew CD, Platzker ACG, Stabile MW, Keens TG. Childhood sequelae of infant lung disease: exercise and pulmonary function abnormalities after bronchopulmonary dysplasia. J Pediatr 1987; 110:693–699.
113. Chan KN, Noble-Jamieson CM, Elliman A, Bryan EM, Silverman M. Lung function in children of low birth weight. Arch Dis Child 1989; 64:1284–1293.
114. McCormick MC, Brooks GU, Workman D. The health and development status of very low-birth-weight children at school age. JAMA 1992; 267:2204–2208.
115. Chan KN, Elliman A, Bryan E, Silverman M. Respiratory symptoms in children of low birth weight. Arch Dis Child 1989; 64:1294–1304.
116. Nickerson BG, Taussig LM. Family history of asthma in infants with bronchopulmonary dysplasia. Pediatrics 1980; 65:1140–1144.
117. Smyth JA, Tabachnik E, Duncan WJ, Reily BJ, Levison H. Pulmonary function and bronchial hyperreactivity in long-term survivors of bronchopulmonary dysplasia. Pediatrics 1981; 68:336–340.
118. Mansell AL, Driscoll JM, James LS. Pumonary follow-up of moderately low brith weight infants with and without respiratory distress syndrome. J Pediatr 1987; 110:111–115.
119. Tay JSH, Ngiam TE, Yip WCL. Birth order of children with bronchial asthma. J Singapore Paediatr Soc 1982; 24:152–155.
120. Åberg N. Birth season variation in asthma and allergic rhinitis. Clin Exp Allergy 1989; 19:643–648.
121. Smith JM, Springett VH. Atopic disease and month of birth. Clin Allergy 1979; 9:153–157.
122. Wright AL. Holberg CJ, Martinez FD, Morgan WJ, Taussig LM, Group Health Medical Associates. Breast feeding and lower respiratory tract illness in the first year of life. Br Med J 1989; 299:946–949.
123. Fergusson DM, Horwood LJ, Shannon FT. Asthma and infant diet. Arch Dis Child 1983; 58:48–51.
124. Taylor B, Wadsworth J, Golding J, Butler N. Breast feeding, eczema, asthma, and hayfever. J Epidemiol Commun Health 1983; 37:95–99.
125. Fergusson DM, Horwood LJ, Shannon FT. Asthma and infant diet. Arch Dis Child 1983; 58:48–51.
126. Gortmaker SL, Walker DK, Jacobs FH, Ruch-Ross H. Parental smoking and the risk of childhood asthma. Am J Public Health 1982; 72:574–579.
127. Neuspiel DR, Rush D, Butler NR, Golding J, Bijur PE, Kurzon M. Parental smoking and post-infancy wheezing in children: a prospective study. Am J Public Health 1989; 79:168–171.
128. Burchfiel CM, Higgins MW, Keller JB, Howatt WF, Butler WJ, Higgins ITT. Passive smoking in childhood: respiratory conditions and pulmonary function in Tecumseh, Michigan. Am Rev Respir Dis 1986; 133:966–973.

129. Fergusson DM, Horwood LJ, Shannon FT, Taylor B. Parental smoking and lower respiratory illness in the first three years of life. J Epidemiol Commun Health 1981; 35:180–184.
130. Chilmonczyk BA, Salmun LM, Megathlin KN, Neveux LM, Palomaki GE, Knight G, Pulkkinen AJ, Haddow JE. Association between exposure to environmental tobacco smoke and exacerbations of asthma in children. N Engl J Med 1993; 328:1665–1669.
131. Taylor B, Wadsworth J. Maternal smoking during pregnancy and lower respiratory tract illness in early life. Arch Dis Child 1987; 62:786–791.
132. Weitzman M, Gortmaker S, Walker DK, Sobol A. Maternal smoking and childhood asthma. Pediatrics 1990; 85:505–511.
133. Murray AB, Morrison BJ. Passive smoking and the seasonal difference of severity of asthma in children. Chest 1988; 94:701–708.
134. Anderson HR, Bland JM, Patel S, Peckham C. The natural history of asthma in childhood. J Epidemiol Commun Health 1986; 40:121–129.
135. Martin AJ, Landau LI, Phelan PD. Asthma from childhood to age 21: the patient and his disease. Br Med J 1982; 284:380–382.
136. Van Niekerk CH, Weinberg EG, Shore SC, Hesse H de V, Van Schlakwyk DJ. Prevalence of asthma: a comparative study of urban and rural Xhosa children. Clin Allergy 1979; 9:319–324.
137. Keeley DJ, Neill P, Gallivan S. Comparison of the prevalence of reversible airways obstruction in rural and urban Zimbabwean children. Thorax 1991; 46:549–553.
138. Aberg N. Asthma and allergic rhinitis in Swedish conscripts. Clin Exp Allergy 1989; 19:59–63.
139. Kaplan BA, Mascie-Taylor CGN. Biosocial factors in the epidemiology of childhood asthma in a British national sample. J Epidemiol Commun Health 1985; 39:152–156.
140. Adams PF, Benson V. Current estimates for the National Health Interview Survey, 1989. National Center for Health Statistics. Vital Health Statist 1990; 10.
141. Pöysä L, Korppi M, Pietikäinen M, Remes K, Juntunen-Backman K. Asthma, allergic rhinitis and atopic eczema in Finnish children and adolescents. Allergy 1991; 46:161–165.
142. Brunekreef B, Dockery DW, Speizer FE, Ware JH, Spengler JD, Ferris BG. Home dampness and respiratory morbidity in children. Am Rev Respir Dis 1989; 140:1363–1367.
143. Dales RE, Zwanenburg H, Burnett R, Franklin CA. Respiratory health effects of home dampness and molds among Canadian children. Am J Epidemiol 1991; 134:196–203.
144. Strachan DP. Damp housing and childhood asthma: validation of reporting of symptoms. Br Med J 1988; 297:1223–1226.
145. Goldstein IF, Landovitz L. Analysis of air pollution patterns in New York City. I. Can one station represent the large metropolitan area? Atmos Environ 1977; 11:47–52.
146. Goldstein IF, Landovitz L. Analysis of air pollutions patterns in New York City. II. Can one aerometric station represent the area surrounding it? Atmos Environ 1977; 11:53–57.

147. Goren AI, Hellman S. Prevalence of respiratory symptoms and diseases in school children living in a polluted and in a low polluted area in Israel. Environ Res 1988; 45:28–37.
148. Whittemore AS, Korn EL. Asthma and air pollution in the Los Angeles area. Am J Public Health 1980; 70:687–696.
149. Richards W, Azen SP, Weiss J, Stocking S, Church J. Los Angeles air pollution and asthma in children. Ann Allergy 1981; 47:348–354.
150. Dawson KP, Allan J, Fergusson DM. Asthma, air pollution and climate: a Christchurch study. NZ Med J 1983; 96:165–167.
151. Ribon A, Glasser M, Sudhivoraseth N. Bronchial asthma in children and its occurrence in relation to weather and air pollution. Ann Allergy 1972; 30:276–281.
152. Dockery DW, Pope AC, Xu X, Spengler JD, Ware JH, Fay ME, Ferris BG, Speizer FE. An association between air pollution and mortality in six U.S. cities. N Engl J Med 1993; 329:1753–1759.
153. Pope III CA. Respiratory disease associated with community air pollution and a steel mill, Utah valley. Am J Public Health 1989; 79:623–628.
154. Pierson WE, Covert DS, Koenig JQ. Air pollutants, bronchial hyperreactivity, and exercise. J Allergy Clin Immunol 1984; 73:717–721.
155. Sheppard D. Sulfur dioxide and asthma: a double-edged sword? J Allergy Clin Immunol 1988; 82:961–964.
156. Neas LM, Dockery DW, Ware JH, Spengler JD, Speizer FE, Ferris BJJ. Association of indoor nitrogen dioxide with respiratory symptoms and pulmonary function in children. Am J Epidemiol 1991; 134:204–219.
157. Ostro BD, Lipsett MJ, Wiener MB, Selner JC. Asthmatic responses to airborne acid aerosols. Am J Public Health 1991; 81:694–702.
158. Koenig JQ, Covert DS, Hanley QS, van Belle G, Pierson WE. Prior exposure to ozone potentiates subsequent response to sulfur dioxide in adolescent asthmatic subjects. Am Rev Respir Dis 1990; 141(2):377–380.
159. Anto JM, Sunyer J, Rodriguez-Roisin R, Suarez-Cervera M, Vazquez L, The Toxicoepidemiological Committee. Community outbreaks of asthma associated with inhalation of soybean dust. N Engl J Med 1989; 320:1097–1102.
160. Carter-Pokras OD, Gergen PJ. Reported asthma among Puerto Rican, Mexican-American, and Cuban-American children, 1982–1984. Am J Public Health 1993; 83:580–582.
161. Gergen PJ, Weiss KB. Changing patterns of asthma hospitalization among children: 1979 to 1987. JAMA 1990; 264:1688–1692.
162. Sly RM. Mortality from asthma in children 1979–1984. Ann Allergy 1988; 60:433–442.
163. Weiss KB, Wagener DK. Changing patterns of asthma mortality: identifying target populations at high risk. JAMA 1990; 264:1683–1687.
164. Wissow LS, Gittelsohn AM, Szklo M, Starfield B, Mussman M. Poverty, race, and hospitalization for childhood asthma. Am J Public Health 1988; 78:777–782.
165. Mitchell EA, Borman B. Demographic characteristics of asthma admissions to hospitals. NZ Med J 1986; 99:576–579.
166. Mitchell EA, Cutler DR. Paediatric admissions to Auckland Hospital for asthma from 1970–1980. NZ Med J 1984; 97:67–70.

167. Mitchell EA. Why are Polynesian children admitted to hospital for asthma more frequently than European children. NZ Med J 1988; 101:446–448.
168. Mitchell EA. Racial inequalities in childhood asthma. Soc Sci Med 1991; 32:831–836.
169. Khot A, Burn R, Evans N, Lenney C, Lenney W. Seasonal variation and time trends in childhood asthma in England and Wales 1975–81. Br Med J 1984; 289:235–237.
170. Goldstein IF, Cuzick J. Daily patterns of asthma in New York City and New Orleans: an epidemiologic investigation. Environ Res 1983; 30:211–223.
171. Greenburg L, Field F, Reed JI, Erhardt CL. Asthma and temperature change. Arch Environ Health 1963; 8:642–647.
172. Beer SI, Kannai YI, Waron MJ. Acute exacerbation of bronchial asthma in children associated with afternoon weather changes. Am Rev Respir Dis 1991; 144:31–35.
173. Salvaggio J, Seabury J, Schoenhardt EA. New Orleans asthma V. Relationship between Charity Hospital asthma admission rates, semiquantitative pollen adn fungal spore counts, and total particulate aerometric sampling data. J Allergy Clin Immunol 1971; 48:96–114.
174. Khot A, Burn R, Evans N, Lenney W, Storr J. Biometeorological triggers in childhood asthma. Clin Allergy 1988; 18:351–358.
175. Charpin D, Kleisbauer J-P, Lanteaume A, et al. Asthma and allergy to house-dust mites in populations living in high altitudes. Chest 1988; 93:758–761.
176. Charpin D, Birnbaum J, Haddi E, et al. Altitude and allergy to house-dust mite. Am Rev Respir Dis 1991; 143:983–986.
177. Vervloet D, Penaud A, Razzouk H, et al. Altitude and house dust mites. J Allergy Clin Immunol 1982; 69:290–296.
178. Spieksma FTHM, Zuidema P, Leupen MJ. High altitude and house-dust mites. Br Med J 1971; 1:82–84.
179. Sly RM, O'Donnell R. Lack of effect of geographic elevation on mortality from asthma. Ann Allergy 1989; 63:495–497.
180. Minor TE, Dick EC, DeMeo AN, Ouellette JJ, Cohen M, Reed CE. Viruses as precipitants of asthmatic attacks in children. JAMA 1974; 227:292–298.
181. Minor TE, Dick EC, Baker JW, Ouellette JJ, Cohen M, Reed CE. Rhinovirus and influenza type a infections as precipitants of asthma. Am Rev Respir Dis 1976; 113:149–153.
182. Tarlo S, Broder I, Spence L. A prospective study of respiratory infection in adult asthmatics and their normal spouses. Clin Allergy 1979; 9:293–301.
183. Minor TE, Baker JW, Dick EC, et al. Greater frequency of viral respiratory infections in asthmatic children as compared with their nonasthmatic siblings. J Pediatr 1974; 85:472–477.
184. Cogswell JJ, Halliday DF, Alexander JR. Respiratory infections in the first year of life in children at risk of developing atopy. Br Med J 1982; 284:1011–1013.
185. McIntosh K. Ellis EF, Hoffman LS, Lybass TG, Eller JJ, Fulginiti VA. The association of viral and bacterial respiratory infections with exacerbations of wheezing in young asthmatic children. J Pediatr 1973; 82:578–590.
186. Rachelefsky GS, Spector SL. Sinusitus and asthma. J Asthma 1990; 27:1–3.

187. Pullan CR, Hey EN. Wheezing, asthma, pulmonary dysfunction 10 years after infection with respiratory syncytial virus in infancy. Br Med J 1982; 284:1665–1669.
188. Konig P. The relationship between croup and asthma. Ann Allergy 1978; 41:227–231.
189. Frick OL, German DF, Mills J. Development of allergy in children. I. Association with virus infections. J Allergy Clin Immunol 1979; 63:228–241.
190. Busse WW. The relationship between viral infections and onset of allergic diseases and asthma. Clin Exp Allergy 1989; 19:1–9.
191. Welliver RC, Wong DT, Sun M, Middleton EJ, Vaughan RS, Ogra PL. The development of respiratory syncytial virus-specific IgE and the release of histamine in nasopharyngeal secretions after infection. N Engl J Med 1981; 305:841–846.
192. Welliver RC, Wong DT, Middleton EJ, Sun M, McCarthy N, Ogra PL. Role of parainfluenza virus-specific IgE in pathogenesis of croup and wheezing subsequent to infection. J Pediatr 1982; 101:889–896.
193. Van Asperen PP. Is asthma really changing? Aust Paediatr J 1987; 23:271–272.
194. Burr ML. Is asthma increasing? J Epidemiol Commun Health 1987; 41:185–189.
195. Buist AS, Vollmer WM. Reflections on the rise in asthma morbidity and mortality. JAMA 1990; 264:1719–1720.
196. Gergen PJ, Weiss KB. The increasing problem of asthma in the United States. Am Rev Respir Dis 1992; 146:823–824.
197. Yunginger JW, Reed CE, O'Connell EJ, Melton III LJ, O'Fallon WM, Silverstein MD. A community-based study of the epidemiology of asthma. I. Incidence rates, 1964–84. Am Rev Respir Dis 1992; 146:888–894.
198. Gortmaker S, Weitzman M, Perrin J, Sobel A. Recent trends in the prevalence and impact of childhood asthma. Am J Dis Child 1992; 146:495.
199. Taylor WR, Newaheck PW. The impact of childhood asthma on health. Pediatrics 1992; 90:657–662.
200. Haahtela T, Lindholm H, Bjorksten F, Koskenvuo K, Laitinen LA. Prevalence of asthma in Finnish young men. Br Med J 1990; 301:266–268.
201. Robertson CF, Heycock E, Bishop J, Nolan T, Olinsky A, Phelan PD. Prevalence of asthma in Melbourne schoolchildren: changes over 26 years. Br Med J 1991; 302:1116–1118.
202. Shaw RA, Crane J, O'Connell TV, Porteous LE, Coleman ED. Increasing asthma prevalence in a rural New Zealand adolescent population: 1975–89. Arch Dis Child 1990; 65:1319–1323.
203. Anderson HR. Is the prevalence of asthma changing? Arch Dis Child 1989; 64:172–175.
204. Weiss KB, Gergen PJ, Wagener DK. Breathing better or wheezing worse? The changing epidemiology of asthma morbidity and mortality. Annu Rev Public Health 1993; 14:491–513.
205. Alderson M. Trends in morbidity and mortality from asthma. Population Trends 1987; 49:18–23.
206. Williams MH. Increasing severity of asthma from 1960 to 1987. N Engl J Med 1989; 320:1015–1016.
207. Wietzman et al. JAMA 1992; 268:2673–2677.

208. Horwood LJ, Dawson KP, Mogridge N. Admission patterns for childhood acute asthma. Christchurch 1974–89. NZ Med J 1991; 104:277–279.

209. Mitchell AE. International trends in hospital admission rates for asthma. Arch Dis Child 1985; 60:376–378.

210. Sears MR. International trends in asthma mortality. Allergy Proc 1991; 12:155–158.

211. Jackson R, Sears M, Beaglehole R, Rea H. International trends in asthma mortality: 1970 to 1985. Chest 1988; 94:914-918.

212. Halfon N, Newacheck PW. Trends in the hospitalization for acute childhood asthma, 1970–84. Am J Public Health 1986; 76:1308–1311.

213. Burney PG. Asthma mortality in England and Wales: evidence for a further increase, 1974–84. Lancet 1986; 2:323–326.

214. Hoffman HJ, Bergsjo P, Denman DW. Trends in birth weight-specific perinatal mortality rates: 1970–83. In: Proceedings of the International Collaborative Effort on Perinatal and Infant Mortality. Vol. II. DHHS, Hyattsville, MD, October, 1988, pp. III-51–III-71.

215. Environmental Protection Agency. National air quality and emissions trends report, 1990: Office of Air Quality Planning and Standards, EPA-450/4-91-023, Research Triangle Park, NC 27711, November 1991.

216. National Center for Health Statistics: Health, United States, 1988. DHHS Pub. No. (PHS)89-1232. Public Health Service. Washington, DC: U.S. Government Printing Office, 1989.

217. Cigarette smoking among adults—United States, 1990. MMWR 1992; 41:354–362.

218. Pierce JP, Fiore MC, Novotny TE, Hatziandreu EJ, Davis RM. Trends in cigarette smoking in the United States: educational differences are increasing. JAMA 1989; 261:56–60.

219. Homebuilders Association Data Report. Washington, DC: National Home Builders Association, 1990.

220. Statistical Highlights: Ten Year Summary. Washington, DC: Gas Appliance Manufacturers Association, 1990.

221. Schwartz J, Gold D, Dockery DW, Weiss ST, Speizer FE. Predictors of asthma and persistent wheeze in a national sample of children in the United States: association with social class, perinatal events, and race. Am Rev Respir Dis 1990; 142:555–562.

222. Weitzman M, Gortmaker S, Sobol A. Racial, social, and environmental risk factors for childhood asthma. Am J Dis Child 1990; 144:1189–1194.

223. Davis P, Jackson R, Pearce N. Asthma mortality. NZ Med J 1985; 98:604.

224. Weiss KB, Gergen PJ, Crain EF. Inner-city asthma: the epidemiology of an emerging US public health concern. Chest 1992; 101:362–367s.

225. Helmick SA, Zimmerman JD. Trends in the distribution of children among households and families. Child Welfare 1984; 63:401–409.

226. Data Sourcebook: Five Million Children. New York: Columbia University National Center for Children in Poverty, 1990:9.

227. Five Million Children: A Statistical Profile of Our Poorest Young Citizens. New York: Columbia University National Center for Children in Poverty, 1990:22.

228. Bosco LA, Knapp DE, Gerstman BB, et al. Asthma drug therapy trends in the United States, 1972 to 1985. J Allergy Clin Immunol 1987; 80:398–402.
229. Gerstman BB, Bosco LA, Tomita DK, Gross TP, Shaw MM. Prevalence and treatment of asthma in the Michigan Medicaid patient population younger than 45 years, 1980–1986. J Allergy Clin Immunol 1989; 83:1032–1039.
230. Inman WHW, Adelstein AM. Rise and fall of asthma mortality in England and Wales in relation to use of pressurized aerosis. Lancet 1969; 2:279–285.
231. Crane J, Flatt A, Jackson R, et al. Prescribed fenoterol and death from asthma in New Zealand, 1981–1983: case-control study. Lancet 1989; 1:917–922.
232. Mullen MC, Mullen B, Carey M. The association between beta-agonist use and death from asthma: a meta-analytic investigation of case-control studies. JAMA 1993; 270:1842–1845.

8

Risk Factors for Sensitization and Development of Allergic Diseases

Bengt Björkstén
University Hospital
Linköping, Sweden
and Tartu University
Estonia

I. INTRODUCTION

The epidemiology of asthma was discussed in Chapter 7. In this chapter the epidemiology of environmental factors influencing the development of asthma and allergy, particularly in early childhood, will be analyzed. For an understanding of this interaction, however, the genetically determined individual propensity to allergy and individual variations in susceptibility over time also have to be discussed in some detail. The underlying immunological concepts concerning primary sensitization are discussed in Chapter 10.

The etiology of allergy is multifactorial and depends on the interaction, in genetically susceptible individuals, between the time and amount of allergen exposure and the presence of nonspecific "adjuvant" factors, including air pollution (Fig. 1). There is epidemiological evidence that the prevalence of allergic diseases is increasing, at least in children and young adults. Unfortunately, however, even when adding all environmental influences that are suspected to increase the prevalence of asthma and allergy, this can explain only a relatively small proportion of the cases. Thus, the reasons for the suspected increase are

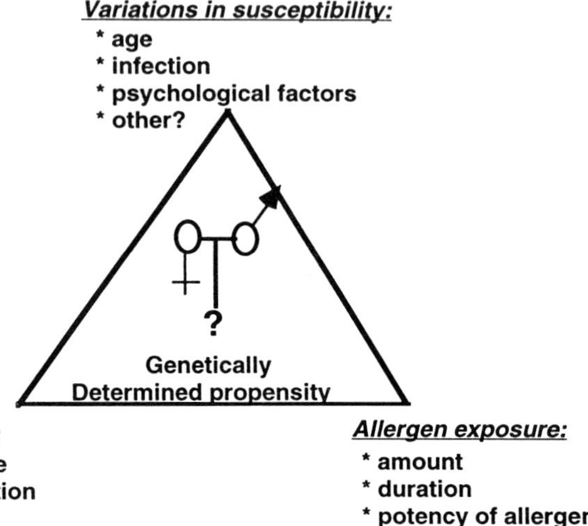

FIGURE 1   Schematic presentation of the interaction between allergen exposure, nonspecific "adjuvant" factors, and genetic propensity.

largely unknown. Recent advances in the understanding of the regulation of IgE antibody formation and the genetics of asthma and allergy, combined with clinical studies, may provide better insight into the epidemiology of asthma and allergy.

Exposure to an allergen is necessary to induce IgE antibody formation. Allergens are present in almost every part of the world but the relative importance of the individual allergens varies locally. In temperate regions, like the Scandinavian countries, house dust mites used to be uncommon (1), but there is now evidence for an increasing prevalence (2,3). This may be due, at least partly, to modern technology used for building houses and energy conservation measures (4,5).

It has traditionally been assumed that air pollution is primarily an outdoor problem. Several studies have shown, however, that indoor concentrations of some pollutants may be far in excess of the outdoor concentrations (6,7). For example, there is probably no air outdoors that is so polluted as that in a room where people are smoking. Outdoor air pollution has decreased over the past decades in many countries, yet the prevalence of allergy seems to be increasing in these countries. Furthermore, there is not clear relationship between air pollution and the prevalence of allergy. On the contrary,Scandinavian studies show a higher prevalence of allergy in the northern, less polluted parts than in the southern, more industrialized regions (8–10). The latter are also more affected by pollution from central Europe. Thus, the relationship between air pollution and allergy is not simple.

There is increasing experimental and clinical evidence that the conditions under which an allergen is encountered in infancy may have consequences for many years, perhaps even for life (11). If this is indeed true, then the search for environmental triggers of allergy should be directed toward infancy, rather than toward factors prevailing at the time of onset of clinical symptoms.

The influence of environmental factors is modified by the genetic susceptibility and individual factors that may vary over time (12). The potential role of a certain environmental influence should therefore be studied in populations that are defined with regard to these individual factors.

II. IDENTIFICATION OF SUSCEPTIBLE INDIVIDUALS

It has long been recognized that a family history of asthma and/or allergy in a young child is strongly associated with an increased risk for the development of allergic disease. Unfortunately, the value of even a carefully obtained family history as a predictive marker is limited because of low specificity (many infants with a positive family history of allergy do not develop disease). It is also often difficult to obtain a reliable family history and almost impossible to do so in an epidemiological study merely using a questionnaire.

There are some clinical findings that may indicate the existence of allergic disease. For example, a dry skin and dermographism in an otherwise healthy infant has been associated with later-appearing allergic manifestations (13). These signs are non-specific, however, and therefore not clinically useful for identification of individuals at risk.

The clinical symptoms of atopy vary with age. Thus, the phenotypic expression of the "allergic genotype" is highly age-dependent. Food allergy and eczema in an infant is often the first manifestation of allergic disease in the atopic individual (Fig. 2). They are therefore predictive of other manifestations of allergy, e.g., asthma (14–16). Thus, even if the prognosis of food allergy in infants and young children is usually good with regard to that particular allergy, such manifestations indicate that the individual is atopic and at risk to develop other allergic manifestations later in life. Wheezing in connection with a respiratory tract infection is commonly encountered in infancy and most of these babies do not develop asthma. In infants with eczema and/or food allergy, however, particularly if there is also a family history of atopy, wheezing may be the first indication of asthma. The "atopic march" then continues in typical cases with more obvious symptoms from the respiratory tract, including asthma after about 2 years of age. At that time the infantile eczema has often resolved, perhaps to return later as atopic dermatitis, typically mainly located on the

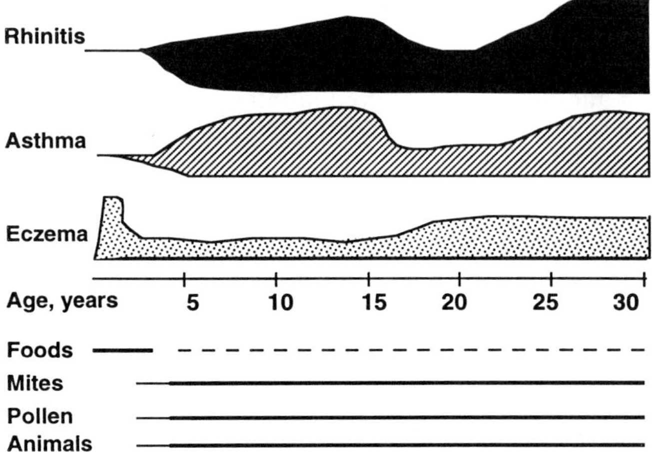

FIGURE 2 The "atopic march" usually begins with dermatitis and allergy to foods in infancy. Later, asthma and allergic rhinitis develop. Food allergy is less common after 3 years of age, and from then, inhaled allergens dominate as sensitizing and triggering agents.

flexural sides of the extremities. From about 5 years of age, rhinoconjunctivitis becomes increasing more common, reaching a peak prevalence in young adults.

Excessive IgE antibody formation is a hallmark of atopy. In the absence of parasitosis and immune deficiency, it bears a strong relationship to various manifestations of allergic disease (17,18). This is particularly true in children and young adults. Thus, the presence of elevated levels of IgE antibodies in serum as proven by various laboratory tests, or in the skin as demonstrated by positive skin prick tests, is strongly associated with manifestations of allergic disease, either at the time of testing or developing subsequently (16,19–21). The serum IgE levels can therefore be used as a screening test for the identification of atopic individuals. Unfortunately, neither the specificity nor the sensitivity is adequate for clinical use or epidemiological studies, the latter being about 50% and the former slightly higher. These and other aspects of IgE antibody determinations are discussed in greater detail in Chapter 10.

Determination of specific IgE antibodies against defined allergens is more clinically useful than the total IgE levels for identification of atopic individuals and the allergens to which they are sensitive. The general conclusion from prospective studies is that the specificity of tests for IgE antibodies is high (a positive test is associated with disease in 85–90%), while the sensitivity is lower (22).

Several reports published from 1976 indicated that an elevated level of IgE in cord blood strongly predicted allergy (23–25). As is often the case with new tests, however, the early enthusiasm was followed by disappointment, as in many subsequent studies the sensitivity was poor, although most of them confirmed a high specificity. The advantages and problems with the determinations have recently been summarized by Kjellman (22), based on a literature survey and his own extensive studies, including an 11-year study comprising 1700 children (16). The conclusion was that an elevated level of IgE in serum is present in less than 30% of infants who will develop allergic manifestations during the first 11 years of life. For this reason, IgE tests are not recommended for screening purposes to identify healthy individuals at risk for later-appearing asthma and allergy. As discussed in Chapter 5, however, the predictive capacity is substantially better for severe atopic manifestations, including asthma, than it is for more trivial and short-lasting symptoms.

In conclusion, the demonstration of IgE antibodies to defined allergens remains so far the most useful predictive marker of asthma or allergy in children and young adults, despite its limitations.

Several other immunological, immunochemical, and biochemical tests have been employed for the identification of subjects at high risk for developing allergy (Table 1). They include determination of IgG anti-IgE antibody complexes in serum (26), lymphocyte tests (27), amniotic fluid analysis (28), leukocyte phosphodiesterase levels (29,30), basophil releasability (31,32), and quantitation of blood eosinophils (32,33). None of these procedures are clinically useful for allergy prediction, however, as they either have a poor sensitivity and specificity and/or are complicated to perform and poorly standardized. They do, however, support the hypothesis that the atopic individual has (a) primary abnormality(-ies) of the immune system (c.f. Chapter 10).

In conclusion, the most reliable predictive test for future allergy so far is the demonstration of IgE antibodies in a clinically healthy infant, either in the skin by skin prick tests or in the serum by various laboratory tests.

III. VARIATIONS IN SUSCEPTIBILITY

A. Genetics

The role of genetic factors is discussed extensively elsewhere in this book. As indicated in the Introduction, the epidemiology of factors influencing the development of asthma and allergies is influenced by the genetic propensity for allergy in the study population. To identify environmental risk factors, the effects on genetically susceptible and nonsusceptible individuals should therefore be analyzed separately. This means that in epidemiological studies, e.g., of the role of environmental influences, the genetics of the individuals in the study population should always be considered.

TABLE 1 Abnormalities in Atopic Individuals and Methods Suggested for Early Identification of Atopic Individuals Before They Have Manifested Asthma and Other Symptoms from the Respiratory Tract

Method	Finding	Primary finding	Clinical documentation
Family history	Present	Yes	Yes[a]
Clinical signs			
Skin texture	E.g., dry	Yes	Poor
Blood tests			
S-IgE	Elevated	Yes	Yes[b]
Specific IgE	Present	Yes	Yes[b]
IgG-anti-IgE	Low	Yes	Unconfirmed
Lymphocyte populations	Low helper[c]	Yes	Yes[c]
Lymphocyte function	Reduced[c]	Yes	Poor[c]
Phosphodiesterase	Elevated	No	Poor
Basophil function	Increased	No	Poor
Eosinophils	Elevated	No	Limited
Skin prick tests	Positive	Yes	Yes[b]

[a]Low specificity (proportion of affected individuals with a positive test) and sensitivity (proportion of healthy individuals with a negative test) limits the clinical use.
[b]Low sensitivity.
[c]Several different tests. Not confirmed in prospective studies. Mostly too complicated for clinical use.

B. Age

The likelihood for sensitization is affected by the time and the conditions under which exposure to allergens take place. There appears to be a period in early life during which the individual is more easily sensitized than later in life (12,34, 35). In a large epidemiological study comprising 40,000 individuals, a Finnish team observed a significantly higher prevalence of allergy to birch and grass pollen in 10-year-old children who were born in the spring, as compared to children who were born at other times of the year (34,36). Subsequently the authors reported that the risk of pollen allergy, as diagnosed at 10 years of age, was affected not only by the month of birth, but also by the intensity of the pollen season the year they were born. The intensity of the first pollen season even had a stronger impact than the intensity of the pollen season when their symptoms first appeared.

Similar results have been reported for grass allergy in British children (37) and for ragweed allergy in individuals born in the United States (38), before and during the peak ragweed pollen season. In a Swedish study it was observed, however, that the relationship between season of birth and allergy development was limited to children with elevated IgE levels in the cord blood, i.e., with a congenital propensity for allergy (39), again supporting the concept that manifestations of disease are the result of an interaction between environmental and genetic factors, as suggested in Figure 1.

Similar to the apparent effects of early exposure to pollen, early contacts with animal epithelia and house dust appear to influence the incidence of allergy. Thus, children born in the autumn, i.e., before the main indoor season, seem to be more prone to sensitization to indoor allergens than babies born at other times of the year (37,40). These observations in pollen-, dander-, and mite-sensitive individuals all indicate that early exposure to an allergen increases the risk for allergy. The possible underlying mechanisms for the propensity toward sensitization in early childhood are discussed in detail in Chapter 10. From the experimental studies discussed in that chapter and the epidemiological observations discussed here, it is reasonable to conclude that a search for environmental factors that influence the development of asthma and allergy should be directed particularly toward factors operating during the first years of life.

Exposure to a not previously encountered allergen that may induce sensitization is not limited to children but also occurs in adults. This may have practical consequences for the design of workplaces, as indicated by a reduced risk for occupational allergy when exposure to occupational allergens is reduced by the introduction of effective air-cleaning devices. A study of sensitization to alcalase clearly demonstrated the interaction between exposure and genetic propensity also in adults (Fig. 3) (41). This enzyme is present in laundry detergents and it is a potent allergen. The prevalence of sensitivity to the allergen was 85% among atopic persons working in a factory where the detergent was produced, as compared to only 2.6% among consumers exposed to the

	Exposure to alcalase	
	Factory workers (High)	**Consumers (Low)**
Atopic	85%	2.6%
Non-atopic	35%	0.2%

FIGURE 3 Relative influence of genetic propensity and amount of exposure to allergen. Persons working in a factory producing alcalase-containing laundry detergent are exposed to much higher levels for longer time periods than consumers using the product. The atopic individuals are much more readily sensitized than the nonatopic persons. (Data from Ref. 41.)

product only occasionally and then at a lower concentration. This demonstrates the role of exposure to high, as compared to low, allergen levels. Figure 3 also shows the role of genetics, as in both groups atopic individuals had the highest prevalence of sensitivity.

In conclusion, although sensitization may occur at any age, the first years of life and the conditions under which the primary encounter with an allergen takes place seem to be particularly important, even if the consequences may not become apparent until many years later.

C. Infections

The role of infections in the respiratory tract as risk factors for the development of childhood allergic disease and asthma is complex. An infection induces an inflammatory reaction in the respiratory mucosa, which in turn modifies the local immune response. To what extent this enhances sensitization to inhaled allergens is not fully understood, although there are studies indicating that this is the case for at least some viruses, e.g., respiratory syncytial virus (42). Animal experiments support the clinical observations, showing an enhanced IgE production in virus-infected dogs after allergen exposure (43,44).

It is well established that infections may trigger and aggravate asthma in already sensitized individuals and that infections increase bronchial hyperreactivity. The presence and absence of infections may explain variations in susceptibility to disease manifestations in the individual over time. Epidemiological studies of the relationship between infections and manifestation of allergic disease are, however, complicated by the fact that symptoms like a runny nose, wheezing, and cough may all be caused by either an infection or an allergic reaction and that the etiology of the symptoms is therefore not always easily identified by patients and researchers.

The understanding of the interaction between infections and sensitization has become even more complicated in light of the experimental studies of the primary sensitization. As discussed in Chapter 10, bacterial infections early in life may enhance the down-regulation of the IgE antibody formation to allergens encountered at the time of the infection. Reports of less atopy among schoolchildren in the formerly socialist countries of Eastern Europe (45–47) lend some support to the clinical relevance of these findings. Furthermore, in a British study it was reported that atopic as compared to nonatopic adults had less respiratory tract infections during childhood (47a). An inverse relationship between the number of siblings (46), particularly older siblings (47b), and atopy has also been reported. In the latter study, there was no significant relationship between atopy and the presence of younger siblings, indicating that many infections during the first year of life could protect against sensitization. Very recently it was observed that the prevalence of positive skin prick tests may be lower in tuberculin-positive than in tuberculin-negative children (J. Hopkins and T. Shirakawa, unpublished), indicating that bacterial infections and vaccinations early in life may possibly enhance the down-regulation of IgE antibody formation to allergens encountered at the time of the infection.

Among the infectious agents, *Bordetella pertussis* is of particular interest, as it is a well-established adjuvant for the induction of IgE antibody formation in experimental animals (48). Furthermore, whooping cough is associated with bronchial hyperreactivity for several months and consequently also with increased likelihood of asthma (49). IgE antibodies to pertussis toxin commonly appear after an infection and after immunization against pertussis (49–51). The latter observation raises the question about a possible role of vaccinations as a risk factor for allergic disease. This notion is further strengthened by the fact that aluminum, which is used as an adjuvant in many vaccines, is also one of the most potent adjuvants for IgE antibody synthesis in animals (52). It is not known to what extent vaccinations actually represent risk factors for asthma and sensitization to environmental allergens. Theoretically, they could act as adjuvants, enhancing sensitization against allergens that the individual is exposed to at the time of vaccination. Properly designed epidemiological studies are needed to clarify a possible relationship between routine immunizations of infants and development of atopic disease.

D. Psychological Factors

Animal studies and clinical observations have indicated that stress alters the immune response, as measured by various laboratory tests of inflammatory responses, immunoglobulin production, and cell-mediated immunity (53,54). Clinical studies also indicate that stress may cause reduced resistance to infections (55,56). It is clinically well established that psychological factors influence the severity of asthmatic symptoms and allergic reactions in affected patients. For example, dysfunctional patterns of interaction and relations are more common in the families of children with severe asthma than in families of children with another severe chronic disease, i.e., diabetes mellitus (57,58). Patterns of low flexibility ("rigidity") and too much closeness ("enmeshment") dominated among the dysfunctional families. Family therapy to such families reduced the severity of the asthma in the affected children.

A recent prospective study addressed the question whether the disturbed family interaction is a primary finding or a consequence of disease. The study included the families of 100 infants with a strong family history of allergy (59). The entire family participated in a standardized family test when the children were 3 and 18 months old, assessing the ability to adjust to demands of the situation ("adaptability") and the balance between emotional closeness and distance ("cohesion"). An unbalanced family interplay was common at 3

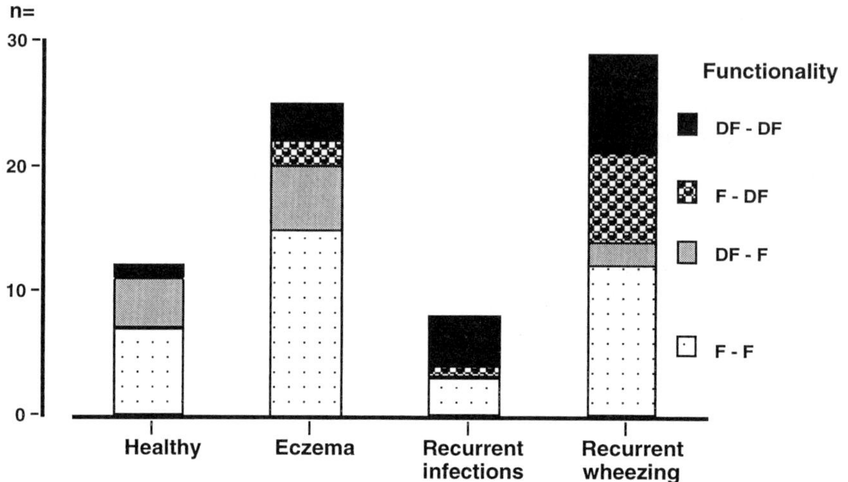

FIGURE 4   Family interaction and subsequent development of asthma and allergy during the first 2 years of life. Many families are temporarily dysfunctional when they have a baby. Most of them then become functional if the child remains healthy. In infants with a wheezing child, however, the family tends to remain or to become dysfunction. (Data from Ref. 59.)

months (37%) but it was not predictive for respiratory illness (Fig. 4). At 18 months a dysfunctional interaction was significantly more common in families of children with eczema and obstructive symptoms, as compared to families of healthy children. The study indicates that a dysfunctional family interaction is the result, rather than a cause, of recurrent wheezing in infancy. Further studies are needed to clarify the role of psychological factors for variations in individual susceptibility to allergic manifestations over time.

IV. NONSPECIFIC ENVIRONMENTAL FACTORS, "ADJUVANTS"

Various environmental factors that do not, like the examples discussed in the previous section, directly influence the host defense may enhance sensitization and also trigger an allergic reaction in a sensitized individual (Table 2) (7,12). While allergy to most of the compounds listed in Table 2 is rare, they do play a role, both in enhancing sensitization to allergens and in eliciting and aggravating clinical symptoms. It is not entirely clear how these adjuvants act. Possibly, an inflammatory reaction is induced in the airways, which in turn facilitates the penetration of allergens or, alternatively, stimulates antigen-

TABLE 2 Adjuvant Factors Suggested to Be Involved in Sensitization and/or Manifestations of Allergic Disease

---

Air pollution and sources
  Tobacco smoke
  Industries and traffic; solid particles, SO_2, NOx
  Combustion by-products; CO_2, CO, SO_2, NO_2, NO, formaldehyde, volatile
    vapors
  Photochemical reactions; ozone, NO_2
  Building materials; formaldehyde, decoration, and paints; solvents
Tight, poorly ventilated homes
Pesticides and consumer products; organic substances, aerosols
Respiratory infections: dual effects depending on circumstances? Cf. Section III.C
Immunizations; aluminum? pertussis?
Allergic reactions (facilitates sensitization to new allergens)

---

presenting cells. Most of these factors are discussed in greater detail in Chapter 7 in relation to asthma.

A. Geographical Differences

The true worldwide prevalence and the regional differences in prevalence of asthma and other allergic diseases are unknown. The reason for this is that epidemiological studies of asthma and/or other allergic manifestations in various countries have only rarely employed identical selection criteria and methodology (60). Soon, epidemiological data will become available, however, allowing such comparisons both for adult populations and for children. In a study sponsored by the European Community, an identical protocol was used in many countries to study the prevalence of asthma and bronchial hyperreactivity among young adults. In the International Study of Asthma and Allergy in Children (ISAAC), at least 40 study sites in over 20 countries are included. Each study population comprises over 3000 13–14-year-old schoolchildren who answered a carefully validated questionnaire. These two large collaborative epidemiological studies will provide, for the first time, accurate comparisons of the worldwide prevalence of asthma and other allergies. The preliminary data clearly demonstrate the existence of major differences in the prevalence, among both children and adults.

    The reported differences between populations are not genetically determined. Rather, they seem to be explained by differences in living conditions. The results of the migrant studies discussed in Chapter 7 demonstrate a higher prevalence of allergic disease in developing countries in people living under privileged conditions than among the poor. Thus a low prevalence of asthma was observed in children migrating to Britain from the West Indies with their parents, while the prevalence of asthma in the younger children in these families, who were born in Britain, was similar to that of the native British children (61,62). A South African study yielded similar results, in that children of the Xhosa tribe who were born in a rural area had much less asthma and other allergies than Xhosa children raised in Cape Town (63).

Environmental differences in the prevalence of allergy are also recorded between urban and rural areas in industrialized countries. As an example, a recent Swedish study showed that the relative risk for a positive skin prick test is 70% higher among 11-year-old children living in a moderately polluted town in northern Sweden than among children living in the neighboring countryside (47,64).

An understanding of the role of environmental factors has, however, become complicated by some recent observations. Air pollution is a major problem in many formerly socialistic countries in central and eastern Europe. Yet, the prevalence of atopy among children is much lower than in western Europe. As an example, the prevalence of positive skin prick tests in Leipzig in eastern Germany is less than half of that among children of the same age living in Munich in western Germany (45,46,65). Similarly, atopic sensitization is much lower in Konin in central Poland and in Estonia than it is in northern Sweden (Table 3), despite much higher levels of SO_2 particles and probably also of NO_2 and other nitrogen compounds in the air in the formerly socialistic countries (47,66,67).

The low prevalence of atopy, as defined by at least one positive skin prick test to common allergens, was not associated with less respiratory disease. Responses to questionnaires given to 2600 11-year-old children revealed that symptoms of bronchial hyperreactivity and wheezing were similar or higher than in Sweden. The diagnosis "asthma" was, however, much more common in Sweden than in Poland and Estonia. Some of the results are summarized in Table 3. The studies show that asthma and bronchial hyperreactivity are common in eastern Europe, but the etiology is not IgE-mediated allergy, as is usually the case for children in Western industrialized countries.

The living conditions in the formerly socialistic countries of Europe are in many respects similar to those that prevailed in western Europe 30–40 years ago, including type of air pollution, panorama of childhood infections and immunizations, building standards, and food. The low prevalence of allergy in these countries supports the general feeling that the prevalence of allergy has increased substantially in the West over the past decades. The nature of the factors associated with the environment and/or changing living conditions is unknown. In all the studies, however, there was an inverse relationship between sensitization and manifestations of allergy, on one hand, and crowded

TABLE 3 Prevalence of Symptoms from the Respiratory Tract and Positive Skin Prick Tests Among 11–12-Year-Old Schoolchildren in Five Locations in the Baltic Sea Region

	Sundsvall, rural	Sweden urban	Poland, Konin	Estonia, Tallinn	Tartu
n	289	351	358	597	637
Respiratory tract symptoms					
Cough after exercise, %	4.1	9.1	8.5	5.7	6.2
Cough >2 weeks, %	5.7	12.0	15.2	18.8	13.8
≤6 infections per year, %	6.3	8.0	14.0	10.4	10.5
Skin prick tests					
≥1 positive, %	24.2	35.3	13.7	12.9	8.3
Crude OR	1	1.71	0.49	0.46[a]	0.28[a]
95% CI		1.2–2.4	0.3–0.7	0.3–0.7	0.2–0.4
Cat, %	12.5	20.9	2.6	6.2	3.6
Timothy, %	13.9	20.0	2.3	4.2	3.6

[a]Odds ratio for ≥1 positive in Tallinn (industrial city) versus Tartu (university town) was 1.81 (95% CI 1.3–2.5).
Source: Data from Refs. 66 and 67.

dwellings and the number of respiratory infections among the children, on the other hand.

These very recent studies in formerly socialistic countries of eastern and central Europe strongly indicate that other factors connected with Western life-style are more important than air pollution for the development of allergy, although the latter also plays an obvious role.

B. Air Pollution

Air pollutants such as ozone, SO_2, and NO_2 may all trigger asthma, as discussed in Chapter 7. They are also associated with increased serum IgE levels, at least in experimental animals (11,68–71). Data are less clear-cut in humans but in an epidemiological survey of 5300 children in Sweden, bronchial hyperreactivity and pollen allergy were both more common in children living near a moderately air-polluting paper factory than among children living in a forested unindustrialized area about 40 km away from the factory (72). If the parents smoked at home, the prevalence of bronchial hyperreactivity and allergy was

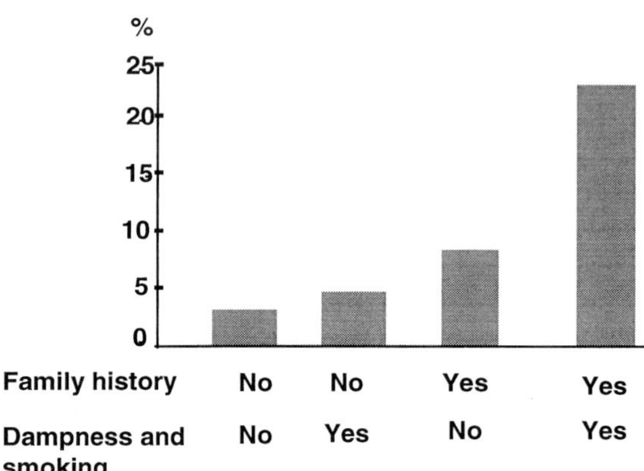

FIGURE 5   Interaction between genetic propensity for asthma (as defined by family history), exposure to tobacco smoke, and increased dampness at home as risk factors for childhood asthma. (Data from Ref. 72.)

further increased, indicating a synergistic effect between the two pollutants (Fig. 5).

As mentioned in the previous section, the prevalence of allergic manifestations is lower in rural than in nearby urban areas in western Europe. The most likely explanation for this is different levels of air pollution. As shown in Table 3, a similar difference was also noted in the formerly Soviet-occupied Estonia. Thus, the prevalence of at least one positive skin prick test was significantly higher in Tallinn, an industrialized coastal city with considerable pollution, than in Tartu, an inland university town.

C. Exposure to Tobacco Smoke

Tobacco smoke is the major indoor air pollutant. Tobacco smoke is strongly associated with allergic sensitization, asthma, and other respiratory diseases. Increased serum IgE levels and an increased prevalence of positive skin tests toward occupational allergens have been shown in numerous studies (14,72–92). Thus, smokers are sensitized more easily to occupational allergens than nonsmokers who are exposed to the allergens to a similar degree.

The effect of tobacco smoke is, however, not limited to active smoking. Children of parents who smoke at home have a significantly earlier onset of allergy, and wheezy bronchitis is about five times more common in them than in children of nonsmoking parents. There is little doubt that exposure to tobacco smoke is the most important environmental risk factor for childhood allergy and respiratory disease that has been identified so far. The long-term effects of childhood exposure to tobacco smoke are unknown.

The effect of tobacco smoke on sensitization to allergens may be explained by a local effect on the airways, or by a direct effect on the immune system. The former notion is supported by the finding that smoking rats exposed to antigen in aerosol develop higher IgE responses than subcutaneously immunized animals and nonsmoking aerosol-immunized controls (93).

In conclusion, passive smoking is by far the best identified risk factor for the development of allergic disease, particularly in early childhood, and this is independent of how "allergy" is defined.

D. Housing

Many children spend at least 90% of their time indoors. It is therefore likely that the indoor environment is even more important than geographical and other macroenvironmental factors. Modern, well-insulated buildings with poor ventilation represent a definite risk factor for allergic sensitization. Many new compounds are used in modern buildings, e.g., plastic material, synthetic paints, and chemical substances with unknown effects on human health. Combined with an efficient insulation and a reduced ventilation, this has created a new indoor climate. In temperate climates, the energy crises and increased interest in energy-conserving measures have resulted in improved building standards, particularly better insulation and reduced ventilation. This in turn has resulted in more "sick buildings," characterized by damage due to dampness, indoor mold growth, and the presence of various symptoms among people dwelling in the houses. At least one well-documented consequence of this is a much increased prevalence of sensitivity to house dust mite allergens in regions with a temperate climate (2,4,5,7). Sensitivity to these allergens used to be rare in a climate with cold and dry winters (1,94), but the creation of a warm and humid "subtropical" indoor climate has changed this.

In an epidemiological survey, it was found that homes with damage due to dampness were associated with both a higher incidence of atopic disease and/or bronchial hyperreactivity in the children. In children living in houses with damage by dampness and whose parents in addition smoked at home, there was a marked increase in allergic asthma and bronchial hyperreactivity, as compared with children exposed to only one of these factors (Fig. 5). The effects of the living conditions were most marked for children with a family history of asthma. This supports the notion that the environmental influences mainly play a particular role in individuals with a genetic susceptibility to allergic disease.

Much more has to be learned about the role of the indoor climate for sensitization and triggering of allergic manifestations. It is, however, reasonable to conclude that a search for environmental factors influencing the development of asthma and allergy should be directed toward factors affecting the indoor climate.

V. PRE- AND PERINATAL RISK FACTORS

As some newborn babies who will develop allergic disease can be identified at birth by an elevated level of IgE in cord blood, the possibility has been discussed that sensitization may take place already during fetal life. This is, however, only rarely the case. The IgE antibodies in cord serum seem more to be the consequence of nonspecific spontaneous IgE synthesis, perhaps lack of suppression, than of antigen stimulation. This notion is supported by the negative outcome of randomized studies of manipulation of the maternal diet during pregnancy (95–98). On the other hand, there are some recent studies, in which antigen-specific T-cell responses were recorded in cord blood (99). These studies did not, however, control for several alternative possibilities and they are therefore not conclusive. The possible importance of intrauterine sensitization therefore remains an open question.

As discussed in Chapter 7, perinatal stress factors are associated with respiratory problems during the first years of life. It has also been suggested that they could increase the risk for sensitization to allergens. These studies (summarized in Ref. 100) were all retrospective, however, and they did not control for various other possibilities. In unpublished studies we could not confirm that prematurity in itself is a risk factor for atopic sensitization.

While there is convincing evidence for an association between exposure to tobacco smoke and childhood allergy, the role of tobacco smoking during pregnancy is less clear. Although there are reports of an association between the two, the studies are still inconclusive owing to their design (101).

Medication with the ß-receptor blocking agent propranolol during pregnancy has been reported to be associated with an increased risk for allergy in the children (102). This observation is interesting, since ß-receptor blockade may enhance IgE antibody formation in animals. The clinical relevance of this observation is limited, however, since the treatment is no longer used during pregnancy.

In conclusion, factors encountered during fetal life are probably not of major importance for the development of asthma and allergy.

VI. EFFECT OF PREVENTIVE MEASURES IN INFANCY

Great interest has been taken over the past 10 years in the possibility of preventing allergic disease, notably asthma, by avoiding primary sensitization in infancy. The efforts have been focused on various procedures to avoid exposure to allergen, including the administration of infant formulae with reduced allergen content and reduction of airborne allergens in the homes of babies.

The original hypothesis for the allergy-preventive efforts was that allergic disease could be avoided by preventing the onset of the "allergic march" in early infancy (Fig. 2). Thus, by preventing the development of food allergy and eczema in early life, the later onset of asthma and then allergic rhinoconjunctivitis would be avoided. Recent prospective studies of infants with a genetic propensity to allergic disease have not confirmed this hypothesis. In these studies, exposure of infants to allergenic foods during the first months of life, notably cow's milk and eggs, was avoided (98,103,104). The mothers of breast-fed babies also adhered to a diet free from cow's milk, eggs, and certain other allergenic foods, as it is well known that nursing infants may be sensitized by minute amounts of foreign proteins that are present in the maternal milk. Any supplementary feeding to the babies was in the form of extensively hydrolyzed products with low allergenicity. The dietary manipulation of breast-feeding mothers for the first 3 months of lactation and the infants for 12 months was associated with a lower incidence of allergic manifestations and demonstrable IgE antibodies to foods. The effect was, however, limited to the first year or possibly 2 years of life and to eczema, while the incidence of respiratory symptoms and later-appearing allergic manifestations was not affected. The results are not surprising in light of the more recent knowledge concerning the primary sensitization discussed in Chapter 10. As discussed in detail in that chapter, experimental studies show that the effects of avoidance of exposure to allergens during the period of particular susceptibility in early life are antigen-specific. Thus, dietary restrictions in infants would not be expected to have an effect on sensitization to inhaled allergens, nor to reduce the incidence of sensitization to any food antigens that are not avoided. The conclusion from a practical point of view would be that the various "hypoallergenic" infant formulae, some of which should not even be regarded as "hypoallergenic" (105), do not represent a major improvement in the search for effective allergy prevention. At best, they would be expected to reduce the incidence of cow's milk allergy in infants, provided truly hypoallergenic preparations are used. To avoid sensitization to other allergens, each of them has to be avoided. Thus, to prevent allergic asthma, all important inhalant allergens and/or adjuvants for sensitization should be avoided. Neither of these goals is easily achieved.

An alternative strategy for primary prevention would be to stimulate tolerance induction in early childhood, as indicated by the recent understanding of the primary immune response to allergens that is discussed in Chapter 10. By this principle, infants at risk for allergy should be identified early in life and then given a high dose of the most important allergens. Such an approach to prevent allergy to inhaled allergens is, however, difficult, as virtually nothing is known about the doses that would be needed in humans or about the optimal mode of administration. Furthermore, the ethical aspects of administration of large amounts of allergens to infants should be carefully considered.

The possible role of maternal diet during pregnancy for the development of allergy has been evaluated in prospective studies comprising families with a history of allergy (95–98). The test diets given to the pregnant women during the last trimester included total avoidance of cow's milk protein and eggs, avoidance of visible amounts of these foods, a normal unrestricted diet, and an unrestricted diet with an intake of at least 1 L of milk and one egg daily. None of the diets had any effects on the incidence of allergic symptoms in the babies or on IgE levels in serum or sensitization, as determined by skin prick tests. Thus, maternal diet during pregnancy does not significantly contribute to the development of allergy, supporting the statement in the previous section that intrauterine sensitization is rare.

In conclusion, avoidance of exposure to tobacco smoke is by far the most important measure to protect young children from the development of sensitization, allergic manifestations, and wheezing. In addition, reduced exposure to potent inhaled allergens may have some effect. Dietary restrictions in infants and their breast-feeding mothers are probably associated with less manifestations of food allergy and infant eczema, but they have no effect on other, later-appearing manifestations of allergic disease.

VII. CONCLUSIONS

Even if it is not conclusively proven, it is likely that the prevalence of atopic disease has increased over the past decades. The likelihood for this to be true is supported by recent studies in formerly socialistic countries of Europe. In these countries the prevalence of allergy is much lower than in western Europe. It is reasonable to suggest that this increase is largely a consequence of changes in the environment that the individual is exposed to early in life, as the life-style in many respects is similar to that in western Europe 30–40 years ago. It is not known whether "Western life-style" is associated with an introduction of new, unknown adjuvants enhancing sensitization, or whether factors necessary for the induction of tolerance have been eliminated. The strategy for primary prevention would be quite different depending on which of these hypotheses is true.

There seems to be a period during which primary sensitization takes place, resulting in allergic manifestations later in life. Although environmental factors undoubtedly play a major role for the development of allergic disease, the mechanisms as well as the individual factors are unknown.

Efforts during infancy toward primary long-term prevention of allergic disease have largely failed and they are probably based on an incorrect hypothesis. It seems likely that avoidance of exposure to allergens is antigen-specific. This means that the avoidance of allergenic foods in infancy would only be expected to result in less allergy to that particular food and not to any reduction of the subsequent "atopic march"; e.g., allergy to inhaled allergens, would not be prevented. Avoidance of certain inhalant allergens, such as house dust mites, for the first years of life may temporarily reduce the incidence of sensitization to that particular antigen. There is, however, no evidence that such avoidance would reduce the general propensity to allergy over a longer time period. Based on recent immunological studies, mainly in experimental animals, an alternative strategy can be envisioned, i.e., an early administration of the most important allergens to induce tolerance. This approach is, however, not yet feasible clinically, as much remains to be learned about doses, routes of administration, and long-term effects in humans.

The only definite measure to reduce the general risk for allergy and asthma is to carefully avoid all exposure of infants and young children to tobacco smoke. The pathogenesis of the atopic sensitization and development of allergic manifestations remains an enigma, although there is considerable circumstantial evidence that the process starts during early childhood, even if clinical symptoms do not appear until later in life.

REFERENCES

1. Turos M. Mites in house dust in the Stockholm area. Allergy 1979; 84:11–18.
2. Wickman M, Nordvall SL, Pershagen G, Sundell J, Schwartz B. House dust mite sensitization in children and residential characteristics in a temperate region. J Allergy Clin Immunol 1991; 88:89–95.
3. Munir A, Einarsson R, Kjellman N-IM, Björkstén B. Mite (Der p I, Der f I) and cat (Fel d I) allergens in homes of babies with a family history of allergy. Allergy 1993; 48:158–163.
4. Munir AKM, Warner A, Ekstrand Tobin A, Kjellman NI-M, Björkstén B. Mite allergen in relation to home conditions and sensitisation of asthmatic children from three climatic zones. Allergy 1995; 50:55–64.
5. Wickman M. Residential characteristics and allergic sensitization in children especially to mites. Medical dissertation, Stockholm, 1993.
6. Sundell J, Andersson B, Andersson K, Lindvall T. Volatile organic compounds in ventilating air at different sampling points in the building and their relationships with the prevalence of occupant symptoms. Indoor Air 1993; 3:82–93.
7. Munir B, Björkstén B. Indoor pollution and allergic sensitisation. In: Knöppel H, Wolkoff P, eds. Chemical Microbiological Health and Comfort: Aspects of Indoor Air Quality. Brussels: ECSC, EEC, 1992:181–199.
8. Abramson M. Air pollution health effects and air quality objectives. Med J Aust 1991; 154:716–717.
9. Åberg N. Asthma and allergic rhinitis in Swedish conscripts. Clin Exp Allergy 1989; 19:59–63.
10. Åberg N, Engström I, Lindberg U. Allergic diseases in Swedish school children. Acta Paediatr Scand 1989; 78:246–252.

11. Holt P. Environmental factors and primary T-cell sensitisation to inhalant allergens in infancy: reappraisal of the role of infections and air pollution. Pediatr Allergy Immunol 1995; 6:1–10.
12. Björkstén B. Risk factors in early childhood for the development of atopic diseases. Allergy 1994; 49:400–407.
13. Kjellman N-IM, Croner S, Fälth Magnusson K, Odelram H, Björkstén B. Prediction of allergy in infancy. Allergy Proc 1991; 12:245–249.
14. Foucard T, Sjöberg O. A prospective 12-year follow-up study of children with wheezy bronchitis. Acta Paediatr Scand 1984; 73:577–583.
15. Kjellman N-IM. Atopic disease in seven-year-old children: incidence in relation to family history. Acta Paediatr Scand 1977; 66:465–471.
16. Croner S, Kjellman N-IM. Development of atopic disease in relation to family history and cord blood IgE levels: eleven-year follow-up in 1654 children. Pediatr Allergy Immunol 1990; 1:14–20.
17. Zetterström O, Johansson S. IgE concentrations measured by PRIST® in serum of healthy adults and in patients with respiratory allergy: a diangostic approach. Allergy 1981; 63:537–543.
18. Johansson S, Bennich H, Berg T. The clinical significance of IgE. Clin Immunol 1972; 1:157–163.
19. van Asperen PP, Kemp AS. The natural history of IgE sensitization and atopic disease in early childhood. Acta Paediatr Scand 1989; 78:239–245.
20. Hattevig G, Kjellman B, Björkstén B, Johansson SGO. The prevalence of allergy and IgE antibodies to inhalant allergens in Swedish school children. Acta Paediatr Scand 1987; 76:349–355.
21. Hattevig G, Kjellman B, Björkstén B. Appearance of IgE antibodies to ingested and inhaled allergens during first 12 years of life in atopic and non-atopic children. Pediatr Allergy Immunol 1993; 4:182–189.
22. Kjellman N-IM. IgE determination in neonates is not suitable for general screening. Pediatr Allergy Immunol 1994; 5:1–4.
23. Kjellman N-IM, Johansson SGO. IgE and atopic allergy in newborns and infants with a family history of atopic disease. Acta Paediatr Scand 1976; 65:601–607.
24. Croner S, Kjellman N-IM, Eriksson B, Roth A. IgE screening in 1701 newborn infants and the development of atopic disease during infancy. Arch Dis Child 1982; 57:364–368.
25. Michel FB, Bousquet J, Greiller P, Robinet-Levy M, Coulomb Y. Comparison of cord blood immunoglobulin E concentrations and maternal allergy for the prediction of atopic disease in infancy. J Allergy Clin Immunol 1980; 65:422–430.
26. Vassella C, Odelram H, Kjellman N-I, Borres M, Vanto T, Björkstén B. High anti-IgE levels at birth are associated with a reduced allergy incidence in early childhood. Clin Exp Allergy 1994; 24:771–777.
27. Björkstén B, Kjellman N-IM. Immunological abnormalities in atopic infants. Allergologie 1989; 12S:176–179.
28. Heiner D. IgE in colostrum, maternal blood, cord blood and amniotic fluid. In: Proc XI International Congress of Allergology and Clinical Immunology. London: Macmillan, 1983:149–150.

29. Heskel NS, Chan SC, Thiel ML, Stevens SR, Casperson LS, Hanifin JM. Elevated umbilical cord blood leukocyte cyclic adenosine monophosphate–phosphodiesterase activity in children with atopic parents. J Am Acad Dermatol 1984; 11:422–426.
30. Odelram H, Björkstén B, Chan SC, Hanifin J, Kjellman N-IM. Neonatal leukocyte cAMP-phosphodiesterase determination is not suitable for allergy prediction. Allergy 1994; 49:677–679.
31. Miadonna A, Tedeschi A, Leggieri E, et al. Cord blood basophil releasability: a predictive marker for allergy? Allerg Immunol (Paris) 1988; 20:45–47.
32. Borres MP. Metachromatic cells and eosinophils in atopic children: a prospective study. Pediatr Allergy Immunol 1991; 2(Suppl):1–24.
33. Foucard T. A follow-up study of children with asthmatoid bronchitis. II. Serum IgE and eosinophil counts in relation to clinical course. Acta Paediatr Scand 1974; 63:129–139.
34. Björkstén F, Suoniemi I, Koski V. Neonatal birch-pollen contact and subsequent allergy to birch pollen. Clin Allergy 1980; 10:585–591.
35. Sporik R, Holgate ST, Platts-Mills TA, Cogswell JJ. Exposure to house-dust mite allergen (Der p I) and the development of asthma in childhood: a prospective study. N Engl J Med 1990; 323:502–507.
36. Björkstén F, Suoniemi I. Time and intensity of first pollen contacts and risk of subsequent pollen allergies. Acta Med Scand 1981; 209:299–303.
37. Morrison-Smith J, Springett VH. Atopic disease and month of birth. Clin Allergy 1979; 9:153–157.
38. Settipane R, Hagy G. Effect of atmospheric pollen on the newborn. Rhode Island Med J 1979; 62:477–482.
39. Croner S, Kjellman N-IM. Predictors of atopic disease: cord blood IgE and month of birth. Allergy 1986; 41:68–70.
40. Björkstén F, Suoniemi I. Early allergen contacts, adjuvant factors and subsequent allergy. In: Kern JW, Ganderton MA, eds. Proc. of the XI International Congress of Allergology and Clinical Immunology. London: Macmillan, 1983:144–148.
41. Zetterström O, Osterman K, Machado L, Johansson SGO. Another smoking hazard: raised serum IgE concentration and increased risk of occupational allergy. Br Med J 1981; 283:1215–1217.
42. Welliver R, Wong D, Sun M, Middleton E, Vaughan R, Ogra P. The development of respiratory syncytial virus-specific IgE and the release of histamine in nasopharyngeal secretions after infection. N Engl J Med 1981; 305:841–846.
43. Frick OL, Brooks DL. Immunoglobulin E antibodies to pollens augmented in dogs by virus vaccines. Am J Vet Res 1983; 44:440–445.
44. Holt P, Vines J, Bilyk N. Effect of influenza virus infection on allergic sensitization to inhaled antigen in mice. Int Arch Allergy Appl Immunol 1988; 86:121–123.
45. von Mutius E, Fritzsch C, Weiland SK, Röll G, Magnussen H. Prevalence of asthma and allergic disorders among children in united Germany: a descriptive comparison. Br Med J 1992; 305:1395–1399.
46. von Mutius E, Martinez FD, Fritzsch C, Nicolai T, Roell G, Thiemann HH. Prevalence of asthma and atopy in two areas of West and East Germany. Am J Respir Crit Care Med 1994; 149:358–364.

47. Bråbäck L, Breborowicz A, Dreborg S, Knutsson A, Pieklik H, Björkstén B. Atopic sensitization and respiratory symptoms among Polish and Swedish schoolchildren. Clin Exp Allergy 1994; 24:826–835.

47a. Strachan D. Hay fever, hygiene and household size. Br Med J 1989; 289:1259–1260.

47b. Strachan D. Epidemiology of hay fever: towards a community diagnosis. Clin Exp Allergy 1995; 25:296–303.

48. Pauwels R, van der Straeten M, Platteu B, Bazin H. The nonspecific enhancement of allergy: in vitro effects of *Bordetella pertussis* vaccine on IgE synthesis. Allergy 1983; 38:239–246.

49. Schuster A, Hofman A, Reinhardt D. Does pertussis infection induce manifestations of allergy? Clin Invest 1993; 71:208–213.

50. Blennow M, Granström M, Björkstén B. Immunoglobulin E response to pertussis toxin after vaccination with acellular pertussis vaccine. In: Manclark CR, ed. Proceedings of the Sixth International Symposium on Pertussis. Bethesda, MD: Department of Health and Human Services, United States Public Health Service, 1990:184–188.

51. Hedenskog S, Björkstén B, Blennow M, Granström G, Granström M. Immunoglobulin E response to pertussis toxin in whooping cough and after immunization with a whole-cell and an acellular pertussis vaccine. Int Arch Allergy Appl Immunol 1989; 89:156–161.

52. Pauwels R, Bazin H, Platteau B, Van Der Straeten M. The influence of different adjuvants on the production of IgD and IgE antibodies. Ann Immunol 1979; 130C:49–58.

53. Husband A, King M, Brown R. Behaviourally conditioned modification of T cell subset ratios in rats. Immunol Lett 1987; 14:91–94.

54. King M, Husband A, Kusnecov. Behavioural conditioning of the immune system: from laboratory to clinical application. In: Sheppard J, ed. Advances in Behavioural Medicine. Sydney: Cumberland College of Health Sciences, 1987:110–117, Vol. 4.

55. Jemmott JI, Borysenko J, Borysenko M, et al. Academic stress, power motivation, and decrease in secretion rate of salivary secretory immunoglobulin A. Lancet 1983; 1:1400–1402.

56. Depression, stress and immunity. Lancet 1987; 1:1467–1468.

57. Gustafsson PA, Kjellman N-IM, Cederblad M. Family therapy in the treatment of severe childhood asthma. J Psychosom Res 1986; 30:369–374.

58. Gustafsson PA, Kjellman N-IM, Ludvigsson J, Cederblad M. Asthma and family interaction. Arch Dis Child 1987; 62:258–263.

59. Gustafsson PA, Björkstén B, Kjellman N-IM. Family dysfunction in asthma—a prospective study of illness development. J Pediatr 1994; 49:508–516.

60. Burr ML. Epidemiology of clinical allergy. In: Hansson L-Å, Shakib F, eds. Monographs in Allergy. Basel: Karger, 1993:130–145, Vol 31.

61. Morrison Smith J. Skin tests and atopic allergy in children. Clin Allergy 1973; 3:269–275.

62. Morrison Smith J, Harding L, Cumming G. The changing prevalence of asthma in school children. Clin Allergy 1971; 1:57–61.

63. van Niekerk C, Weinberg E, Shore S, de V Heese H, van Schalkwyk D. Prevalence of asthma: a comparative study of urban and rural Xhosa children. Clin Allergy 1979; 9:319–324.
64. Bråbäck L, Kälvesten L. Urban living as a risk factor for atopic sensitization in Swedish schoolchildren. Pediatr Allergy Immunol 1991; 2:14–19.
65. von Mutius E, Martinez FD, Fritzsch C, Nicolai T, Reitmeir P, Thiemann HH. Skin test reactivity and number of siblings. Br Med J 1994; 308:692–695.
66. Bråbäck L, Breborowicz, Julge K, Knutsson A, Riikjärv M-A, Vasar M, Björkstén B. Risk factors for respiratory symptoms and atopic sensitization in the Baltic area. Arch Dis Child 1995; 72:487–493.
67. Riikjärv MA, Julge K, Vasar M, Bråbäck L, Knutsson A, Björkstén B. The prevalence of atopic sensitization and respiratory symptoms among Estonian schoolchildren. Clin Exp Allergy 1995; 25:1198–1204.
68. Osebold J, Chung Zee Y, Gershwin L. Enhancement of allergic lung sensitization in mice by ozone inhalation. Proc Soc Exp Biol Med 1988; 188:259–264.
69. Holt P, McMenamin C. Defence against allergic sensitization in the healthy lung: the role of inhalation tolerance. Clin Exp Allergy 1989; 19:255–262.
70. Holt P. Immune and inflammatory function in cigarette smokers. Thorax 1987; 42: 241–249.
71. Nilsson L, Björkstén B, ed. Factors which promote or prevent allergy. In: Burr ML, ed. Epidemiology of Clinical Allergy. Monogr Allergy 1993; 31:190–210.
72. Andrae S, Axelson O, Björkstén B, Fredriksson M, Kjellman N-IM. Symptoms of bronchial hyperreactivity and asthma in relation to environmental factors. Arch Dis Child 1988; 63:473–478.
73. Arshad SH, Matthews S, Gant C, Hide DW. Effect of allergen avoidance on development of allergic disorders in infancy. Lancet 1992; 339:1493–1497.
74. Barbee RA, Halonen M, Kaltenborn W, Lebowitz M, Burrows B. A longitudinal study of serum IgE in a community cohort: correlations with age, sex, smoking, and atopic status. J Allergy Clin Immunol 1987; 79:919–927.
75. Brunekreef B, Groot B, Hoek G. Pets, allergy and respiratory symptoms in children. Int J Epidemiol 1992; 2:338–342.
76. Burr ML, Miskelly FG, Butland BK, Merrett TG, Vaughan WE. Environmental factors and symptoms in infants at high risk of allergy. J Epidemiol Commun Health 1989; 43:125–132.
77. Cogswell JJ, Mitchell EB, Alexander J. Parental smoking, breast feeding and respiratory infection in development of allergic disease. Arch Dis Child 1987; 62: 338–344.
78. Dahlström A, Lundell B, Curvall M, Thapper L. Nicotine and cotinine concentrations in the nursing mother and her infant. Acta Pædiatr Scand 1990; 79:142–147.
79. Ekwo E, Weinberger M, Lachenbruch P, Huntley W. Relationship of parental smoking and gas cooking in respiratory disease in children. Chest 1983; 84:662–668.
80. Fergusson D, Horwood L, Shannon F. Parental smoking and respiratory illness in infancy. Arch Dis Child 1980; 55:358–361.
81. Frischer T, Kuehr J, Meinert R, et al. Maternal smoking in early childhood: a risk factor for bronchial responsiveness to exercise in primary-school children. J Pediatr 1992; 121:17–22.

82. Gortmaker SL, Klein Walker D, Jacobs F, Ruch-Ross H. Parental smoking and the risk for childhood asthma. Am J Public health 1982; 72:574–579.

83. Halonen M, Barbree R, Lebowitz M, Burrows B. An epidemiological study of the relationship of the total serum immunoglobulin IgE, allergy skin-test reactivity and eosinophilia. J Allergy Clin Immunol 1982; 69:221–228.

84. Halken S, Høst A, Husby S, Hansen LG, Østerballe O, Nyboe J. Recurrent wheezing in relation to environmental risk factors in infancy. Allergy 1991; 46:507–514.

85. Kunz B, J R, Dirschedl P. Effect of maternal smoking during pregnancy on the development of atopic disease in the child. J Invest Dermatol 1989; 92:465.

86. Landau L. Smoking and childhood asthma. Med J Aust 1991; 154:715–716.

87. Martinez F, Antognoni G, Macri F, et al. Parental smoking enhances bronchial responsiveness in nine-year-old children. Am Rev Respir Dis 1988; 138:518–523.

88. Murray A, Morrison B. The effect of cigarette smoke from the mother on bronchial responsiveness and severity of symptoms in children with asthma. J Allergy Clin Immunol 1986; 77:575–581.

89. Murray A, Morrison B. Passive smoking and the seasonal difference in severity of asthma in children. Chest 1988; 94:701–708.

90. Ronchetti R, Macri F, Ciofetta G, et al. Increased serum IgE and increased prevalence of eosinophilia in 9-year-old children of smoking parents. J Allergy Clin Immunol 1990; 86:400–407.

91. Rugtveit J. Environmental factors in the first months of life and the possible relationship to later development of hypersensitivity. Allergy 1990; 45:154–156.

92. Sennhauser FH, Guntert BJ. Prevalence of bronchial asthma in childhood in Switzerland: significance of symptoms and diagnosis. Schweiz Med Wochenschr 1992; 122:189–193.

93. Zetterström O, Nordvall SL, Björkstén B, Ahlstedt S, Stelander M. Increased IgE antibody responses in rats exposed to tobacco smoke. J Allergy Clin Immunol 1985; 75:594–598.

94. Nordvall S, Eriksson M, Rylander E, Schwartz B. Sensitization of children in the Stockholm area to house dust mite. Acta Paediatr Scand 1988; 77:716–720.

95. Fälth-Magnusson K, Öman H, Kjellman N-IM. Maternal abstention from cow milk and egg in allergy risk pregnancies: effect on antibody production in the mother and the newborn. Allergy 1987; 42:64–73.

96. Fälth-Magnusson K, Kjellman N-IM. Allergy prevention by maternal elimination diet during late pregnancy—a 5-year follow-up of a randomized study. J Allergy Clin Immunol 1992; 89:709–713.

97. Lilja G, Dannæus A, Foucard T, Graff-Lonnevig V, Johansson S, Öman H. Effects of maternal diet during late pregnancy and lactation on the development of atopic diseases in infants up to eighteen months of age—in vivo results. Clin Exp Allergy 1989; 19:473–479.

98. Zeiger R, Heller S, Mellon M, Helsey J, Hamburger R, Sampson H. Genetic and environmental factors affecting the development of atopy through age 4 in children of atopic parents: a prospective randomized study of food allergen avoidance. Pediatr Allergy Immunol 1992; 3:110–127.

99. Tang M, Kemp A, Thorburn J, Hill D. Reduced IFNg secretion in neonates and subsequent development of atopy. Lancet 1995; 344:983–985.

100. Björkstén B, Kjellman N-IM. Perinatal factors influencing the development of allergy. Clin Rev Allergy 1987; 5:339–347.
101. Magnusson CG. Cord serum IgE in relation to family history and as predictor of atopic disease in early infancy. Allergy 1988; 43:241–251.
102. Björkstén B, Finnström O, Wichman K. Intrauterine exposure to the beta-adrenergic receptor-blocking agent metoprolol and allergy. Int Arch Allergy Appl Immunol 1988; 87:59–62.
103. Hattevig G, Kjellman B, Sigurs N, Björkstén B, Kjellman N-IM. Effect of maternal avoidance of eggs, cow's milk and fish during lactation upon allergic manifestations in infants. Clin Exp Allergy 1989; 19:27–32.
104. Hattevig G, Kjellman B, Sigurs N, Grodzinsky E, Hed J, Björkstén B. The effect of maternal avoidance of eggs, cow's milk, and fish during lactation on the development of IgE, IgG, and IgA antibodies in infants. J Allergy Clin Immunol 1990; 85:108–115.
105. Businco L, Dreborg S, Einarsson R, et al. Hydrolysed cow's milk formulae: allergenicity and use in treatment and prevention: an ESPACI position paper. Pediatr Allergy Immunol 1993; 4:101–111.

9

Specific Immune Responses to Purified Allergens

David G. Marsh, Thorunn Rafnar, Balaram Ghosh, and Shau-Ku Huang
Johns Hopkins Asthma and Allergy Center
Johns Hopkins University School of Medicine
Baltimore, Maryland

I. INTRODUCTION

This chapter presents a resume of the current status of our knowledge of the molecular genetic basis of specific immune responsiveness to inhaled allergens, focusing on a group of model allergens, the Amb 5 homologs from various species of ragweed pollen. Most allergenic complexes, such as pollen grains, contain large numbers of components that have been shown to be antigenic in animals. Figure 1 presents a crossed immunoelectrophoretic (CIE) analysis of short ragweed (*Ambrosia artemisiifolia*) pollen extract and emphasizes the complexity of the antigenic profile within a single matrix. Through this and other studies, we have found that more than 60 distinct antigens (Ags) can be detected in ragweed pollen extracts using hyperimmune animal antisera (1,2). Of these, we found at least 22 components to be allergenic by crossed radioimmunoelectrophoretic (CRIE) analysis of a group of 37 ragweed-allergic subjects (3). Importantly, the sera of different ragweed-allergic sub-

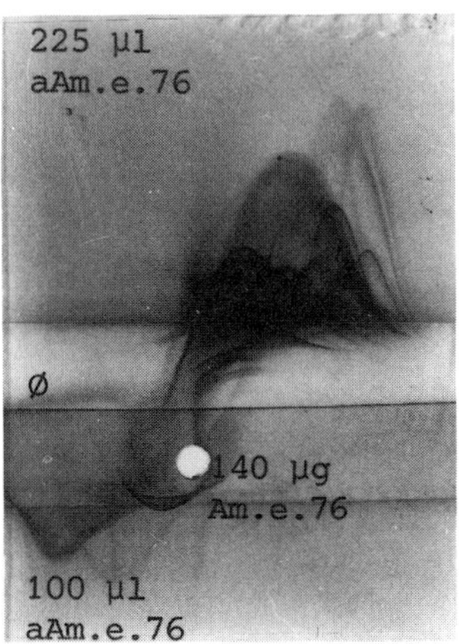

FIGURE 1   CIE analysis of a whole extract of short ragweed (*Ambrosia artemisiifolia*) pollen (Am.e. 76) against a hyperimmune rabbit antiserum pool (aAm.e. 76) raised toward the whole pollen extract. The extract was separated by agarose gel electrophoresis in the first dimension (anode to the right) and by electrophoresis into an agarose gel containing the antibody in the second dimension (anode at the top).

jects were found to contain detectable IgE antibodies (Abs) toward different combinations of these Ags. These and other studies show that individual atopic subjects possess characteristic differences in their "allergic fingerprints" toward the various ragweed components (4,5). Based on considerations to be discussed below, it seems probable that the immune recognition of these ragweed components will be more complex, in that a number of different epitopes (and combinations of epitopes) will be recognized by different individuals' immune systems, at both the T- and B-cell levels. We believe that this immune recognition is determined by the complex interaction of numerous genetic and environmental factors (5–9).

II. MOLECULAR BASIS OF IMMUNE RECOGNITION

We have been studying two aspects of the genetic control of immune responsiveness to inhaled allergens, namely, overall IgE production and specific IgE Ab responsiveness (5–9). We will focus on specific immune responsiveness and, particularly, how genes of the *HLA-D* region of the human major histocompatibility complex (MHC) determine this responsiveness. One of the early events in the induction of a specific IgE Ab response involves the interaction of a B cell with an inhaled Ag via its specific surface Ab receptor. The resultant Ag-Ab complex is endocytosed and the Ag is "processed" (i.e., broken down by enzymatic degradation) into peptides. One of these peptide "T-cell epitopes" may bind with sufficient affinity to a compatible *HLA-D*-encoded class II molecule within the endosomal compartment of the B cell, resulting in a

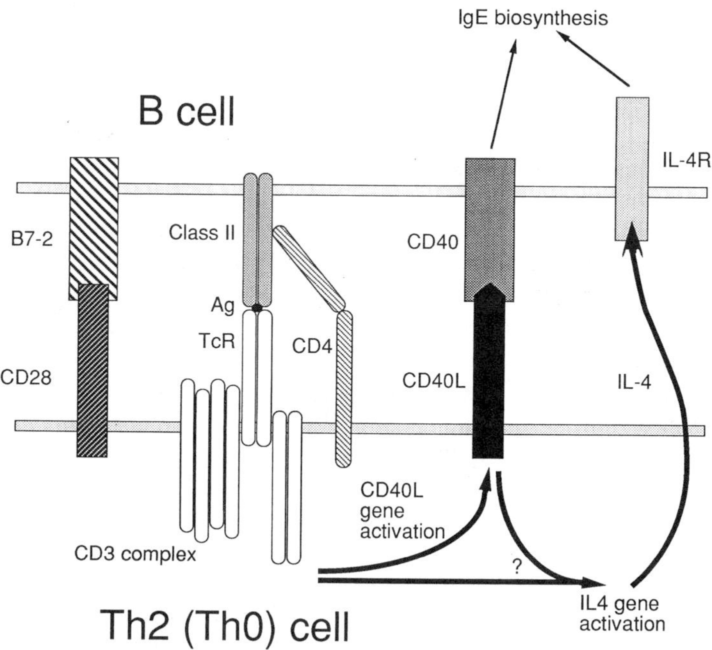

FIGURE 2   Schematic representation of the cellular events that may lead to a specific IgE Ab response. Not shown: The allergen interacts with a specific immunoglobulin molecule on the surface of a B cell and is "processed" into peptides within the endosomal compartment of the B cell, where it interacts with a compatible MHC class II molecule. Shown: The class II molecule, along with the associated antigen fragment (Ag), is transported to the surface of the B cell where the class II–Ag complex interacts with a specific TcR on a Th2 (or Th0) cell. This interaction initiates a series of signaling events that lead to the expression of cell-surface molecules CD28 and CD40L. These molecules interact with their receptors on the B cell, thereby facilitating T-cell activation. The activation, transcription, and translation of the IL-4 gene result from these activation steps (via mechanisms not yet clearly understood). IL-4, released from the T cell, interacts with the IL-4R on the B cell and leads to one of the two signals necessary for IgE biosynthesis. The second signal results from the interaction of CD40L with CD40.

stable class II–Ag fragment complex. This complex is then transported to the cell surface where it interacts with a high-affinity T-cell receptor (TcR) on a helper T cell (Fig. 2). The type of T cell normally involved in the allergic response is a Th2 (or Th0) cell, which is capable of secreting the cytokine IL-4 (10). The release of IL-4 from the T cell induces the immunoglobulin production (within the interacting B cell) to be switched to IgE (11). This process eventually leads to a specific IgE Ab response against the Ab originally endocytosed by the B cell (see legend to Fig. 2 and Refs. 10–12 for further details).

III. RATIONALE

In general, low-molecular-weight allergens would be expected to produce fewer peptides compatible with available class II molecules than high-molecular-weight allergens. Thus, one might anticipate that immune responsiveness to high-molecular-weight allergens would be more complex and could potentially involve interactions of allergen peptides with several different class II molecules in different atopic subjects. Conversely, responsiveness to very-low-molecular-weight allergens could potentially involve a single major T-cell epitope interacting with a single class II molecule. Thus, to analyze the molecular basis of immune responsiveness in the outbred human population, we have elected to use a series of low-molecular-weight "model" allergens that have either a single major T-cell epitope or a very limited number of epitopes.

To understand further the molecular basis of specific atopic responsiveness, it is appropriate to analyze the different trimolecular complexes comprising class II molecules, Ag fragments, and TcRs that are involved in the initiation of specific immune responses to a wide array of allergens. For analysis of the molecular basis of class II molecular interaction, we have investigated the sequences of the various polymorphic *HLA-D* genes that encode the α chains and β chains of class II molecules that are implicated in Ag presentation, namely,

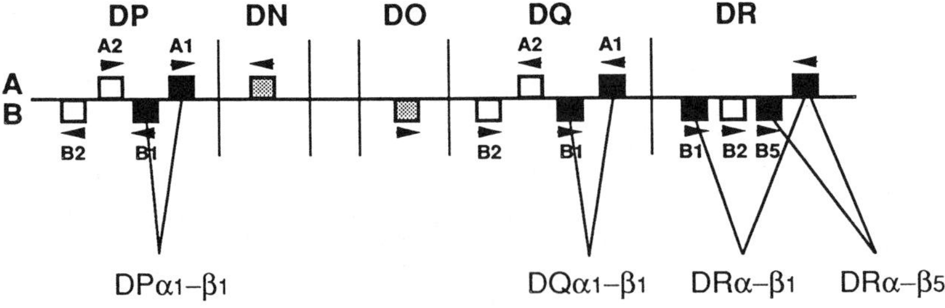

FIGURE 3   MHC class II molecules expressed by HLA-DR2 haplotypes.

TABLE 1 Associations of HLA with Specific Antibody Responsiveness Toward Highly Purified Amb 5 Ragweed Pollen Allergens Atopic for U.S. Caucasoid Subjects Living in the Baltimore Area

Allergen	M_r	Major HLA Association	Westinghouse subjects[a]		Clinic patients		Overall p values[c]
			+ve[b]	–ve[b]	+ve	–ve	
Amb a V	5000	DR2/Dw2	9/9 (100%)	20/83 (24%)	27/29 (93%)	10/56 (18%)	$<10^{-9}$
Amb t V	4400	DR2/Dw2	3/4 (75%)	0/13 (0%)	3/3 (100%)	1/7 (14%)	$<10^{-3}$

[a]Atopic subjects from an epidemiologic study of 92 Westinghouse Electric Corporation employees.
[b]Positive (+ve) or negative (–ve) with respect to the patient having detectable serum IgE Ab prior to immunotherapy, except in the case of *Amb t* V where the data refer to serum IgG Ab in patients who had received immunotherapy with extracts containing giant ragweed in the past.
[c]p values by Fisher's exact test for analysis of the combined groups of Westinghouse and clinic subjects.

HLA-DR β, DQα, DQβ, DPα, and DPβ (Fig. 3): DRα need not be studied since it is nonpolymorphic. Then, we have examined the specific Ag peptide sequences that interact with both the class II molecule and the TcR. Third, we are in the process of determining the sequences of the TcR α and β chains that bind to the specific Class II–Ag fragment complex. Finally, we feel that it will be appropriate to investigate the three-dimensional (3D) structures of the class II–Ag and class II–Ag–TcR complexes to clarify the molecular basis of the interactions. Such analyses are now feasible, based on the recent studies of Wiley and his collaborators (13), who have obtained crystalline structures of class II molecules bound to specific Ag fragments.

IV. ANALYSIS OF MHC CLASS II MOLECULES INVOLVED IN ANTIGEN PRESENTATION

In unrelated allergic subjects, we have analyzed the statistical associations between specific Ab responsiveness (primarily IgE) and specific HLA-D types. Our early observations (2,14,15) and similar findings of other laboratories (16–18) showed striking associations between HLA-DR2 and Dw2* (DR2.2) and immune responsiveness to Amb a 5 from short ragweed pollen (Table 1). Amb 5 and its homologs from other ragweed species are the smallest pollen allergens that have been defined to date. They each contain single basically charged

---

*The mixed lymphocyte reaction (MLR) specificity most commonly associated with HLA-DR2 in Caucasian populations.

polypeptide chains (Mr = 4400–5000) containing 40–45 amino acids with no detectable carbohydrate or lipid (15,16,19). The most common variants contain eight cysteine residues, all of which are disulfide-bonded. Genetic analysis of immune responsiveness to Amb t 5 and Amb p 5 (from giant and western ragweeds, respectively) also revealed significant associations with DR2.2 (15,16, 20; Table 1). These consistent DR2.2 associations with responsiveness to all three Amb 5 species suggest that single, related major T-cell epitopes/agretopes are present on the different Amb 5 molecules. Furthermore, these findings also suggested that the Amb 5 homologs would provide the first simple model allergens for molecular and cellular analysis of the human immune response.

For further analysis of the HLA-D specificities involved in responsiveness to the Amb 5 homologs, we amplified the polymorphic second exons of the *HLA-D* genes in responder and nonresponder subjects using the polymerase chain reaction (PCR). We employed sequence-specific oligonucleotides (SSOs) and dot-blot analysis, as well as sequencing, to examine the regions of the *HLA-D* genes that encode the Ag-binding regions of the class II molecules (21,22). This allowed us to define more precisely the HLA class II specificity likely to be involved in "presenting" the major T-cell epitopes of the Amb 5 molecules to specific TcRs. Our analyses showed that, in Caucasians, the most likely candidate was a class II molecule encoded either by DRA and DRB1 or by DRA and DRB5 genes of *DR2.2*. These particular class II molecules are known as DR(α,β1*1501) and DR(α,β5*0101), respectively.

To investigate further which class II molecule is actually involved in the presentation of the major Amb a 5 peptide epitope, we isolated a series of Amb a 5–specific human T-cell clones from Amb a 5–atopic subjects having the DR2.2 phenotype (23). These T cells express Th2-associated cytokines and are able to induce Amb a 5–specific IgE synthesis in vitro (23a). In experiments using Amb a 5 and DR2.2$^+$ Ag-presenting cells (APCs), all of these clones showed clear evidence of Amb a 5–induced proliferation. (Representative experiments using three clones from DR2.2$^+$ subject AP are shown in Fig. 4.) When monoclonal Abs (MAbs) directed against HLA-DQ or DP were included in the stimulation assays, we found no evidence of inhibition of T-cell proliferation relative to the Ag control (Fig. 4a and b). However, with the addition of a MAb to DR, there was clear evidence of inhibition. These experiments confirmed that an HLA-DR molecule is involved in the presentation of Amb a 5 to the T cells. To resolve the issue of whether the DR $\alpha\beta$5 class II molecule was involved, we used MAb Hu30, which is specific for DR($\alpha\beta$1*15) groups [(DRα,β1*1501) and DR(α,β1*1502)].* This MAb strongly inhibited

---

*DR(α,β1*1502) is associated with DR2 and with the MLR typing Dw12. This specificity is found more commonly in Orientals than in Caucasians.

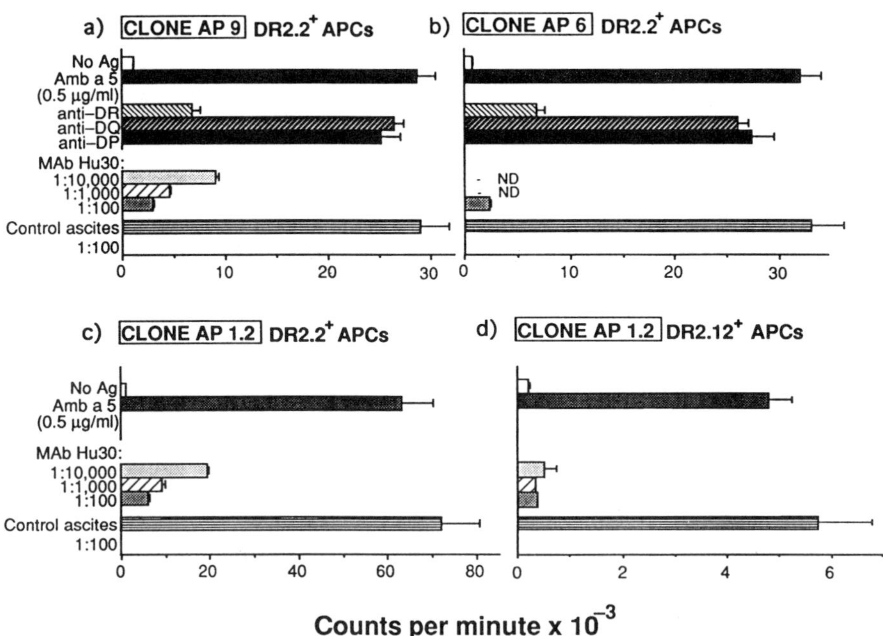

FIGURE 4   Inhibition of Amb a 5–induced proliferation of human T-cell clones AP9, AP6, and AP1.2 by anti-HLA-DR, DQ, and DP MAbs. MAb Hu30, which is specific for the DR(α,β1*1501) and DR(α,β1*1502) class II molecules, was also used in all experiments. T-cell proliferation was measured by the uptake of ^{3}H-thymidine. Autologous APCs from the HLA-DR2.2$^+$ donor were used in experiments a, b, and c; APCs from an HLA-DR2.12 donor were used for experiment d. (From Ref. 23 with permission of the copyright owners.)

T-cell proliferation (Fig. 4a, b, and c), clearly showing that the DR$\alpha$$\beta$1 molecule is involved in Amb a 5 presentation to these T-cell clones.

Further experiments using DR2.12 cells from another donor as APCs showed that DR(α,β1*1502) is also able to present Amb a 5 to the T-cell clones, and that T-cell stimulation in this case could be also be inhibited by Hu30 (Fig. 4d). However, the class II molecules of other HLA-DR2 subspecificities DR(α,β1*1601) and DR(α,β1*1602), that are associated with Dw21 and Dw22 MLR types, respectively, were unable to present Amb a 5 to these T-cell clones (23). The only difference between DR(α,β1*1501) and DR(α,β1*1502) is at position 86 of the respective β1 polypeptides where there is a valine-to-glycine difference (Fig. 5). However, for the other two DR2 β1 specificities, 1601 and 1602 (associated with DR2.21 and DR2.22, respectively),

	DRβ1			
Amino Acid Residue	**1501 (DR2.2)**	**1502 (2.12)**	**1601 (2.21)**	**1602 (2.22)**
67	Ile	Ile	Phe	Leu
70	Gln	Gln	Asp⁻	Asp⁻
71	Ala	Ala	Arg⁺	Arg⁺
86	Val	Gly	Gly	Gly

FIGURE 5   The various amino acid residues within HLA-DRβ1 subtypes. Positively or negatively charged residues (at neutral pH) are indicated.

there are differences at residues 67, 70, and 71: notably, two neutral amino acid residues at positions 70 and 71 (glutamine and alanine) are replaced by two charged residues (aspartic acid and arginine, respectively). Thus, it would appear that certain amino acid residues in the β-polypeptide chain of class II molecules are critical in determining immune responsiveness versus nonresponsiveness to Amb a 5. Further experiments using Amb t 5 and Amb p 5 as inhibitors of Amb a 5–induced T-cell proliferation of these clones suggested that responsiveness to these Amb 5 homologs is also determined by this same structural requirement (24).

V. ANALYSIS OF T-CELL EPITOPES

We have used the aforementioned Amb a 5–specific human T-cell clones primarily for the analysis of Amb a 5 T-cell epitopes (24,25). Three Amb 5 homologs, Amb a 5, Amb t 5, and Amb p 5, were used in these experiments (sequences of representative isoforms of these allergens are shown in Fig. 6). We found that Amb t 5 and Amb p 5 were not able to stimulate the T-cell clones directly, but were able to inhibit, in a dose-dependent manner, the stimulation of the T cells by Amb a 5 (24). These findings suggest that the T-cell-binding portions of the epitopes of the Amb t 5 and Amb p 5 molecules are different, whereas the ability to inhibit suggests that the portions of these epitopes that bind to the class II molecule (the so-called "agretopes") are similar. To define the epitopes more precisely, Huang and Marsh (24) synthesized a series of synthetic peptides that were derived from overlapping regions of the Amb a 5 sequence, but where alanine residues replaced the cysteine residues. Each of these peptides was tested for its ability to stimulate the Amb a 5–specific T cells directly, or to inhibit the stimulation of these cells by Amb a 5. The results of these studies indicated that a peptide spanning amino acids 31–44 in Amb a 5 was able to block presentation of Amb a 5 to the T cells but could not stimulate the T cells directly. This result suggests that the alanine-substituted peptide can bind to DR(α,β1*1501) and that either the cysteine

```
                   1           5              10              15
Amb a 5.0101:    L  L  P  C  A  W  A  G  N  V  C  G  E  K  R
Amb p 5.0203:    V  M  A  C  Y  A  A  G  S  I  C  G  E  K  R
Amb t 5:      D  D  G  L  C  Y  -  E  G  T  N  C  G  K  V  G

                   16          20             25              30
Amb a 5.0101:    A  Y  C  C  S  D  P  G  R  Y  C  P  W  Q  V
Amb p 5.0203:    G  Y  C  C  T  N  P  G  R  Y  C  P  W  Q  V
Amb t 5:         K  Y  C  C  S  P  I  G  K  Y  C  -  -  -  -

                   31          35             40              45
Amb a 5.0101:    V  C  Y  E  S  S  E  I  C  S  K  K  C  G  K
Amb p 5.0203:    V  C  Y  E  S  R  K  I  C  A  K  N  A  A  K
Amb t 5:         V  C  Y  D  S  K  A  I  C  N  K  N  C  T
```

FIGURE 6 Comparison of the sequences of common forms of three Amb 5 homologs, Amb a 5 (variant 0101, formerly *Amb a* VA1), Amb t 5 (formerly *Amb t* V) and Amb p 5 (variant 0203, formerly *Amb p* VB3). Amino acid residues in Amb p 5.0203, and Amb t 5 that are identical to those in Amb a 5.0101 are shown in bold. Residues that are identical or closely similar are boxed. (See Refs. 15, 16, 19, and 26–28 for details.) The allergen nomenclature is as recommended by the Allergen Nomenclature Sub-Committee (37).

residues are required for T-cell recognition or a part of the T-cell epitope lies N-terminally to the peptide. More recently, a second synthetic peptide (without alanine substitutions), which spans amino acid residues 26–39 of Amb a 5, was found to stimulate the Amb a 5–specific T-cell clones to an extent equal to or greater than the native molecule (25). Taken together, these results indicate that at least one of the Amb a 5 residues between positions 26 and 30 is crucial for T-cell recognition. Comparison of the amino acid sequence of Amb a 5 with that of Amb t 5 (which cannot stimulate the Amb a 5-specific T cells) supports this hypothesis (Fig. 6), especially since amino acids 27–30 in Amb a 5 have no counterparts in Amb t 5. At present, we are trying to determine exactly which amino acid residues are critical for binding to the DR(α,β1*1501) class II molecule using synthetic peptides, as well as Amb 5 mutants prepared by recombinant DNA technology (see below).

VI. ANALYSIS OF B-CELL EPITOPES

We have also examined the B-cell epitopes of Amb a 5, Amb t 5, and Amb p 5. Amb t 5 is the odd one out in that there is essentially no cross-reactivity between this Ag and Amb a 5 and Amb t 5 using either IgE or IgG Abs. We have cloned and sequenced all three Amb 5 homologs (26–28) and have expressed them as β-glutathione (GST) fusion proteins in the pGEX vector grown in *Escherichia coli* (29). The fusion proteins were purified by affinity chromatography, and each allergen was then cleaved from the GST using thrombin and purified by high-performance liquid chromatography (HPLC). These recombinant allergens can be used just like the native proteins in T-cell assays (where 3D conformation is not critical for activity). In assays of Ag-binding (B-cell assays), recombinant Amb t 5 is indistinguishable for the native Amb t 5, but recombinant Amb a 5 and Amb p 5 are somewhat less active, presumably the result of different protein folding than in their native configurations.

The high degree of sequence homology among the Amb 5 allergens suggests that the molecules adopt similar 3D folding patterns in their native forms. This has been verified experimentally. In collaboration with Drs. William Metzler and Luciano Mueller of Bristol Myers–Squibb, we determined the NMR structures of both Amb t 5 and Amb a 5 (30,31; Fig. 7), and we have obtained the structure of Amb p 5 by computer modeling based on the Amb a 5 structure (28). The molecules each contain a small segment of antiparallel

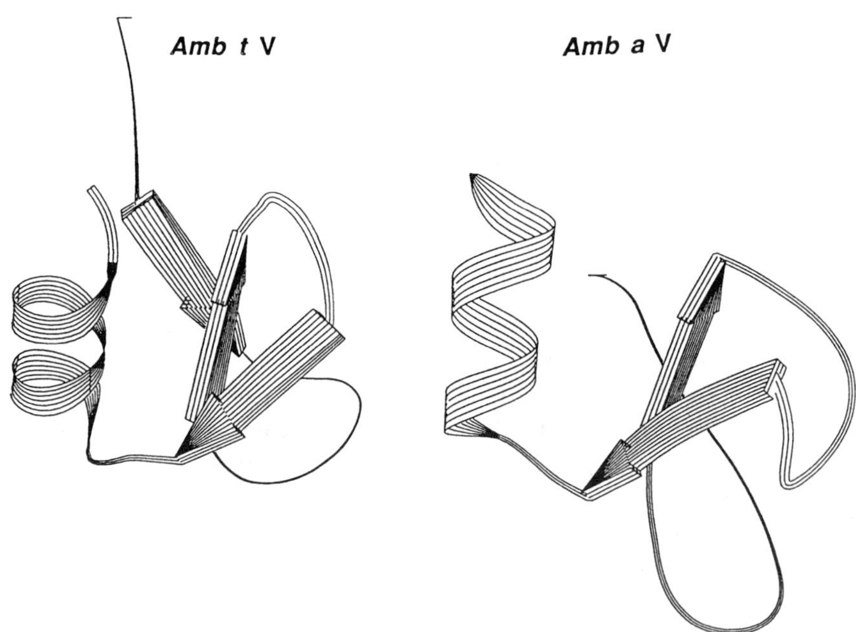

FIGURE 7   Ribbon diagrams of the 3D structures of Amb t 5 and Amb t 5 obtained by two-dimensional NMR spectroscopy. (See Refs. 30 and 31 for further details.) (Provided by Dr. W. Metzler.)

β-pleated sheet, a C-terminal α-helix, and several loops (Fig. 7a). At the interface of the helix and sheet is a rigid core, comprised mainly of hydrophobic residues and two disulfide bonds. In Amb t 5, there was clear evidence of three strands of a β-pleated sheet, but in Amb a 5, a more flexible molecule, there was convincing evidence for only two of these β strands, perhaps resulting from inclusion of the larger loop comprising residues 27–30 in Amb a 5 (Fig. 6), which leads to greater flexibility in the molecule.

It has been observed that immunodominant B-cell epitopes tend to lie primarily on the surface of native molecules in regions subject to the most rapid evolutionary change (32). Examination of the structures of Amb a 5 and Amb t 5, which are antigenically non-cross-reactive, indicates that the less conserved residues tend to be located at the exposed surfaces. From the NMR structures, we were able to predict the B-cell epitopes, which were located in three surface loop structures (Fig. 7b). Using recombinant DNA technology, we are now in the process of mutating residues in each of the loops in the Amb t 5 structure, converting them to the respective Amb a 5 residues (e.g., Asn_{10} of Amb t 5 to Val_{10} of Amb a 5). Our preliminary results suggest that these loop regions of the two molecules contain important B-cell epitopes as predicted from the computer-modeling studies (33). So far, we have found that mutation of certain Amb t 5 to Amb a 5 residues results in the loss of Ag-binding activity. Provided we can make the correct mutations, we hope that it may be possible to observe a concomitant gain in Amb a 5–binding activity. Thus, it should be possible to define quite precisely the principal B-cell epitopes on these Amb 5 molecules.

VII. CONCLUSIONS AND FUTURE DIRECTIONS

The Amb 5 homologs serve as models for molecular genetic and cellular studies of Ag-specific immune responsiveness. In the future, it will be important to extend these studies to major allergenic proteins, including those that have been implicated in asthma. We are at present involved in analyzing data from a large International HLA and Allergy Study (34). We have recently examined the HLA-D associations with IgE Ab responsiveness to the major allergens of allergenic complexes that have been associated with the expression of asthma, namely, Der p 1, Fel d 1, Asp f 1, and Alt a 1 from the house-dust mite (*Dermatophagoides pteronyssinus*), cat dander, and the molds *Aspergillus* and *Alternaria*, respectively. In three ethnically different populations, we have evidence that various HLA-DR4 subtypes are associated with IgE Ab responsiveness to each of these allergens. In the future, it will be important to define more fully the various class II molecules, T-cell epitopes, and TcRs involved in initiation of the immune responses toward these much more complex major allergens. B-cell epitopes that are involved in the specific IgE Ab responses should also be studied. Such studies, which are already underway in a number of laboratories (35,36), will enhance our knowledge of the molecular basis of immune responsiveness and its relationship to the expression of atopic diseases, including asthma.

ACKNOWLEDGMENTS

We wish to thank Drs. William Metzler and Luciano Mueller for their collaboration with the NMR studies. This work was supported by NIH Grants AI19727 and 20059.

REFERENCES

1. Løwenstein H, Marsh DG. Antigens of *Ambrosia elatior* (short ragweed) pollen. I. Crossed immunoelectrophoretic analysis.
2. Marsh DG, Hsu SH, Roebber M, Kautzky EE, Freidhoff LR, Meyers DA, Pollard MK, Bias WB. HLA-Dw2: a genetic marker for human immune response to short ragweed pollen allergen Ra5. I. Response resulting primarily from natural antigenic exposure. J Exp Med 1982; 155:1439–1451.
3. Løwenstein H, Marsh DG. Antigens of *Ambrosia elatior* (short ragweed) pollen. III. Crossed radioimmunoelectrophoresis of ragweed-allergic patients' sera with special attention to quantification of IgE responses. J Immunol 1983; 130:727–731.
4. Marsh DG. Defining human immune response fingerprints toward ultra-pure allergens: immunochemical and genetic aspects of responsiveness toward the *Amb* V (Ra5) homologues. In: Reed CE, ed. Proc. XII Internatl. Congress Allergol. Clin. Immunol., Washington, D.C., 1985. J Allergy Clin Immunol 1986; 78 (Suppl): 242–248.
5. Marsh DG. Immunogenetic and immunochemical factors determining immune responsiveness to allergens: studies in unrelated subjects. In: Marsh DG, Blumenthal MN, eds. Genetic and Environmental Factors in Clinical Allergy. Minneapolis: University of Minnesota Press, 1990:97–123.
6. Huang S-K, Marsh DG. Genetics of allergic diseases. Ann Allergy 1993; 70:347–359.
7. Ghosh B, Marsh DG. Molecular, cellular and genetic studies of atopic disease. In: Barnes PJ, Stockley RA, eds. Molecular Biology of Lung Disease. Oxford: Blackwell Scientific Publ, 1994:300–313.
8. Rafnar T, Metzler WJ, Marsh DG. The *Amb* V allergens from ragweed. In: Mohapatra S, Knox B, eds. Pollen Biotechnology: Genes, Allergens and Development. New York: Chapman and Hall (in press).
9. Marsh DG. Genetics of atopy and IgE. In: Frank MM, Austen KF, Claman HN, Unanue ER, eds. Samter's Immunological Diseases, 5th ed. Boston: Little, Brown (in press).
10. Romagnani S. Human Th1 and Th2: doubt no more. Immunol Today 1991; 12: 256–257.

11. Gauchat J-F, Lebman DA, Coffman RL, Gascan H, De Vries JE. Structure and expression of germline ε transcripts in human B cells induced by interleukin 4 to switch to IgE production. J Exp Med 1990; 172:463–473.

12. June CH, Bluestone JA, Nadler LM, Thompson CB. The B7 and CD28 receptor families. Immunol Today 1994; 15:321–331.

13. Stern LJ, Brown JH, Jardetzky TS, et al. Crystal structure of the human class II MHC protein HLA-DR1 complexed with an influenza virus peptide. Nature 1994; 368:215–221.

14. Marsh DG, Meyers DA, Friedhoff LR, Kautzky EE, Roebber M, Norman PS, Hsu SH, Bias WB. HLA-Dw2: a genetic marker for human immune response to short ragweed pollen allergen Ra5. II. Response after ragweed immunotherapy. J Exp Med 1982; 155:1452–1463.

15. Roebber M, Klapper DG, Goodfriend L, Bias WB, Hsu SH, Marsh DG. Immunochemical and genetic studies of *Amb t* V (Ra5G), an Ra5 homologue from giant ragweed pollen. J Immunol 1985; 134:3062–3069.

16. Goodfriend L, Choudhury AM, Klapper DG, Coulter KM, Dorval G, DelCarpio J, Osterland CK. Ra5G, a homologue of Ra5 in giant ragweed pollen: isolation, HLA-DR-associated activity and amino acid sequence. Mol Immunol 1985; 22: 899–906.

17. Coulter KM, Yang WH, Dorval GD, Drouin MA, Osterland CK, Goodfriend L. Specific IgE antibody responses to ragweed allergens Ra5S and Ra5G associated with distinct HLA-DR β genes. Mol Immunol 1987; 24:1207–1210.

18. Blumenthal MN, Marcus-Bagley D, Awdeh Z, Johnson B, Yunis EJ, Alper CA. HLA-DR2, [HLA-B7, SC31, DR2], and HLA-B8, SC01, DR3] haplotypes distinguish subjects with asthma from those with rhinitis only in ragweed pollen allergy. J Immunol 1992; 148:411–416.

19. Mole LE, Goodfriend L, Lapkoff CB, Kehoe JM, Capra JD. The amino acid sequence of allergen Ra5. Biochemistry 1975; 14:1216–1220.

20. Marsh DG, Zwollo P, Freidhoff L, Golden DBK, Ansari AA, Kautzky EE, Meyers DA, Holland CL. Studies of human immune response to the *Amb* V (Ra5) homologues. J Allergy Clin Immunol 1990; 85:201 (abstract).

21. Marsh DG, Zwollo P, Huang SK, Ghosh B, Ansari AA. Molecular studies of human response to allergens. Cold Spring Harbor Symp Quant Biol 1990; 54:459–470.

22. Zwollo P, Ehrlich-Kautzky E, Ansari AA, Scharf SJ, Erlich HA, Marsh DG. Molecular studies of human immune response genes for the short ragweed allergen, *Amb a* V: Sequencing of HLA-D second exons in responders and non-responders. Immunogenetics 1991; 33:141–151.

23. Huang SK, Zwollo P, Marsh DG. Class II MHC restriction of human T-cell responses to short ragweed allergen, *Amb a* V. Eur J Immunol 1991; 21:1469–1473.

23a. Shinomiya N, Kumai M, Marsh DG, Huang SK. Secretion of specific IgE-secreting cells using an enzyme-linked immunospot assay. J Allergy Clin Immunol 1993; 92:479–487.

24. Huang SK, Marsh DG. Human T-cell responses to ragweed allergens: *Amb* V homologues. Immunology 1991; 73:363–365.

25. Rafnar T, Huang S-K, Ghosh B, Kumai M, Marsh DG. Identification of a dominant T-cell epitope on the short ragweed allergen *Amb a* V. J Allergy Clin Immunol 1993; 91:337 (abstract).
26. Ghosh B, Perry MP, Marsh DG. Cloning the cDNA encoding the *Amb t* V allergen from giant ragweed (*Ambrosia trifida*) pollen. Gene 1991; 101:231–238.
27. Ghosh B, Perry MP, Rafnar T, Marsh DG. Cloning and expression of immunologically active recombinant *Amb a* V allergen from short ragweed (*Ambrosia artemisiifolia*) pollen. J Immunol 1993; 150:5391–5399.
28. Ghosh B, Rafnar T, Perry MP, Bassolino-Klimas D, Metzler WJ, Klapper DG, Marsh DG. Immunologic and molecular characterization of *Amb p* V allergens from *Ambrosia psilostacha* (Western ragweed) pollen. J Immunol 1994; 152:2882–2889.
29. Rafnar T, Ghosh B, Metzler WJ, Huang S-K, Perry MP, Mueller L, Marsh DG. Expression and analysis of recombinant *Amb a* V and *Amb t* V allergens: comparison with native proteins by immunological analysis and NMR spectroscopy. J Biol Chem 1992; 267:21119–21123.
30. Metzler WJ, Valentine K, Roebber M, Friedrichs M, Marsh DG, Mueller L. Solution structures of ragweed allergen *Amb t* V. Biochemistry 1992; 31:5117–5127.
31. Metzler WJ, Valentine K, Roebber M, Marsh DG, Mueller L. Proton resonance assignments and three-dimensional solution structure of the ragweed allergen *Amb a* V by nuclear magnetic resonance spectroscopy. Biochemistry 1992; 31:8697–8705.
32. Benjamin DC, Berzofsky JA, East IJ, et al. The antigenic structure of proteins: a reappraisal. Annu Rev Immunol 1984; 2:67–101.
33. Rafnar T, Metzler WJ, Brummet ME, Marsh DG. Characterization of allergenic epitopes at the molecular level. FASEB J 1994; 8:Λ762.
34. Marsh DG, Blumenthal MN, Ishikawa T, Ruffilli A, Sparholt S, Friedhoff LR. HLA and specific immune responsiveness to allergens. In: Tsuji K, Aizawa M, Sasazuki T, eds. HLA 1991: Proc. 11th Internat. Histocompatibility Workshop and Conference. Oxford: Oxford University Press, 1992:765–771.
35. O'Hehir RE, Garman RD, Greenstein JL, Lamb JR. The specificity and regulation of T-cell responsiveness to allergens. Annu Rev Immunol 1991; 9:67–95.
36. Kapsenberg ML, Jansen HM, Bos JD, Wierenga EA. Role of type 1 and type 2 T helper cells in allergic diseases. Curr Opin Immunol 1992; 4:788–793.
37. King TP, Hoffman DR, Lowenstein H, et al. Allergen nomenclature. Bull WHO (in press).

10

Regulation of IgE Synthesis In Vitro and In Vivo

Christine McMenamin and Patrick G. Holt
TVW Telethon Institute for Child Health Research
West Perth, Western Australia, Australia

I. INTRODUCTION

The central role of IgE in the pathogenesis of allergic diseases, including atopic asthma, is becoming increasingly more apparent. In particular, a series of recent clinical studies have clearly demonstrated a direct relationship between the occurrence of asthma and positive IgE-mediated skin test reactivity to common aeroallergens, as well as between asthma and high total serum IgE levels (1–3). In addition, bronchial hyperreactivity in children has also been found to be significantly associated with elevated total serum IgE levels (4).

Accordingly, it may be postulated that the genetic and environmental factor(s) that regulate the "tonus" of IgE responses within individuals are important determinants of susceptibility to the induction and expression of allergic respiratory disease. Our current understanding of the cellular and molecular mechanism(s) underlying IgE immunoregulation, derived from experimental animal and human model systems, is summarized in this chapter.

II. CELLULAR AND MOLECULAR MECHANISMS IN IgE REGULATION: IN VITRO STUDIES

A. Heterogeneity Among T-Helper Cells

Following immunization of experimental animals with a soluble protein antigen, different types of effector CD4$^+$ T cells are produced. On the basis of the restricted range of cytokines they secrete in vitro, these T-cell subpopulations have been designated T-helper 1 (TH1) and T-helper 2 (TH2) (5) although other types such as TH0, which exhibit an apparently unrestricted cytokine profile, have also been described (6). TH1 cells secrete IL-2 and IFN-γ and are important in the induction of cell-mediated immunity (7). TH2 cells do not synthesize IL-2 or IFN-γ but instead produce IL-4, IL-5, IL-6, IL-10, and IL-13 and induce immunoglobulin synthesis, particularly of the IgE isotype (8,9), as well as supporting growth of mast cells, basophils, and eosinophils. Thus TH1 and TH2 cells appear to correspond to the two poles in the spectrum of immune responses. On recognition of different classes of antigens and pathogens, the appropriate type of T-helper cell may be selectively activated and expanded, resulting in the production of a restricted range of cytokines, which favors the generation of a specific type of immune response. In addition, CD8$^+$ T cells may also be activated and exert regulatory effects on CD4$^+$ T cells through cytokine production.

Analysis of the cytokine profiles of isolated CD4$^+$ T-cell clones from atopic and normal individuals suggests specific compartmentalization of the response to allergens, in that cytokine production is skewed toward IL-4 (TH2-like) in the atopic versus IFN-γ (TH1-like) in the normals (10,11). Thus in allergic individuals, allergen exposure results in development of TH2 cells that produce IL-4 and IL-5, which in turn activate B cells to produce IgE and additionally stimulate mast cell and eosinophil proliferation. However, in nonallergic individuals, exposure to the same allergen results in an entirely different type of immune response, in which the T cells that are activated produce IFN-γ and other factors that inhibit IgE synthesis and mast cell/eosinophil proliferation.

The nature of the allergen may also play a role in determining the cytokine production phenotype of T cells. Allergen-specific T cells derived from atopic donors produced high levels of IL-4 but no IFN-γ whereas bacterial antigen-specific T-cell clones established from the same donors produced predominantly IFN-γ but not IL-4 (12).

B. The Role of Cytokines in IgE Production

Cytokines are essential for B-cell proliferation and differentiation; they not only determine immunoglobulin secretion quantitatively but also direct immunoglobulin isotype switching (13,14).

1. IgE-Promoting Cytokines

a. IL-4. Coffman and colleagues first reported that the T-cell-derived lymphokine IL-4 was able to induce IgE production in vitro by costimulation of murine B-cell blasts (15). The IgE-inducing effect of IL-4 initially observed in vitro was confirmed by in vivo studies showing that administration of an IL-4 monoclonal antibody inhibited 99% of the primary IgE response (16). Direct evidence linking IL-4 to the allergic response was provided by Tepper et al. (17), when the IL-4 gene was fused to an immunoglobulin promoter-enhancer and incorporated into a transgenic mouse model. Overexpression of IL-4 resulted in a marked increase in serum IgE levels and histopathological features seen in typical allergic reactions. The reverse case, in which the IL-4 gene had been disrupted leading to the complete absence of circulating IgE, also confirmed its importance (18) in IgE regulation.

Supporting evidence that IL-4 plays a key role in the regulation of IgE synthesis was soon provided by additional in vitro studies using human T-cell clones (19,20). The "helper" function of individual T-cell clones for IgE synthesis was strongly related to the ability of the clones to produce IL-4. In addition, further experiments demonstrated that recombinant IL-4 was able to induce IgE synthesis in mononuclear or B-cell-enriched suspensions in a dose-dependent fashion. More importantly, the addition of anti-human IL-4 antibody inhibited IgE synthesis induced by recombinant IL-4, and also that stimulated by T-cell clones and their supernatants.

IL-4-induced IgE synthesis reflects isotype switching and is not due to a selective outgrowth of a few B cells committed to IgE synthesis. Switching to ε in both murine and human B cells is preceded by the induction of germline ε RNA synthesis, and these transcripts have been shown to be important in the ε switch process (21–23). However, the growth-promoting activity as well as the activating effect of IL-4 on T cells and T-cell clones are equally important functions of this cytokine (24,25), since the delivery of costimulatory signals by T cells is required for B-cell proliferation and differentiation (see below).

b. IL-13. Although it had been thought that IL-4 was the only cytokine capable of inducing IgE synthesis, a non-IL-4-producing T-cell clone has been identified that can induce germline transcription in purified B cells, indicating that an IL-4-independent pathway of induction of germline ε transcription is operational (21,22). This activity has been ascribed to another TH2-cell-derived cytokine, IL-13 (26). IL-13-induced IgE production is independent of IL-4, since IL-13 induced synthesis of IgE by highly purified B cells in the absence of exogenous IL-4. In addition, anti-IL-4 antibodies, which efficiently blocked IL-4-induced IgE synthesis, failed to affect IL-13-induced IgE production.

Despite similarities between IL-4 and IL-13 in their effects on B cells, such as the induction of germline ε RNA synthesis, the up-regulation of class

II MHC antigens, and the significant expression of CD23 (FcεRII) (26), the functions of IL-4 and IL-13 are not identical. No additive or synergistic effects were observed when IL-4 and IL-13 were added together at optimal concentrations, suggesting that IL-4 and IL-13 may use a common signaling pathway for induction of IgE switching (26). Indeed, recent studies have shown that receptors for IL-13 and IL-4 share a common subunit that functions in signal transduction. However, IL-13 does not bind to cells bearing the 130-kDa IL-4 receptor, indicating it does not act through this IL-4-binding protein. The levels of IgE produced in response to IL-13 are generally lower than those induced by IL-4. Moreover, IL-13 does not act on T cells or T-cell clones either as an activator or as a growth promoter. Thus, the lack of T-cell-activating-inducing activity on the part of IL-13 may partially explain why maximal IL-13-induced IgE synthesis by B cells is lower than that induced by IL-4.

    *c. **Other IgE-Promoting Cytokines.*** There are a number of other cytokines which act synergistically with IL-4, but which are ineffective at inducing synthesis of IgE in their own right.

    In addition to its role as a growth and differentiation factor for eosinophils, IL-5 is effective in enhancing IgE synthesis induced by IL-4 in murine LPS-activated purified B cells, as well as in human B cells (19,27), but is not effective on its own. Thus IL-5 contributes to the maintenance of type I hypersensitivity reactions through mechanism(s) unrelated to its role in regulating eosinophils.

    Endogenous IL-6 plays an obligatory role in the IL-4-dependent induction of IgE synthesis in human peripheral blood mononuclear cells, since a neutralizing anti-IL-6 antibody completely inhibited IgE synthesis in the presence of IL-4 (28). However, restoration of the response was achieved by addition of recombinant IL-6 (29). IL-6 seems to be involved in the amplification of IgE by coordinated transcriptional activation, selective accumulation of mRNA for the secreted form of IgE, and possibly differential mRNA stabilization, as has been shown for IgG (30).

    More recently, the IgE-potentiating activity of another T-cell-derived cytokine, IL-9, has been described (31). This cytokine does not induce IgE production by B cells independently. However, IL-9 is capable of potentiating IgE production by B cells following induction by suboptimal levels of IL-4. In addition, the frequency of IgE-secreting cells was enhanced in the presence of IL-9. The target for this cytokine appears to be the B cells themselves and involves the initial steps in IgE synthesis, i.e., activation and proliferation of B cells, and is not related to an enhanced release of IL-4 by non-B, non-T cells or T cells. Along with the potentiating effect on IgE production, IL-9 also promotes the growth of mucosal mast cells (32); thus this cytokine contributes to the regulation of allergic reactions on a number of fronts.

TNF-α has been found to activate B cells and to enhance IL-4-dependent IgE synthesis (21,33). The membrane-bound form of TNF-α is transiently expressed after T-cell activation and can act as a costimulatory signal required for IL-4-dependent induction of IgE synthesis (34). In addition, in the absence of T cells, germline ε transcription is enhanced by TNF-α; thus this cytokine is capable of affecting IgE production by modulation of germline ε RNA synthesis in B cells (21).

2. IgE-Inhibiting Cytokines

a. Interferon-γ (IFN-γ).   As early as 1986, Coffman et al. (15) provided data suggesting that IgE production in experimental animals could be inhibited by IFN-γ. In subsequent years, Pène and colleagues showed that IFN-γ can inhibit IL-4-mediated IgE production by normal human lymphocytes in vitro (19). IFN-γ specifically antagonizes the activity of IL-4 for the induction of IgE antibody production (13,16). The cellular target for the effects of IFN-γ vary depending on the model system used. Gauchat et al. (22) reported that inhibition of functional C_ε mRNA transcripts by IFN-γ in IL-4-induced peripheral blood lymphocytes required the presence of T cells. In contrast, IL-4-induced IgE synthesis by purified human B cells infected with Epstein-Barr virus can be suppressed by IFN-γ (35). Thus the capacity of human and mouse T cell clones to induce IgE synthesis is directly related to their relative rates of secretion of IL-4 and IFN-γ.

A number of studies involving patients with atopic dermatitis (AD) have revealed the importance of this balance between IL-4 and IFN-γ in vivo. Results from a number of independent studies indicate that after mitogenic stimulation, PBMCs from patients with AD secrete decreased levels of IFN-γ and increased amounts of IL-4 compared to nonatopic donors (36–38). A dualistic mechanism may be operative in AD resulting in increased IL-4 and decreased IFN-γ production. Excessive production of IL-4 may contribute to the decreased secretion of IFN-γ per cell (39,40); however, there is also a lower overall frequency of IFN-γ-producing cells in atopic versus nonatopic patients. Supernatants from the PBMCs of AD patients induce significantly greater levels of IgE synthesis than supernatants from healthy controls. Indeed, supernatants from control subjects were unable to induce the production of IgE unless an anti-IFN-γ antibody was present (38). These studies support the notion that IFN-γ plays a critical role in down-regulating IgE synthesis, and further that this mechanism functions suboptimally in AD.

Recent studies have demonstrated that the in vivo administration of recombinant IFN-γ to AD patients results in decreased spontaneous production of IgE by PBMCs, as well as decreased clinical severity of skin lesions (41–43).

b. Interferon*-α *(IFN-*α*).   IFN-α blocks the IL-4-dependent formation of IgE by PBMCs (19,44). Like IFN-γ, IFN-α functionally antagonizes the switch of B cells to IgE. The timing of the action of IFN-α is crucial in that it must act within 48 hr of onset of culture to inhibit IgE synthesis. This spans the same time period in which IL-4 exerts its stimulatory effect, indicating its direct functional antagonistic effect on the IL-4-induced switch (45). One important implication is that cells other than T cells, e.g., macrophages, may also regulate B-cell activity with regard to IgE production. Again, IFN-α has been used clinically to reduce serum IgE levels in AD patients and leads to transient clinical improvement (46).

3. Other IgE-Inhibiting Cytokines

IL-8 was initially characterized and cloned as a neutrophil chemotactic and activating agent (47). However, its effects are far more pleotropic than first thought. It has been demonstrated that IL-8 selectively inhibits IgE production in mononuclear cells stimulated with IL-4 (48). Inhibition by IL-8 was specific, since it could be blocked by anti-IL-8 antibody. IL-8 inhibits the early activation step during IL-4 stimulation, since inhibition could only occur when it was added at the initiation of the culture. The inhibitory effect of IL-8 was not mediated by IFN-γ, since the inhibition could not be blocked by addition of anti-IFN-γ. It should be noted that IL-8 could inhibit IL-4-induced IgE production in both T-cell-dependent and -independent systems. Thus, IL-8 acts directly both on the B cell and on the costimulatory accessory cells necessary for IgE synthesis. As for many of the other IgE-inhibiting cytokines, IL-4 inhibits the production of IL-8 by monocytes (49).

   IL-10 is a cytokine produced by several cell types after activation, including TH0-, TH1-, and TH2-like CD4$^+$ T-cell subsets, a proportion of CD8$^+$ T cells, B cells, and monocytes (50–54). It shares several, but not all, activities with an open reading frame in the EBV genome, BCRF1, now designated v-IL-10 (55–57). IL-10 is an important suppressor factor for immunoproliferative and inflammatory responses through reducing the antigen-presentation capacity of monocytes by modulation of the expression of class II MHC molecules on these cells (56,58,59). IL-10 and v-IL-10 inhibit IgE synthesis by unfractionated PBMCs but not by highly purified B cells cultured with activated T-cell clones. Thus the inhibitory effect of IL-10 is indirect and mediated through inhibition of the accessory cell function of monocytes (60).

   The pattern of IL-10 secretion represents a notable (and rare) difference between the murine and human systems. In the murine model IL-10 is an exclusive product of TH2 cells, which through down-regulation of IFN-γ production favors development of TH2 pathways (61)—in contrast, human IL-10 is produced by TH0, TH1, and TH2 cells (50) and efficiently prevents Ag-specific activation of T-cell clones with these phenotypes. Thus, reduced levels of

IL-10 production may lead to activation and proliferation of allergen-specific T cells in atopic patients. Since IL-4 is a major product of TH2 cells and has been shown to inhibit production of IL-10, this could lead to enhanced synthesis of IgE. On the other hand, down-regulation of IL-10 may result in enhanced IFN-γ production and inhibition of IgE synthesis. The time course of IL-10 production is much later following activation of cells compared to IL-4 production implying that IL-4 can be functional before IL-10 becomes active. The way in which IL-4 and IL-10 cross-regulate each other's synthesis and activities remains to be determined.

Picomolar concentrations of recombinant IL-12 markedly inhibit the synthesis of IgE by IL-4-stimulated PBMCs. The suppression of IgE is observed at the protein and mRNA levels and is completely overridden by neutralizing antibodies to IL-12 (62). IL-12 induces the production of significant amounts of IFN-γ; however, further mechanisms of IgE suppression seem to be operative in this case. Neutralizing antibodies to IFN-γ failed consistently to overcome the IL-12-mediated suppression of IgE synthesis. In addition, IL-12 was able to markedly inhibit IgE synthesis by neonatal lymphocytes costimulated with IL-4 and hydrocortisone; these neonatal lymphocytes do not produce detectable levels of IFN-γ (62), indicating that the effects of IL-12 in this system are clearly IFN-γ-independent. Nevertheless, the effect of IL-12 appears to be indirect and requires the presence of T cells, monocytes, or NK cells, since IgE synthesis by highly purified B cells stimulated with IL-4 and anti-CD40 (see below) could not be inhibited by the addition of IL-12.

Transforming growth factor β (TGF-β) also has an inhibitory effect on the IL-4-dependent IgE production (21). TGF-β affects the production of IgE directly by modulation of germline ε RNA synthesis (21). However, through the suppression of TH2 cells and the loss of production of IL-4 and other IgE-promoting cytokines (63), TGF-β can also be indirectly responsible for the inhibition of IgE.

C. Cognate Signals Involved in IgE Production

In addition to cytokines, contact-mediated signals delivered by CD4$^+$ T cells are required for B-cell proliferation and immunoglobulin synthesis. Although IL-4 is the major inducer of IgE synthesis, it has been demonstrated that a second signal provided by T cells is required, since IL-4 failed to induce IgE synthesis by highly purified B cells.

1. TcR, CD4, and Class II MHC Molecules

It has been demonstrated that human B cells can be induced to switch to IgE production following a contact-mediated signal provided by activated CD4$^+$ T-cell clones and IL-4 (19,64,65). The signal was antigen-nonspecific, indicating that the TcR/CD3 complex was not involved in the T-B interaction. The CD4$^+$ clones could be replaced by plasma-membrane-enriched fractions from the activated T-cell clones. Induction of IgE synthesis by B cells cocultured with clones or membrane preparations could be blocked by anti–class II MHC and anti-CD4 monoclonal antibodies (66). Murine L cells or EBV-LCL transfected with CD4 could not replace CD4$^+$ T-cell clones. These results indicate that, although CD4 and class II MHC antigens are required for productive T-cell-clone–B cell interactions, an additional signal, provided by a membrane-associated protein(s) that is induced by activation of CD4$^+$ T cells, is needed for induction of IgE production in the presence of IL-4. It is interesting to note that the pro-IgE cytokines IL-4 and IL-13 both enhance class II MHC expression.

2. CD40 and CD40 Ligand (CD40L)

The CD40 surface molecule is expressed on B lymphocytes, epithelial cells, and some carcinoma cell lines. Cloning of the CD40 gene has revealed that CD40 is closely related to the receptors for nerve growth factor (67) and TNF-α (68). Monoclonal antibodies against CD40 mediate a variety of effects on B cells, including proliferation (69–71) and differentiation (29,72), indicating that CD40 could be the receptor for a ligand with important functions in B-cell development and activation.

It was shown that anti-CD40 antibodies, in the absence of T cells but in the presence of IL-4, could costimulate B cells to synthesize IgE (29). Anti-CD40 antibodies have synergistic effects on germline ε mRNA induction by IL-4 and both signals are required for induction of productive ε transcripts and IgE synthesis (73).

CD40L is expressed on activated T cells (74), mast cells, and basophils (75). The biological activities of CD40L in both proliferation of B cells and secretion of IgE fulfilled predictions made for the functional effects of the ligand, based on the previously described activity of the anti-CD40 antibody (29,69–72). The mitogenic activity of CD40L is likely to be dependent on its expression as a cell-membrane molecule, as immobilized (but not soluble) CD40 antibody provides a similar proliferative signal (71). A variety of factors that control IgE production also regulate CD40L expression (20), and T-cell-mediated stimulation of IgE synthesis can be inhibited by soluble forms of CD40 (76).

3. CD23

CD23 is the low-affinity receptor for IgE (Fc$_\varepsilon$RII). It is expressed on B cells and also other hemopoietic cells such as monocytes, macrophages, and eosinophils, as well as T cells and epidermal Langerhans cells. CD23 is poorly expressed on resting B cells but is induced by IL-4 and IL-13 as an early and transient activation marker. This expression can be inhibited by IFN-γ. The association between IL-4 induction and IFN-γ inhibition of CD23 expression and the production/nonproduction of IgE implies an involvement for CD23 in the control of IgE synthesis (19). Further support was lent to this hypothesis by the finding that in vivo administration of an anti-CD23 antibody to experimental animals resulted in up to 90% inhibition of antigen-specific IgE synthesis (77). In addition, the frequency of CD23$^+$ B cells is increased in allergic diseases associated with high IgE levels (78,79).

It has been proposed that CD23 acts as an adhesion molecule in cell-cell interactions that are necessary for complete differentiation of IgE-committed B cells. The principal evidence supporting this claim comes from the finding that CD23 on T cells interacts with CD21 on B cells (80,81). In this context it has been demonstrated that triggering of CD21 by anti-CD21 antibody, recombinant soluble CD23 (82), or EBV (35) enhances IgE production even in the absence of T cells. In addition, IL-4 and specific allergen induce CD23 on T cells (83).

CD23 also exists in a non-membrane-bound form as soluble CD23 (sCD23) and acts as an IgE-binding factor (84). IL-4 and IL-13 also induce the formation and release of sCD23, and the appearance of sCD23 is already observed after 48-hr incubation of MNC in these cytokines (26). CD23 expression as well as sCD23 production by B cells precedes IL-4/IL-13-induced ε switching.

D. Allergic Inflammatory Responses

It has been known for many years that IgE molecules that are bound to high-affinity Fc receptors (Fc$_\varepsilon$RI) on mast cells mediate type I immediate hypersensitivity responses. Exposure to allergen results in crosslinking of these allergen-specific IgE molecules on mast cells and leads to a cascade of events that include the degranulation of the mast cell and the release of a host of inflammatory mediators that initiate the allergic reaction. Although histamine released from mast cells plays a prominent role in the immediate phase of allergic reactions, other mediators and lymphokines released from mast cells (as noted above) and other cell types that are attracted to sites of allergic reactions play equally important roles in the genesis of the allergic inflammatory response, as well as being able to sustain the response once initiated.

IgE synthesis can be induced by the interaction of B cells with mast cells and basophils in the presence of IL-4. Mast cells and basophils can express CD40L, which is known to be able to provide, in conjunction with IL-4, the minimal signals required to induce IgE production. In addition, both cells types are capable of producing a pattern of cytokines analogous to TH2 cells. The fact that inhalation of relevant allergen results in the activation of allergen-

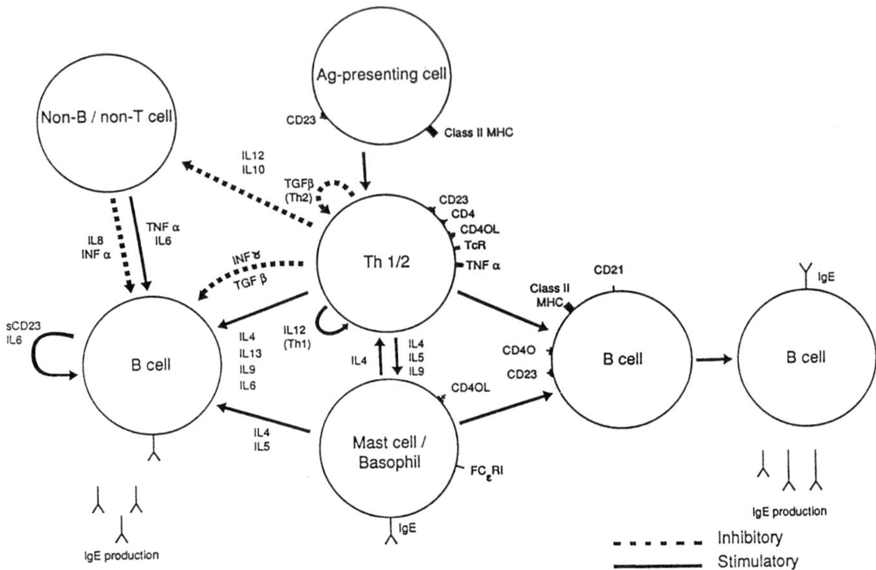

FIGURE 1   The regulation of IgE synthesis within central lymphoid organs and mucosal surfaces involves a complex network of cell-cell interactions, which are modulated by both negative and positive signals from soluble mediators.

specific Th2 lymphocytes in the airway mucosa of patients with allergic disorders (85–87) suggests that all three cells types are likely to play an important role in the induction and maintenance of allergic reactions at mucosal sites.

Thus, the regulation of IgE synthesis within central lymphoid organs and mucosal surfaces involves a complex network of cell-cell interactions, which are modulated by both negative and positive signals from soluble mediators (Fig. 1).

III. CONTROL OF IGE PRODUCTION IN VIVO: REGULATION OF IGE RESPONSES TO ANTIGEN DELIVERED TO MUCOSAL SURFACES

IgE responder phenotype in both humans and experimental animals is genetically determined, but the in vivo expression of phenotype is modulated by a range of host and environmental factors. The experimental literature indicates that protection against primary allergic sensitization to both inhalant and dietary allergens is provided principally via "tolerance/immune deviation" mechanisms, which are based on the cytokine pathways described above. The efficiency of these protective mechanisms varies over a range of 10^4-fold between animals at the extremes of the IgE-response range, and cross-breeding experiments indicate that high efficiency for tolerogenesis is coinherited.

These experimental models provide the basis for interpretation of the existing human seroepidemiological literature relating to IgE, and for speculation on mechanisms of primary allergic sensitization in humans, as discussed below.

A. Primary Immune Responses in Immunologically Naïve Experimental Animals

1. Protection Against Sensitization to Dietary Antigens

The prime function of the immune system in the gastrointestinal tract (GIT) is protection against infection by enteric pathogens. On a quantitative basis, physical exclusion mechanisms operating in tandem with the process of peristalsis prevent the penetration of the majority of potential pathogens below the gastric epithelium. The efficiency of this process is greatly enhanced by local secretory antibody production. Pathogens that broach these defenses trigger adaptive immune mechanisms that operate both locally and systemically, to limit the spread of infection.

The mucosal immune system in the GIT generally performs these functions at a high level of efficiency, as evidenced by the relative rarity of clinically significant enteric infections in most individuals, attesting to the effectiveness of the mechanisms involved in surveillance for pathogenic antigens that broach the gastric epithelium.

However, while exposure to antigens associated with potentially pathogenic microorganisms is relatively frequent within the GIT, encounters with inert (nonpathogenic) antigens comprising dietary proteins and carbohydrates are much more frequent, and the maintenance of local immunological homeostasis necessitates accurate discrimination of the latter from genuine pathogenic (viz. microbial) antigens. Failure to make this discrimination and to instead mount adaptive immune responses to inert dietary antigens is believed to be the basis for a variety of immunologically mediated enteropathies, including food allergy.

Our current understanding of how the mucosal immune system performs this delicate "balancing act" as based on the seminal experiments of Wells and Osborne, which date back to 1911 (88). These researchers demonstrated a phenomenon in guinea pigs that was subsequently termed oral tolerance, the salient features of which were as follows:

1. When immunologically naive animals were repeatedly fed a protein (egg albumin) to which they had not previously been exposed, a high proportion developed symptoms of gastric hypersensitivity, and a small number died of apparent anaphylaxis.
2. The surviving animals, with continuing exposure, progressively lost all symptoms.
3. Upon subsequent reexposure to the same antigen weeks or months later in the life of the animals, they never again developed hypersensitivity symptoms and had apparently developed a form of protection ("tolerance") against such pathogenic immune responses to the antigen, which was lifelong.

This tolerance process was subsequently demonstrated to be universal among experimental animals species (89), and the underlying mechanisms responsible for tolerogenesis have been the focus of intense research, particularly over the last 20 years. While the precise cellular and molecular mechanisms are still unclear, key elements in the process include the development of populations of antigen-specific regulatory T cells ("suppressor" cells) in primary lymphoid organs of tolerized animals, which are capable of transferring this immunological state to naïve animals (90), and the preferential nature of the tolerance for certain aspects of the immune response. In particular, while immediate and delayed hypersensitivity mechanisms become rapidly "tolerized" (89), local secretory IgA responses are usually preserved (91), suggesting that the underlying mechanism involves "selection" as opposed to simple "suppression" of antigen-specific immune responses to the eliciting antigens.

Recent research suggests that the molecular basis for this selection process involves in part the preferential stimulation of subsets of antigen-specific T cells that secrete cytokines such as IFN-γ (92) and TGF-β (63), which are known to inhibit the expansion of T-cell clones of the TH2 phenotype.

2. Evasion of Oral Tolerance Mechanisms

It is clear from work in many laboratories that a range of host and environmental factors can influence the development of oral tolerance in experimental animals. In particular, coexposure of the gastric mucosa to proinflammatory irritants can inhibit tolerogenesis and promote sensitization (89). In addition, disturbance to host hormonal status or reticuloendothelial function, or deliberate drug-induced immunosuppression, can achieve the same effects (89). But most important, developmental status appears to be a key factor: if animals are exposed to dietary proteins in the very early postnatal period, they are at high risk for primary T-cell sensitization, which manifests as hypersensitivity upon reexposure to the same antigens in later life (93,94). This suggests that failures in local barrier exclusion mechanisms and/or deficient immunological functions in early infancy can predispose to sensitization as opposed to tolerance.

It has also been demonstrated that genetic factors, notably those that influence overall IgE responder phenotype, are important determinants of sensitivity to oral tolerance. This manifests as log-scale variations between different inbred strains of animals, in the dose-response curve for tolerance induction to dietary antigens such as egg albumin, with immunologically "normal" low-IgE-responder strains demonstrating much more efficient induction mechanisms compared to their phenotypically high-IgE-responder counterparts (95).

3. Tolerance to Inhalant Antigens

While the phenomenon of oral tolerance was first described in 1911, evidence that similar processes operate at other mucosal sites, in particular in the respiratory tract, was not forthcoming until over 60 years later. The first indication that exposure of respiratory mucosal surfaces to nonmicrobial antigens induced "negative" immune responses came from experiments of Parker and Turk (96) involving intratracheal instillation of chemical haptens into guinea pigs. This process appeared to dampen systemic immune responses of the animals to subsequent parenteral challenge with the same haptens, but it was not clear whether the mechanisms simply involved "regurgitation" of the antigen into the GIT (a common consequence of the inoculation procedure employed) and hence indirect induction of oral tolerance, or instead resulted from local immunological processes.

A subsequent series of experiments from our laboratories, employing protein antigens delivered via aerosol to mimic natural exposure of humans to inhalant (environmental) allergens, demonstrated a phenomenon that has much in common with oral tolerance to dietary antigens. Thus, repeated exposure of immunologically naïve rats or mice to aerosolized ovalbumin (OVA) inhibited the capacity of the animals to mount OVA-specific IgE responses to subsequent parenteral challenge with the same antigen, regardless of the route of challenge (97–99). This "tolerance" process was preferentially directed against immediate (IgE) and delayed (DTH) components of the immune response to the eliciting antigen (95,100), as aerosol-exposed animals often manifested residual low-grade IgG and IgA reactivity and maintained a "memory" pool of OVA-reactive T cells (detectable by in vitro challenge) in central lymphoid organs (101).

As noted above for oral tolerance, sensitivity to tolerogenesis via antigen inhalation is genetically determined, high susceptibility being coinherited with low-IgE-responder phenotype (95). The magnitude of the differences in sensitivity between low- and high-IgE-responder inbred strains is extremely large, varying over a range of up to 104-fold: inhaled antigen doses in the low-nanogram range (in the order of human exposure to common inhalant allergens) are sufficient to "protect" immunologically normal low-IgE-responders, whereas dosages up to the microgram-to-milligram zone (unlikely to be encountered in nature) are required to tolerize genetically hyper-IgE-responsive strains (95,102). In addition, the selectivity of the process varied markedly with background genetics, immunologically normal strains exhibiting across-the-board tolerance in IgE, DTH, IgG, and IgA (95,103) whereas some strains failed to tolerize for DTH and IgG. Virtually all strains maintained at least a small pool of antigen-specific T-memory cells, and, as noted earlier for oral tolerance (89), antigen-specific B-memory cell populations remained normal, indicating that the target for this regulatory process was $CD4^+$ T-helper cells (103). It is important to note that this tolerance phenomenon functions with all types of inert inhaled antigens, including powerful inhalant allergens such as purified Der p I for the house dust mite (104).

A series of adoptive transfer studies has established that the principal mechanism mediating this form of tolerance involves the activation of a population of long-lived antigen-specific suppressor T cells, which express the surface phenotype of $CD3^+$ $CD4^-$ $CD5^+$ $CD8^+$ (105). The nature of the T-cell receptors on the effector cells is currently under investigation; it appears that more than one population may potentially be involved, in particular a subset of IFN-γ-secreting $CD8^+$ T cells related to the CTL (cytokine T lymphocyte) pool associated with antiviral immunity [(106,107); see further discussion below], and/or $CD8^+$ Tγ/δ cells (108,109).

The efficiency with which these $CD8^+$ T cells are activated in response to allergen inhalation is directly related to genetically determined IgE responder phenotype, notably, in low responders they appear rapidly in regional lymph nodes and inhibit the expansion of IL-2-secreting TH2 cells (107); a comparable $CD8^+$ population appears during the early stages of the induction of oral tolerance to fed antigen and these secrete IFN-γ (92) and TGF-β (63). It has clearly been established that neither antibody feedback via IgG (105) nor "barrier protection" via local antigen-specific secretory IgA (101) plays a significant role in this process.

The suppressor T-cell populations mediating tolerance to inhalant allergens are initially activated in the regional lymph nodes draining the upper respiratory tract (the site of most intense antigenic stimulation by inhaled antigens) and subsequently spread to central lymphoid organs (105), analogous to the situation described for oral tolerance (89). It is significant that antigen delivered directly to the peripheral lung via intratracheal intubation is relatively inefficient in tolerance induction (110), highlighting the importance of airway mucosal components of the respiratory tract immune system in the phenomena. This finding, together with localization of the upper respiratory tract regional lymph nodes (RLN) as the initial site of suppressor T-cell activation, suggests that an important component of this process is translocation of inhaled antigen from the airway lumen to T-cell zones in the RLN. Recent studies from our laboratory have demonstrated that the key cell population here are airway intraepithelial dendritic cells (DC), which play a dominant role in local antigen surveillance and subsequent "signaling" to T cells after migration to RLN (111–116). A similar role appears likely for equivalent DC populations in the GIT, which transport dietary antigens from the gut wall to the mesenteric lymph nodes (117).

4. Modulation of Genetic Potential for IgE Reactivity to Inhalant Allergens: Promotion of Primary Allergic Sensitization by Environmental Factors

Analogous to oral tolerance, a variety of environmental factors appear capable of interfering with normal tolerance induction to inhaled antigens (100). The most potent are local inflammatory irritants, targeted at the airway epithelium or its draining lymph nodes. The agents may be chemical (e.g., oxides of nitrogen) or microbial (e.g., respiratory viral infections or exposure to pertussis toxins)—concomitant exposure of the airway mucosa to any of these agents together with inhaled antigen can "prime" for IgE responses (95). Additionally, disturbance of endocrine function, in particular via administration of estradiol at dosages that affect reticuloendothelial activity (95), can abrogate tolerance induction and promote sensitization.

Exposure of animals to histamine aerosols either together with or immediately before inhalant allergen can also stimulate primary IgE responses (95), suggesting that "bystander" allergic reactions in the airways to other allergens constitute risk factors for sensitization. The microbial status of animals additionally modulates the efficiency of tolerance induction, notably, the process operates less efficiently in specific pathogen-free animals than in genetically identical animals carrying a conventional (mixed) commensal flora (95). This suggests that stimulation of the host immune system by microbial products can be protective via selective enhancement of immune function(s) associated with tolerance induction as opposed to priming; as discussed below, these findings may now be interpretable in terms of microbial stimulation of cytokines by mononuclear phagocytes that favor activation of CD4$^+$ TH1 cells as opposed to TH2 cells (118).

B. Immune Responses to Environmental Antigens in Neonates

In the experimental models reported thus far in the literature, the tolerance processes described above are operative only at or around the time of initial exposure of immunologically naïve adult animals to "new" antigens not previously encountered. The option for tolerance induction appears only open to the immune system prior to the establishment of a stable pool of T-memory cells specific for individual allergens. Depending on the intensity of allergenic stimulation, the "window" for tolerance induction in animals appears open only for a matter of weeks.

During this period, animals under continuous aeroallergen or dietary allergen exposure manifest heterogeneous immune reactivity, which (depending on genetic background) may include the full range of IgE, DTH, IgG, and IgA responses, in some circumstances accompanied by the symptoms of immediate and/or delayed hypersensitivity (88) and bronchial hyperreactivity (119). Under ideal ("normal") circumstances, IgE and DTH reactivity is progressively deleted ("suppressed"), leaving variable vestiges of IgG and IgA antibody production, which evoke no clinical symptoms.

In most situations, initial exposure of humans to ubiquitous environmental allergens, both dietary and airborne, occurs during infancy, and hence it is of interest to examine how these tolerance phenomena function during this critical life period. The available evidence indicates that the process is markedly different in the neonate.

With respect to dietary antigens, exposure of animals in the immediate postnatal period does not induce oral tolerance and instead can "prime" the immune system for subsequent responses in later life (93,94). The capacity for oral tolerance induction does not develop adult-equivalent levels of efficiency until around the time of weaning (94). Our laboratory has reported similar findings for tolerance induction to inhaled allergens (120). Tolerogenesis to foreign antigens delivered by other routes operates with high efficiency in these same animals; indeed the high susceptibility of neonates to peripheral tolerance induction constitutes one of the longest-standing experimental models employed in basic immunology research. This indicates that key elements of mucosal immune function exhibit delayed postnatal maturation, relative to analogous mechanisms operative in other tissues.

C. Primary Allergic Sensitization to Environmental Allergens in Humans

While the de novo onset of allergy to environmental allergens clearly does occur in adults, infancy and early childhood appears to be the most common life period during which initial sensitization occurs, although the sensitization may not produce overt disease until later life. This notion is supported by a wide range of epidemiological literature, in particular retrospective seroepidemiological studies that demonstrate associations between high levels of exposure to inhalant allergens in infancy and the subsequent development of respiratory allergy in later childhood and/or adulthood (reviewed in Ref. 121).

A key feature of the human seroepidemiological literature relating to both dietary and inhalant allergy is the clear evidence indicating that active immune "recognition" of ubiquitous environmental allergens is essentially universal, and not restricted to individuals with the genetic potential for atopy. This has been provided by studies indicating that all children manifest serum IgG response to environmental allergens during infancy (e.g., see Ref. 122), and further that low-level IgE assays detect significant IgE titers to both dietary (123) and inhalant (124) allergens in the majority of subjects. Importantly, these low-grade IgE responses are transient in children at low genetic risk for atopy and typically wane by 1 year of age in the case of food allergens and by year 4 or 5 for inhalants. IgG responses (albeit of low titer) often remain detectable into adulthood in nonatopics, and this is paralleled by the presence of varying levels of allergen-specific CD4$^+$ TH1 reactivity in peripheral blood (11,125).

This pattern precisely parallels the findings from the experimental animal models above and suggests that the basis for normal protection against allergic disease involves a cognate immunological process involving antigen-driven "selection" for TH1 reactivity.

In addition, current epidemiological evidence suggests that a similar range of environmental factors to those described in the animals models above as risk factors for promotion of sensitization, notably inhaled airborne irritants and respiratory infections (121), appear capable of stimulating IgE response to inhalant allergens in humans at the time of initial exposure. However, recent comparative studies on genetically comparable populations in Germany, contrasting children living under disparate socioeconomic conditions, indicate that such environmental risk factors do not necessarily operate within a simple linear dose-response framework. Thus, children resident in the former German Democratic Republic, living under conditions of high exposure to environmental air pollution, display markedly *lower* levels of skin test reactivity to inhalant allergens than their counterparts in environmentally "cleaner" West Germany (126). This is despite the clear positive relationship between air pollution and IgE response to inhalant allergens in countries such as Sweden and Austria (127,128). However, the East German children additionally display markedly higher frequency of bronchitis (129). Rates of day-care attendance are up to 10-fold higher in the latter group, suggesting the likelihood of higher respiratory infection rates (129).

Comparable findings have been reported in studies comparing pediatric populations in Sweden with highly polluted areas in Poland and Estonia; i.e., the children living in highly polluted areas in the former Eastern block display low levels of allergic sensitization, but high rates of respiratory infection and bronchitis (130,131).

Thus, while low-moderate levels of air pollution may be significant in promoting allergic sensitization in healthy, well-nourished children, they may not be similarly effective in populations where background levels of respiratory mucosal stimulation (in particular resulting from infection) are relatively high. These findings parallel the earlier literature on the generally low levels of allergy in indigenous pediatric populations in underdeveloped countries throughout the world and provide important clues to the etiology of allergic disease (further discussion below).

D. Kinetics of Postnatal Maturation of Immune Function in Infancy and Early Childhood: A Major Determinant of Susceptibility to Primary Allergic Sensitization?

The newborn of different mammalian species display varying levels of immunological "immaturity" at birth and rely to different degrees on transfer of maternal immunity for protection against challenge by foreign antigens. Recent studies in both human and experimental animals (reviewed in Ref. 132) suggest that the functional capacity of T cells in neonates is low relative to adults, and matures during the preweaning period. The initial suggestion from our laboratory that genetic "risk" for atopy is associated with sluggish postnatal T-cell maturation (133), particularly in regard to capacity to secrete IFN-γ, has subsequently received support from several independent sources (134–136).

Additionally, systemic antigen-presenting cell (APC) functions are low in the neonate (137,138), and this appears partly related to suboptimal surface expression of the class II MHC (Ia) glycoproteins involved in presentation of processed antigen to the T-cell receptor (139).

In rodents, postnatal maturation of local mucosal immune function(s), in particular at the level of responses to antigens impinging on the airway mucosa (120), appears to lag behind systemic immune function. Research in our laboratory indicates that this maturation deficiency in respiratory mucosal immune function is associated with low-level Ia expression on airway intra-epithelial DC populations responsible for the delivery of (inhaled) antigenic signals to T cells in the draining lymph nodes (121,140), and also with the hyporesponsiveness of these DC to activation signals from cytokines (141). The airway DC in the neonatal animals express normal levels of class I MHC, which is employed for presentation of antigens to CD8[+] cells that produce IFN-γ after activation. This suggests that immune reactivity in young animals may be skewed to selectively favor CD8[+] T-cell induction, as a result biasing subsequent "selection" of allergen-specific T-cell reactivity toward CD4[+] T cells, which can survive within lymph node microenvironments rich in IFN-γ, i.e., TH1 as opposed to TH2 cells (107). Work is in progress to determine whether a parallel situation exists in humans.

Thus, it appears that the two key cell populations involved in immune responses to inhaled environmental allergens, both the CD4$^+$ T lymphocytes, which either help or suppress IgE responses, and the antigen-presenting DC, which regulate their activation, may be undergoing major developmental changes during the period of initial exposure to allergens. It can thus be logically hypothesized that factors (both host and environmental) that affect their maturation kinetics may play an important role in the development of "memory" for T help or T suppression for IgE reactivity.

E. Modulation of Allergic Sensitization to Inhalant Allergens by Environmental Factors: Dualistic Effects of Inflammation?

Inflammation at the level of the airway mucosa appears potentially the most important environmental factor in this sensitization process. In relation to the postnatal development of DC function, airway inflammation plays a key role in stimulating "seeding" of bone-marrow-derived precursors into the airway epithelium and in subsequent up-regulation of their Ia expression (140). High levels of Ia expression on airway DC in rodents are observed first in the nasal turbinates, sites of maximal stimulation by inhaled particulates, at a stage in early postnatal life when their counterparts in the epithelium of the conducting airways are Ia^{low}; expression is progressively up-regulated throughout the respiratory tree over subsequent weeks (140). This process can be accelerated by administration of cytokines and retarded by local exposure to inhaled topical steroid (140).

Exposure of the respiratory mucosa to infectious agents appears likely to exert a range of effects on immune responses to locally delivered antigens, which may vary with the agent and with intensity of exposure. On the one hand, airway infection may enhance epithelial permeability to "bystander" antigens, and in some cases [such as *Bordetella pertussis*, through the action of pertussigen toxin (see discussion in Ref. 95)] may provide selective "adjuvant" help for IgE-potentiating T-cell subsets. Low-level aerosol exposure to bacterial cell wall products has also been shown to increase the traffic of DC through the airway epithelium, thus potentially enhancing the delivery of inhaled antigens to T cells in the regional lymph node, and at the same time stimulating their expression of the surface Ia required for presentation of the antigens to T cells (115,141). Low-level exposure to inhaled chemical irritants is also known to enhance epithelial permeability to antigen and may exert similar effects in neonates.

On the other hand, more vigorous stimulation of the local respiratory mucosal immune system may exert different effects. In particular, stimulation of macrophages in vitro via microbial products has been demonstrated to trigger activation and subsequent secretion of high levels of IFN-α and IL-12; these cytokines directly (both directly and indirectly via stimulation of IFN-γ release by adjacent NK cells) inhibit TH2 expansion and accordingly "select" for TH1, thus suppressing IgE responses (118). For this to occur efficiently in vivo, it is likely that relatively high levels of exposure are required, sufficient to mobilize enough airway mucosal macrophages to effect the downstream cytokine milieu within the T-cell zones in the draining lymph nodes, where the activation and subsequent proliferation of inhalant allergen-reactive CD4$^+$ T cells occurs. We hypothesize that this level of microbial stimulation is more likely to be attained in the context of the infection-prone, but allergy-free, East German children described above, as opposed to their Western counterparts (126). If so, the subtly enhanced inward "leakage" of allergens through the airway epithelium in response to air pollution may not be as significant in the East German population, as the immunological milieu within the lymph nodes would effectively be preset to translate incoming antigenic signals (regardless of intensity) into IgE-suppressive TH1 immunity.

The major predictions of this model are testable both in experimental animals models and by further human epidemiological studies.

ACKNOWLEDGMENT

The authors are supported by the National Health and Medical Research Foundation of Australia.

REFERENCES

1. Smith J. In: Middleton E, Reed CE, Ellis EF, Adkinson NF, Yunginger JW, eds. Allergy: Principles and Practice. St. Louis: CV Mosby, 1988:891–929.
2. Friedhoff L. In: Marsh D, Blumenthal M, eds. Genetic and Environmental Factors in Clinical Allergy. Minneapolis: University of Minnesota Press, 1990:53–72.
3. Burrows B, Martinez F, Halonen M, Barbee R, Cline M. Association of asthma with serum IgE levels and skin-test reactivity to allergens. N Engl J Med 1989; 320:271–277.
4. Sears M, Burrows B, Flannery E, Herbison G, Hewitt C, Holdaway M. Relation between airway responsiveness and serum IgE in children with asthma and in apparently normal children. N Engl M Med 1991; 325:1067–1071.
5. Mosmann TR, Cherwinski H, Bond MW, Giedlin MA, Coffman RL. Two types of murine helper T cell clone. I. Definition according to profiles of lymphokine activities and secreted proteins. J Immunol 1986; 136:2348–2357.
6. Firestein GS, Roeder WD, Laxer JA, Townsend KS, Weaver CT, Hom JT, Linton J, Torbett BE, Glasebrook AL. A new murine CD4$^+$ T cell subset with an unrestricted cytokine profile. J Immunol 1989; 143:518–525.
7. Cher DJ, Mossman TR. Two types of murine helper T cell clone. II. Delayed-type hypersensitivity is mediated by Th-1 clones. J Immunol 1987; 138:3688.

8. Coffman RL, Seymour BW, Lebman DA, Hiraki DD, Christiansen JA, Shrader B, Cherwinski HM, Savelkoul HF, Finkelman FD, Bond MW, et al. The role of helper T cell products in mouse B cell differentiation and isotype regulation. Immunol Rev 1988; 102:5–28.

9. DeKruyff RH, Turner T, Abrams JS, Palladino MJ, Umetsu DT. Induction of human IgE synthesis by CD4$^+$ T cell clones. Requirement for interleukin 4 and low molecular weight B cell growth factor. J Exp Med 1989; 170:1477–1493.

10. Wierenga EA, Snoek M, Bos JD, Jansen HM, Kapsenberg ML. Comparison of diversity of house dust mite-specific T-lymphocyte clones from atopic and nonatopic donors. Eur J Immunol 1990; 20:1519–1526.

11. Wierenga EA, Snoek M, de Groot C, Chrétien I, Bos JD, Jansen HM, Kapsenberg ML. Evidence for compartmentalization of functional subsets of CD2$^+$ T lymphocytes in atopic patients. J Immunol 1990; 144:4651–4656.

12. Parronchi P, Macchia D, Biswas M-P, Simonelli C, Maggi E, Ricci M, Ansari AA, Romagnani S. Allergen- and bacterial-antigen-specific T-cell clones established from atopic donors show a different profile of cytokine production. Proc Natl Acad Sci USA 1991; 88:4538–4542.

13. Snapper CM, Paul WE. Interferon-γ and B cell stimulatory factor-1 reciprocally regulate Ig isotype production. Science 1987; 236:944–946.

14. Lutzker S, Rothman P, Pollock R, Coffman R, Alt FW. Mitogen- and IL-4-regulated expression of germ-line Ig gamma 2b transcripts: evidence for directed heavy chain class switching. Cell 1988; 53:177–184.

15. Coffman RL, Ohara J, Bond MW, Carty J, Zlotnik A, Paul WE. B cell stimulatory factor 1 enhances the IgE response to lipopolysaccharide-activated B-cells. J Immunol 1986; 136:4538–4541.

16. Finkelman FD, Katona IM, Urban JFJ, Snapper CM, Ohara J, Paul WE. Suppression of in vivo polyclonal IgE responses by monoclonal antibody to the lymphokine B-cell stimulatory factor 1. Proc Natl Acad Sci USA 1986; 83:9675–9678.

17. Tepper RI, Levinson DA, Stanger BZ, Campos-Torres J, Abbas AK, Leder P. IL-4 induces allergic-like inflammatory disease and alters T cell development in transgenic mice. Cell 1990; 62:457–467.

18. Kühn R, Rajewsky K, Müller W. Generation and analysis of interleukin-4 deficient mice. Science 1991; 254:707–710.

19. Pène J, Rousset F, Brière F, Chrétien I, Bonnefoy JY, Spits H, Yokota T, Arai N, Arai K, Banchereau J, de Vries J. IgE production by normal human lymphocytes is induced by interleukin 4 and suppressed by interferons γ and α and prostaglandin E$_2$. Proc Natl Acad Sci USA 1988; 85:6880–6884.

20. Del Prete G, Maggi E, Parronchi P, Chrétien I, Tiri A, Macchia D, Ricci M, Banchereau J, de Vries J, Romagnani S. IL-4 is an essential factor for the IgE synthesis induced in vitro by human T cell clones and their supernatants. J Immunol 1988; 140:4193–4198.

21. Gauchat J-F, Aversa G, Gascan H, de Vries JE. Modulation of IL-4 induced germline epsilon RNA synthesis in human B cells by tumor necrosis factor-alpha, anti-CD40 monoclonal antibodies or transforming growth factor-beta correlates with levels of IgE production. Int Immunol 1992; 4:397–406.

22. Gauchat J-F, Lebman DA, Coffman RL, Gascan H, de Vries JE. Structure and expression of germline ε transcripts in human B cells induced by interleukin 4 to switch to IgE production. J Exp Med 1990; 172:463–473.

23. Rothman P, Lutzker S, Cook W, Coffman R, Alt FW. Mitogen plus interleukin 4 induction of Cε transcripts in B lymphoid cells. J Exp Med 1988; 168:2385–2389.

24. Paliard X, Malefijt RW, de Vries JE, Spits H. Interleukin-4 mediates CD8 induction on human CD4$^+$ T-cell clones. Nature 1988; 335:642–644.

25. Spits H, Yssel H, Takebe Y, Arai N, Yokota T, Lee F, Arai K, Banchereau J, de Vries JE. Recombinant interleukin 4 promotes the growth of human T cells. J Immunol 1987; 139:1142–1147.

26. Punnonen J, Aversa G, Cocks BG, McKenzie ANJ, Menon S, Zurawski G, De Waal Malefyt R, De Vries JE. Interleukin 13 induces interleukin 4-independent IgG4 and IgE synthesis and CD23 expression by human B cells. Proc Natl Acad Sci USA 1993; 90:3730–3734.

27. Pène J. Regulatory role of cytokines and CD23 in the human IgE antibody synthesis. Int Arch Allergy Appl Immunol 1989; 90:32–40.

28. Vercelli D, Jabara HH, Arai K, Yokota T, Geha RS. Endogenous interleukin 6 plays an obligatory role in interleukin 4–dependent human IgE synthesis. Eur J Immunol 1989; 19:1419–1424.

29. Jabara HH, Fu SM, Geha RS, Vercelli D. CD40 and IgE: synergism between anti-CD40 monoclonal antibody and interleukin 4 in the induction of IgE synthesis by highly purified human B cells. J Exp Med 1990; 172:1861–1864.

30. Raynal MC, Liu ZY, Hirano T, Mayer L, Kishimoto T, Chen KS. Interleukin 6 induces secretion of IgG1 by coordinated transcriptional activation and differential mRNA accumulation. Proc Natl Acad Sci USA 1989; 86:8024–8028.

31. Dugas B, Renauld JC, Pene J, Bonnefoy JY, Petit-Frere C, Braquet P, Bousquet J, Van Snick J, Mencia-Huerta JM. Interleukin-9 potentiates the interleukin-4-induced immunoglobulin (IgG, IgM and IgE) production by normal human B lymphocytes. Eur J Immunol 1993; 23:1687–1692.

32. Moeller J, Hultner L, Schmitt E, Breuer M, Dormer P. Purification of MEA, a mast cell growth-enhancing activity, to apparent homogeneity and its partial amino acid sequencing. J Immunol 1990; 144:4231–4234.

33. Kehrl JH, Miller A, Fauci AS. Effect of tumor necrosis factor alpha on mitogen-activated human B cells. J Exp Med 1987; 166:786–791.

34. Aversa G, Punnonen J, de Vries JE. The 26-kD transmembrane form of tumor necrosis factor alpha on activated CD4+ T cell clones provides a costimulatory signal for human B cell activation. J Exp Med 1993; 177:1575–1585.

35. Thyphronitis G, Tsokos GC, June CH, Levine AD, Finkelman FD. IgE secretion by Epstein-Barr virus infected purified human B lymphocytes is stimulated by interleukin-4 and suppressed by interferon-γ. Proc Natl Acad Sci USA 1989; 86: 5580–5584.

36. Reinhold U, Wehrmann W, Kukel S, Kreysel W. Evidence that defective interferon-gamma production in atopic dermatitis patients is due to intrinsic abnormalities. Clin Exp Immunol 1990; 79:374–379.

37. Rousset F, Robert J, Andary M, Bonnin JP, Souillet G, Chretien I, Briere F, Pene J, de Vries JE. Shifts in interleukin-4 and interferon-gamma production by T cells

of patients with elevated serum IgE levels and the modulatory effects of these lymphokines on spontaneous IgE synthesis. J Allergy Clin Immunol 1991;87:58–69.

38. Jujo K, Renz H, Abe J, Gelfand EW, Leung DYM. Decreased interferon gamma and increased interleukin-4 production in atopic dermatitis promotes IgE synthesis. J Allergy Clin Immunol 1992; 90:323–331.

39. Peleman R, Wu J, Fargeas C, Delespesse G. Recombinant interleukin-4 suppresses the production of interferon γ by human mononuclear cells. J Exp Med 1989; 170: 1751–1757.

40. Vercelli D, Jabara HH, Lauener RP, Geha RS. IL-4 inhibits the synthesis of IFN-γ and induces the synthesis of IgE in human mixed lymphocyte cultures. J Immunol 1990; 144:570–573.

41. Boguniewicz M, Jaffe H, Izu A, Sullivan MJ, York D, Geha RS, Leung DY. Recombinant gamma interferon in treatment of patients with atopic dermatitis and elevated IgE levels. Am J Med 1990; 88:365–370.

42. Parkin JM, Eales L-J, Galazka AR, Pinching AJ. Atopic manifestations in the acquired immune deficiency syndrome response to recombinant interferon gamma. Br Med J 1987; 294:1185–1186.

43. Hanifin JM, Schneider LC, Leung DY, Ellis CN, Jaffe HS, Izu AE, Bucalo LR, Hirabayashi SE, Tofte SJ, Cantu Gonzales G, et al. Recombinant interferon gamma therapy for atopic dermatitis. J Am Acad Dermatol 1993; 28:189–197.

44. Delespesse G, Sarfati M, Peleman R. Influence of recombinant IL-4, IFN-alpha and IFN-gamma on the production of IgE-binding factor (soluble CD23). J Immunol 1989; 142:134–138.

45. Thyphronitis G, Banchereau J, Heusser C, Tsokos GC, Levine AD, Finkelman FD. Kinetics of interleukin-4 induction and interferon-gamma. Cell Immunol 1991; 133:408–419.

46. Souillet G, Rousset F, de Vries JE. Alpha-interferon treatment of a patient with hyper IgE syndrome. Lancet 1989; 1:1384.

47. Lindley I, Aschauer H, Seifert JM, Lam C, Brunowsky W, Kownatzki E, Thelen M, Peveri P, Dewald B, von Tscharner V, Walz A, Baggiolini M. Synthesis and expression in *Escherichia coli* of the gene encoding monocyte-derived neutrophil-activating factor: biological equivalence between natural and recombinant neutrophil-activating factor. Proc Natl Acad Sci USA 1988; 85:9199–9203.

48. Kimata H, Yoshida A, Ishioka C, Lindley I, Mikawa H. Interleukin 8 (IL-8) selectively inhibits immunoglobulin E production induced by IL-4 in human B cells. J Exp Med 1992; 176:1227–1231.

49. Standiford TJ, Streiter RM, Chensue SW, Westwick J, Kashara K, Kunkel SL. IL-4 inhibits the expression of IL-8 from stimulated human monocytes. J Immunol 1990; 145:1439.

50. Yssel H, de Waal Malefyt R, Roncarlo M-G, Abrams JS, Lahesmaa R, Spits H, de Vries JE. IL-10 is produced by subsets of human CD4$^+$ T cell clones and peripheral blood T cells. J Immunol 1992; 149:2378–2384.

51. Fiorentino DF, Ziotnik A, Vieira P, Mosmann TR, Howard M. Moore KW, O'Garra A. IL-10 acts on the antigen presenting cell to inhibit cytokine production by Th1 cells. J Immunol 1991; 146:3444–3451.

52. O'Garra A, Stapleton G, Char V, Pearce M, Schumacher J, Rugo H, Barbis D, Stall A, Cupp J, Moore KW, et al. Production of cytokines by mouse B cells: B lymphomas and normal B cells produce interleukin 10. Int Immunol 1990; 2:821–832.

53. De Waal Malefyt R, Abrams JS, Bennett B, Figdor CG, de Vries JE. Interleukin 10 (IL-10) inhibits cytokine synthesis by human monocytes: an autoregulatory role of IL-10 produced by monocytes. J Exp Med 1991; 147:1209–1220.

54. Fiorentino DF, Ziotnik A, Mosmann TR, Howard M, O'Garra A. IL-10 inhibits cytokine production by activated macrophages. J Immunol 1991; 147:3815–3822.

55. Hsu DH, de Waal Malefyt R, Fiorentino DF, Dang M-N, Vieira P, de Vries JE, Spits H, Mosmann TR, Moore KW. Expression of interleukin-10 activity by Epstein-Barr virus protein BCRF1. Science 1990; 250:830–832.

56. De Waal Malefyt R, Haanen J, Spits H, Roncarolo M-G, Te Velde A, Figdor C, Johnson K, Kastelein R, Yssel H, De Vries JE. Interleukin 10 (IL-10) and viral IL-10 strongly reduce antigen-specific human T cell proliferation by diminishing the antigen-presenting capacity of monocytes via downregulation of class II major histocompatibility complex expression. J Exp Med 1991; 174:915–924.

57. De Waal Malefyt R, Yssel H, Roncarolo MG, Spits H, de Vries JE. Interleukin-10. Curr Opin Immunol 1992; 4:314–320.

58. Ding L, Shevach EM. IL-10 inhibits mitogen-induced T cell proliferation by selectively inhibiting macrophage costimulatory function. J Immunol 1992; 148:3133–3139.

59. Taga K, Tosato G. IL-10 inhibits human T cell proliferation and IL-2 production. J Immunol 1992; 148:1143–1148.

60. Punnonen J, De Waal Malefyt R, Van Blasselaer P, Gauchat J-F, De Vries JE. IL-10 and viral IL-10 prevent IL-4-induced IgE synthesis by inhibiting the accessory cell function of monocytes. J Immunol 1993; 151:1280–1289.

61. Fiorentino DF, Bond MW, Mosmann TR. Two types of mouse helper T cells. IV. Th2 clones secrete a factor that inhibits cytokine production by Th1 clones. J Exp Med 1989; 170:2081–2095.

62. Kiniwa M, Gately M, Gubler U, Chizzonite R, Fargeas C, and Delespesse G. Recombinant interleukin-12 suppresses the synthesis of immunoglobulin E by interleukin-4 stimulated human lymphocytes. J Clin Invest 1992; 90:262–266.

63. Miller A, Lider O, Roberts AB, Sporn MB. Suppressor T cells generated by oral tolerization to myelin basic protein suppress both in vitro and in vivo immune responses by the release of TGF-β following antigenic specific triggering. Proc Natl Acad Sci USA 1992; 89:421–425.

64. Maggi E, Del Prete G, Macchia D, Parronchi P, Tiri A, Chretien I, Ricci M, Romagnani S. Profiles of lymphokine activities and helper function for IgE in human T cell clones. Eur J Immunol 1988; 18:1045–1050.

65. Pène J, Rousset F, Briére F, Chrétien I, Paliard X, Banchereau J, Spits H, de Vries JE. IgE production by normal human B cells induced alloreactive T cell clones is mediated by IL-4 and suppressed by IFN-γ. J Immunol 1988; 141:1218–1224.

66. Gascan H, Aversa GG, Gauchat J-F, Van Vlasselaer P, Roncarolo M-P, Yssel H, Kehry M, Spits H, de Vries JE. Membranes of activated CD4+ T cells expressing

T cell receptor (TcR) αβ or TcR γδ induce IgE synthesis by human B cells in the presence of interleukin-4. Eur J Immunol 1992; 22:1133–1141.

67. Stamenkovic I, Clark EA, Seed B. A B-lymphocyte activation molecule related to the nerve growth factor receptor and induced by cytokines in carcinomas. EMBO J 1989; 8:1403–1410.

68. Smith CA, Davis T, Anderson D, Solam L, Beckmann MP, Jerzy R, Dower SK, Cosman D, Goodwin RG. A receptor for tumor necrosis factor defines an unusual family of cellular and viral proteins. Science 1990; 248:1019–1023.

69. Clark EA, Ledbetter JA. Activation of human B cells mediated through two distinct cell surface differentiation antigens, Bp35 and Bp50. Proc Natl Acad Sci USA 1986; 83:4494–4498.

70. Paulie S, Rosen A, Ehlin Henriksson B, Braesch Andersen S, Jakobson E, Koho H, Perlmann P. The human B lymphocyte and carcinoma antigen, CDw40, is a phosphoprotein involved in growth signal transduction. J Immunol 1989; 142: 590–595.

71. Banchereau J, de Paoli P, Valle A, Garcia E, Rousset F. Long-term human B cell lines dependent on interleukin-4 and antibody to CD40. Science 1991; 251:70–72.

72. Zhang K, Clark EA, Saxon A. CD40 stimulation provides an IFN-gamma-independent and IL-4-dependent differentiation signal directly to human B cells for IgE production. J Immunol 1991; 146:1836–1842.

73. Gascan H, Gauchat J-F, Aversa G, van Vlasselaer P, de Vries JE. Anti-CD40 monoclonal antibodies or CD4$^+$ T cell clones and IL-4 induce IgG4 and IgE switching in purified human B cells via different signalling pathways. J Immunol 1991; 147:8–13.

74. Armitage RJ, Fanslow WC, Strockbine L, Sato TA, Clifford KN, Macduff BM, Anderson DM, Gimpel SD, Davis-Smith T, Maliszewski CR, et al. Molecular and biological characterization of a murine ligand for CD40. Nature 1992; 357:80–82.

75. Gauchat J-F, henchoz S, Mazzei G, Aubry JP, Brunner T, Blasey H, Life P, Talabot D, Florex-Romo L, Thompson J, Kishi K, Butterfield J, Bahinden C, Bonnefoy J-Y. Induction of human IgE synthesis in B cells by mast cells and basophils. Nature 1993; 365:340–343.

76. Fanslow WC, Anderson DM, Grabstein KH, Clark EA, Cosman D, Armitage RJ. Soluble forms of CD40 inhibit biologic responses of human B cells. J Immunol 1992; 149:655–660.

77. Flores-Romo L, Shields J, Humbert Y, Grabler P, Aubry J-P, Gauchat JF, Ayla G, Allet B, Chavez M, Bazin H, Capron M, Bonnefoy J-Y. Inhibition of an in vivo antigen-specific IgE response by antibodies to CD23. Science 1993; 26:1038–1041.

78. Defrance T, Aubry JP, Rousset F, Vandervliet B, Bonnefoy JY, Arai N, Takebe Y, Yokota T, Lee F, Arai K, de Vries JE, Banchereau J. Human recombinant interleukin 4 induces Fc epsilon receptors (CD23) on normal human B lymphocytes. J Exp Med 1987; 165:1459–1467.

79. Rousset F, Malefijt RW, Slierendregt B, Aubry JP, Bonnefoy JY, Defrance T, Banchereau J, de Vries JE. Regulation of Fc receptor for IgE (CD23) and class II MHC antigen expression on Burkitt's lymphoma cell lines by human IL-4 and IFN-gamma. J Immunol 1988; 140:2625–2632.

80. Fischer E, Delibrias C, Kazatchkine MD. Expression of CR2 (the C3dg/EBV receptor, CD21) on normal human peripheral blood T lymphocytes. J Immunol 1991; 146:865–869.

81. Pochon S, Graber P, Yeager M, Jansen K, Bernard AR, Aubry JP, Bonnefoy JY. Demonstration of a second ligand for the low affinity receptor for immunoglobulin E (CD23) using recombinant CD23 reconstituted into fluorescent liposomes. J Exp Med 1992; 176:389–397.

82. Bacon K, Gauchat JF, Aubry JP, Pochon S, Graber P, Henchoz S, Bonnefoy JY. CD21 expressed on basophilic cells is involved in histamine release triggered by CD23 and anti-CD21 antibodies. Eur J Immunol 1993; 23:2721–2724.

83. Prinz JC, Baur X, Mazur G, Rieber EP. Allergen-directed expression of Fc receptors for IgE (CD23) on human T lymphocytes is modulated by interleukin 4 and interferon-gamma. Eur J Immunol 1990; 20:1259–1264.

84. Sarfati M, Nakajima T, Frost H, Kilccherr E, Delespesse G. Purification and partial biochemical characterization of IgE-binding factors secreted by a human B lymphoblastoid cell line. Immunology 1987; 60:539–545.

85. Hamid Q, Azzawi M, Ying S, Moqbel R, Wardlaw AJ, Corrigan CJ, Bradley B, Durham SR, Collins JV, Jeffery PK, Quint DJ, Kay AB. Expression of mRNA for interleukin-5 in mucosal bronchial biopsies from asthma. J Clin Invest 1991; 87: 1541–1546.

86. Robinson DS, Hamid Q, Ying S, Tsicopoulos A, Barkans J, Bentley AM, Corrigan C, Durham SR, Kay AB. Predominant TH2-like bronchoalveolar T-lymphocyte population in atopic asthma. N Engl J Med 1992; 326:298–304.

87. Del Prete GF, de Carli M, D'Elios MM, Maestrelli P, Ricci M, Fabbri L, Romagnani S. Allergen exposure induces the activation of allergen-specific Th2 cells in the airway mucosa of patients with allergic respiratory disorders. Eur J Immunol 1993; 23:1445–1449.

88. Wells HG, Osborne TB. The biological reactions of the vegetable proteins. I. Anaphylaxis. J Infect Dis 1911; 8:66–124.

89. Mowat AM. The regulation of immune responses to dietary protein antigens. Immunol Today 1987; 8:93–98.

90. MacDonald TT. Immunosuppression caused by antigen feeding II. Suppressor T cells mask Peyer's patch B cell priming to orally administered antigen. Eur J Immunol 1983; 13:138–142.

91. Challacombe SJ, Tomasi TJ. Systemic tolerance and secretory immunity after oral immunization. J Exp Med 1980; 152:1459–1472.

92. Zhang Z, Michael JG. Orally inducible immune unresponsiveness is abrogated by IFN-γ treatment. J Immunol 1990; 144:4163–4165.

93. Hanson DG. Ontogeny of orally induced tolerance to soluble proteins in mice. I. Priming and tolerance in newborns. J Immunol 1981; 127:1518–1524.

94. Strobel S, Ferguson A. Immune responses to fed protein antigens in mice. 3. Systemic tolerance or priming is related to age at which antigen is first encountered. Pediatr Res 1984; 18:588–594.

95. Holt PG, Britten D, Sedgwick JD. Suppression of IgE responses by antigen inhalation: studies on the role of genetic and environmental factors. Immunology 1987; 60:97–102.

96. Parker D, Turk JL. Delay in the development of allergic response to metals following intratracheal instillation. Int Arch Allergy Appl Immunol 1978; 57:289–293.
97. Holt PG, Batty JE, Turner KJ. Inhibition of specific IgE responses in mice by pre-exposure to inhaled antigen. Immunology 1981; 42:409–417.
98. Holt PG, Leivers S. Tolerance induction via antigen inhalation: isotype specificity, stability, and involvement of suppressor T cells. Int Arch Allergy Appl Immunol 1982; 67:155–160.
99. Sedgwick JD, Holt PG. Induction of IgE-isotype specific tolerance by passive antigenic stimulation of the respiratory mucosa. Immunology 1983; 50:625–630.
100. Holt PG, McMenamin C. Defence against allergic sensitization in the healthy lung: the role of inhalation tolerance. Clin Exp Allergy 1989; 19:255–262.
101. Holt PG, Reid M, Britten D, Sedgwick J, Bazin H. Suppression of IgE responses by passive antigen inhalation: dissociation of local (mucosal) and systemic immunity. Cell Immunol 1987; 104:434–440.
102. Sedgwick JD, Holt PG. Suppression of IgE responses in inbred rats by repeated respiratory tract exposure to antigen: responder phenotype influences isotype specificity of induced tolerance. Eur J Immunol 1984; 14:893–897.
103. Sedgwick JD, Holt PG. Downregulation of immune responses to inhaled antigen: studies on the mechanism of induced suppression. Immunology 1985; 56:635–642.
104. Stewart GA, Holt PG. Immunogenicity and tolerogenicity of a major house dust mite allergen, *Der p* I from *Dermatophagoides pteronyssinus*, in mice and rats. Int Arch Allergy Appl Immunol 1987; 83:44–51.
105. Sedgwick JD, Holt PG. Induction of IgE-secreting cells and IgE isotype-specific suppressor T cells in the respiratory lymph nodes of rats in response to antigen inhalation. Cell Immunol 1985; 94:182–194.
106. McMenamin C, Oliver J, Girn B, Holt BJ, Kees UR, Thomas WR, Holt PG. Regulation of T-cell sensitization at epithelial surfaces in the respiratory tract: suppression of IgE responses to inhaled antigens by CD3+ Tcr alpha-/beta- lymphocytes (putative gamma/delta T cells). Immunology 1991; 74:234–239.
107. McMenamin C, Holt PG. The natural immune response to inhaled soluble protein antigens involves major histocompatibility complex (MHC) class I–restricted CD8+ T cell–mediated but MHC class II–restricted CD4+ T cell–dependent immune deviation resulting in selective suppression of IgE production. J Exp Med 1993; 178:889–899.
108. McMenamin C, Pimm C, McKersey M, Holt PG. Regulation of IgE responses to inhaled antigen in mice by antigen-specific gamma delta T cells. Science 1994; 265:1869–1871.
109. McMenamin C, McKersey M, Kuhnlein P, Hunig T, Holt PG. γ/δ T-cells downregulate primary IgE responses in rats to inhaled soluble protein antigens. J Immunol 1995; 154:4390–4394.
110. Holt PG. The role of immunological tolerance mechanisms in protection against allergic sensitisation in the respiratory tract: contrasting effects of aeroallergen exposure in adult versus newborn animals. In: Johansson SGO, ed. IgE-Mediated

Allergy in Childhood. Stockholm: Pharmacia Allergy Research Foundation, 1989: 5–11.

111. Holt PG, Schon-Hegrad MA, Oliver J. MHC class II antigen–bearing dendritic cells in pulmonary tissues of the rat: regulation of antigen presentation activity by endogenous macrophage populations. J Exp Med 1988; 167:262–274.

112. Holt PG, Schon-Hegrad MA, Phillips MJ, McMenamin PG. Ia-positive dendritic cells form a tightly meshed network within the human airway epithelium. Clin Exp Allergy 1989; 19:597–601.

113. Holt PG, Schon-Hegrad MA, Oliver J, Holt BJ, McMenamin PG. A contiguous network of dendritic antigen-presenting cells within the respiratory epithelium. Int Arch Allergy Appl Immunol 1990; 91:155–159.

114. Holt PG, Oliver J, McMenamin C, Schon-Hegrad MA. Studies on the surface phenotype and functions of dendritic cells in parenchymal lung tissue of the rat. Immunology 1992; 75:582–587.

115. Schon-Hegrad MA, Oliver J, McMenamin PG, Holt PG. Studies on the density, distribution, and surface phenotype of intraepithelial class II major histocompatibility complex antigen (Ia)-bearing dendritic cells (DC) in the conducting airways. J Exp Med 1991; 173:1345–1356.

116. Holt PG. Regulation of antigen-presenting cell function(s) in lung and airway tissues. Eur Respir J 1993; 6:120–129.

117. Mayrhofer G, Holt PG, Papadimitriou JM. Functional characteristics of the veiled cells in afferent lymph from the rat intestine. Immunology 1986; 58:379–387.

118. Romagnani S. Induction of T_H1 and T_H2 responses: a key role for the "natural" immune response? Immunol Today 1992; 13:379–381.

119. Renz H, Smith HR, Henson JE, Ray BS, Irvin CG, Gelfand EW. Aerosolised antigen exposure without adjuvant causes increased IgE production and increased airways responsiveness in the mouse. J Allergy Clin Immunol 1992; 89: 1127–1138.

120. Nelson D, McMenamin C, Wilkes L, Holt PG. Postnatal development of respiratory mucosal immune function in the rat: regulation of IgE responses to inhaled allergen. Pediatr Allergy Immunol 1991; 4:170–177.

121. Holt PG, McMenamin C, Nelson D. Primary sensitisation to inhalant allergens during infancy. Pediatr Allergy Immunol 1990; 1:3–13.

122. Mariani F, Price JF, Kemeny DM. The IgG subclass antibody response to an inhalant antigen (*Dermatophagoides pteronyssinus*) during the first year of life: evidence for early stimulation of the immune system following natural exposure. Clin Exp Allergy 1992; 22:29–33.

123. Hattevig G, Kjellman B, Björkstén B. Clinical symptoms and IgE responses to common proteins and inhalants in the first 7 years of life. Clin Allergy 1987; 17: 571–578.

124. Hattevig G, Kjellman, B, Björkstén B. Appearance of IgE antibodies to ingested and inhaled allergens during the first 12 years of life in atopic and non-atopic children. Pediatr Allergy Immunol 1993; 4:182–186.

125. Romagnani S. Regulation and deregulation of human IgE synthesis. Immunol Today 1990; 11:316–321.

126. Magnussen H, Jorres R, Nowak D. Effect of air pollution on the prevalence of asthma and allergy: lessons from the German reunification. Thorax 1993; 48: 879–881.
127. Popp W, Zwick H, Streyrer K, et al. Sensitization to aeroallergens depends on environmental factors. Allergy 1989; 44:572–575.
128. Andrae S, Axelson O, Björkstén B. Symptoms of bronchial hyperreactivity and asthma in relation to environmental factors. Arch Dis Child 1988; 63:473–478.
129. Von Mutius E, Martinez FD, Fritzsch C, Nicolai T, Roell G, Theimann H. Prevalence of asthma and atopy in two areas of West and East Germany. Am J Respir Crit Care Med 1994; 149:358–364.
130. Bråbäck L, Breborwicz A, Dreborg S, Knutsson A, Pieklik H, Björkstén B. Atopic sensitisation and respiratory symptoms among Polish and Swedish school children. Clin Exp Allergy 1994; 24:826–835.
131. Björkstén B. Risk factors in early childhood for the development of atopic diseases. Allergy 1994; 49:400–407.
132. Holt PG. Postnatal maturation of immune competence during infancy and early childhood. Pediatr Allergy Immunol 1995; 6:59–70.
133. Holt PG, Clough JB, Holt BJ, Baron-Hay MJ, Rose AH, Robinson BWS, Thomas WR. Genetic "risk" for atopy is associated with delayed postnatal maturation of T-cell competence. Clin Exp Allergy 1992; 22:1093–1099.
134. Warner JA, Miles EA, Jones AC, Quint DJ, Colwell BM, Warner JO. Is deficiency of interferon gamma production by allergen triggered cord blood cells a predictor of atopic eczema? Clin Exp Allergy 1994; 24:423–430.
135. Rinas U, Horneff G, Wahn V. Interferon-γ production by cord-blood mononuclear cells is reduced in newborns with a family history of atopic disease and is independent from cord blood IgE-levels. Pediatr Allergy Immunol 1993; 4:60–64.
136. Tang M, Kemp A, Varigos G. IL-4 and interferon-gamma production in children with atopic disease. Clin Exp Immunol 1993; 92:120–124.
137. Taylor S, Bryson YJ. Impaired production of γ-interferon by newborn cells in vitro is due to a functionally immature macrophage. J Immunol 1985; 134:1493–1498.
138. Wilson CB, Westall J, Johnston L, Lewis DB, Dover SK, Apert AR. Decreased production of interferon gamma by human neonatal cells: intrinsic and regulatory deficiencies. J Clin Invest 1986; 77:860–867.
139. Stiehm ER, Sztein MB, Oppenheim JJ. Deficient DR antigen expression on human cord blood monocytes: reversal with lymphokines. Clin Immunol Immunopathol 1984; 30:430–436.
140. Nelson DJ, McMenamin C, McWilliam AS, Brenan M, Holt PG. Development of the airway intraepithelial dendritic cell network in the rat from class II MHC (Ia) negative precursors: differential regulation of Ia expression at different levels of the respiratory tract. J Exp Med 1994; 179:203–212.
141. McWilliam AS, Nelson D, Thomas JA, Holt PG. Rapid dendritic cell recruitment is a hallmark of the acute inflammatory response at mucosal surfaces. J Exp Med 1994; 179:1331–1336.

11

Inflammation

Penelope A. Lympany and Tak H. Lee
Guy's Hospital
London, England

I. INTRODUCTION

Considerable investigative resources over the past decade have been devoted to the study of the production of inflammatory mediators and the recruitment of inflammatory cells into the airway. The purpose of this chapter is to discuss recent findings related to the role of the inflammatory response with particular reference to atopy and asthma and to outline the way in which molecular biological techniques have been employed in such studies. The techniques themselves will not be discussed in great depth since they are well described, both in the references cited in this chapter and in the current literature.

Asthma is characterized clinically by wheeze, breathlessness, and cough; functionally by reversible airways obstruction; and pathologically by inflammation of the airways, desquamation of the epithelium, and eosinophil infiltration (Fig. 1). Inflammation of the airways is an important feature of asthma, and bronchoconstriction may therefore be part of the sequelae of the inflammatory cascade.

The term "atopy" is most often used to describe a general predisposition to allergic disease as shown by either a positive skin prick test to common inhaled allergens, a raised allergen-specific IgE, or a raised total IgE. Atopy

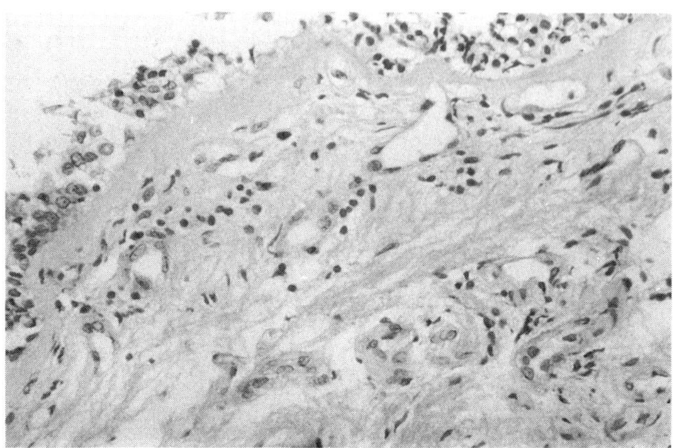

(a)

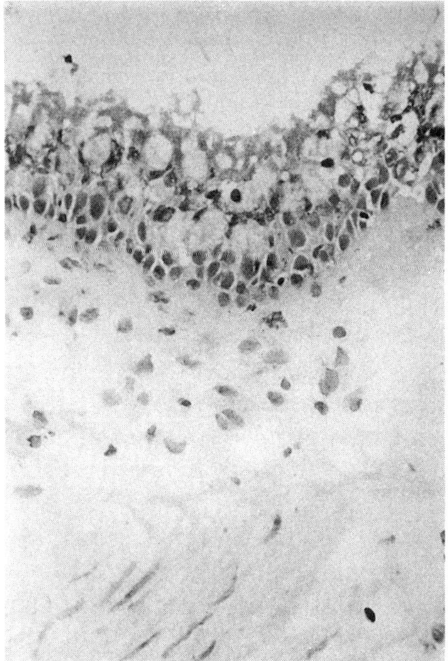

(b)

FIGURE 1 (a) Bronchial biopsy taken from an asthmatic subject, stained with hematoxylin and eosin, showing shedding of the epithelium, basement membrane thickening, and an intense inflammatory cell infiltrate in the submucosa. (b) Bronchial biopsy from a control subject stained by the same method, showing the epithelium intact and decreased numbers of inflammatory cells in the submucosa.

plays an important role in the etiology of allergic disease. Some individuals do not appear to respond to an allergen while the same exposure leads to an "allergic" reaction in other people that manifests as rhinitis, asthma, atopic dermatitis, or anaphylaxis.

Inflammation is the reactive change that occurs in response to tissue injury and consists of a series of events occurring following that injury. In general terms, there is an initial capillary constriction followed by vasodilatation and increased blood flow. There is also edema formation and migration of inflammatory cells to the region. Acute inflammation is the local response of tissue to an injury that is not sufficient to destroy its structure or vitality and is associated with neutrophil infiltration and exudate formation. Chronic inflammation is predominantly associated with macrophages, plasma cells, eosinophils, and mast cells and is thought to modify bronchial smooth muscle, bronchial epithelium, and autonomic systems through the production of inflammatory mediators including histamine, leukotrienes, and cytokines. There is now evidence that T cells are also implicated in chronic inflammation.

The extent of the genetic control of the inflammatory response is still poorly understood, although recent work has attempted to address this issue. It was initially suggested that MHC class II molecules play an important role in determining the allergic response to specific allergens. This view was later supplemented with data that suggested that a region of chromosome 11q was involved in the allergic response and, more recently, that regions close to the cytokine genes on chromosome 5q are important in determining the allergic response. These hypotheses are described in detail in other chapters in this book. However, it is now becoming clear that allergy and asthma are polygenic diseases.

Inflammation is an integral part of asthma and atopy, and a study in mice has suggested that the inflammatory response is polygenically controlled (1). Acute inflammation was induced in mice by the injection of a neutral substrate, and the cell and serum protein concentration of the local exudate was measured. The pattern of alleles controlling the high or low response was different in each parental strain, and a large, continuous range of responses was obtained in different inbred strains of mice, which suggested that the inflammatory response was under polygenic control. Intercrossing of the inbred strains studied resulted in a genetically heterogeneous F3 generation, which presented highly variable responses. Later, the same workers studied the genetic regulation of the acute inflammatory reaction in mice giving a maximal and a minimal inflammatory response (2). The extent of inflammation was measured as previously, and the cell numbers and serum protein concentration were positively correlated and presented a normal frequency distribution. A genetically heterogeneous foundation population was produced by the intercrossing of inbred strains of mice, and selective breeding was carried out by assorted matings of extreme phenotypes. The response to selection in 11 consecutive generations was highly asymmetrical, showing an increase in the maximum and no change in the minimal acute inflammatory response, indicating the importance of a genetic propensity to develop an inflammatory response. If this investigation also serves as a paradigm for the human inflammatory condition, it seems reasonable to suppose that there is a genetic component to the development of an inflammatory response.

It has also been suggested that chronic inflammation may result from the dysregulation of the transcription of the inflammatory mediators, resulting in the characteristic cytokine pattern and cellular infiltration seen in the inflammatory process in the lungs. Proto-oncogenes that are present in normal cells are involved in the regulation and growth of nonmalignant cells as well as the transformation of malignant cells. c-*fos* is a proto-oncogene that regulates the transcription of many genes and may be involved in the regulation of inflammation in asthma. Very low levels of c-*fos* are detectable in most human cells and its expression is rapidly and transiently increased by inflammatory mediators such as histamine, eicosanoids, and cytokines. The presence of c-fos protein and the immunoreactivity of a cell proliferation marker, proliferating cell nuclear antigen (PCNA), were examined by Demoly et al. (3) in bronchial biopsies obtained from asthmatic and normal subjects. c-*fos* was induced only in the epithelial cells of the asthmatic subjects and PCNA immunoreactivity was observed only in one asthmatic and one control subject and was not related to c-*fos* expression. These results suggested that the role for c-*fos* was in cell activation rather than in proliferation. It may therefore be of interest to study the mechanisms by which inflammatory cells become activated such that we may detect any dysfunction in the process that may lead to persistent cell activation and, consequently, a state of chronic inflammation.

II. EVIDENCE FOR INFLAMMATION IN ASTHMA

Asthma is an example of a lung disease in which inflammation of the airways is present and may be a central mechanism in the pathophysiology of the disease. Early studies of patients who died from status asthmaticus revealed marked inflammation of the bronchial tree. Airway edema and inflammation are now recognized as cardinal features of asthma, resulting from increased microvascular permeability of the bronchial circulation with the exudation of plasma and inflammatory cells into the airway lumen. Resistance to airflow is increased and the epithelium is disrupted either directly or by cytotoxic products such as platelet-activating factor (PAF), leukotrienes, and histamine produced by migrating inflammatory cells.

The development of the technique of bronchoalveolar lavage (BAL) has enabled more detailed examination of the inflammatory response in the airways. Using BAL to study the inflammatory response in primate lungs, it was demonstrated that neutrophils accumulated in the lungs in response to the production of chemotactic agents, probably from alveolar macrophages (4). Similarly, it has been shown, using BAL in humans, that there is an increase in the number of ciliated cells, eosinophils, macrophages, and monocytes in the bronchoalveolar lavage fluid (BALF) taken from asthmatic subjects when compared with nonasthmatic subjects (5,6).

Histological examination of airway biopsies has demonstrated the infiltration of a variety of inflammatory cells including neutrophils, eosinophils, and lymphocytes. In a study of bronchial biopsies taken from asthmatic subjects, it was shown by Poston et al. (7) that there was a significant increase in the numbers of activated eosinophils, macrophages, and T cells (Fig. 2). This was the first demonstration of significantly increased numbers of macrophages in biopsies from asthmatic airways. Many of these macrophages showed the phenotypic characteristics of monocytes, which suggested active recruitment of these cells from the bloodstream. Poulter et al. (8) showed that nasal mucosal biopsies taken from asthmatic subjects had similar inflammatory infiltrates to those seen in bronchial biopsies. In this study, immunostaining of bronchial biopsies taken from atopic asthmatic subjects showed an increase both in the numbers of secreting eosinophils and in IL-2 receptor (IL-2R)-positive cells after allergen challenge when compared to those after diluent challenge (9). Although there were no significant differences in the total numbers of leukocytes, neutrophils, macrophages, or mast cells, there was a significant increase in the number of cells expressing mRNA for IL-5 and GM-CSF after allergen challenge. There was also increased expression of MHC class II molecules on the epithelial cells, macrophages, and other infiltrating cells. These findings suggest the importance of inflammatory cells and cytokine production in bronchial asthma.

Antigen-induced and neurogenic inflammation, generated by immunoglobulin E (IgE) and neuropeptides, respectively, may also contribute to edema formation. Sensory nerves synthesize tachykinins and calcitonin-gene-related peptide and package these neuropeptides together in synaptic vesicles. Stimulation of these nerve fibers by a range of chemical and physical factors results in the local release of neuropeptides through the axonal reflex. In the airways, sensory neuropeptides act on bronchial smooth muscle, the mucosal vasculature, and submucosal glands to promote airflow obstruction, increased microvascular permeability, and mucus hypersecretion. In addition, tachykinins potentiate cholinergic neurotransmission and, when released from airway sensory nerves, may also cause bronchoconstriction, vasodilatation, plasma exudation, and mucus secretion, whereas calcitonin may contribute to hyperemia of inflammation. Airway epithelial damage in asthma exposes sensory nerves that may become sensitized by inflammatory products so that neuropeptides

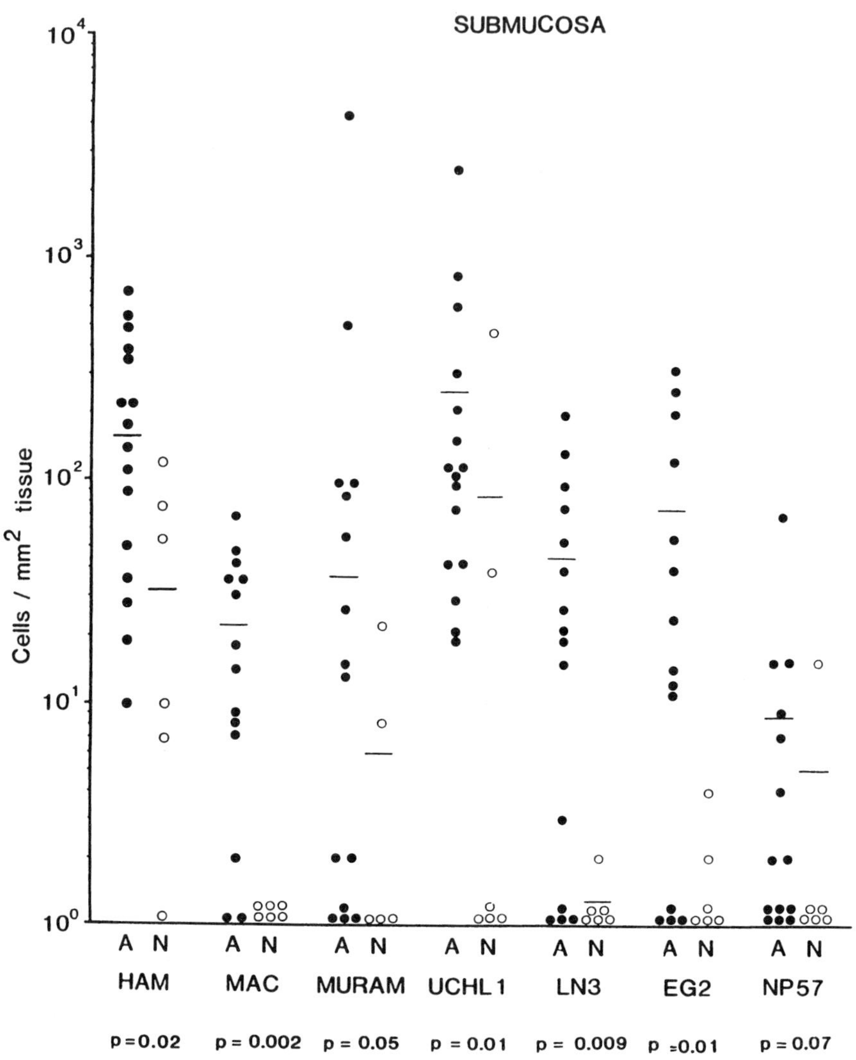

FIGURE 2 Comparison of the cell counts in the submucosa of biopsies taken from asthmatic (A) and normal (N) subjects. HAM = Ham56 (a panmacrophage monoclonal antibody); MAC = monoclonal antimonocyte monoclonal antibody; MURAM = polyclonal antimuramidase antibody; UCHL1 = antimemory T-cell monoclonal antibody; LN3 = anti-HLA-DR monoclonal antibody; EG2 = antieosinophil cationic protein monoclonal antibody; NP57 = antineutrophil elastase monoclonal antibody. The *p* values given were obtained using the Mann-Whitney U test. (From Am Rev Respir Dis 1993; 145:918–921.)

are released via a local reflex trigger such as bradykinin, resulting in inflammation. The effects of tachykinins may be amplified further by loss of the major degrading enzyme, neutral endopeptidase, from epithelial cells. Proinflammatory effects of tachykinins also promote the recruitment, adherence, and activation of granulocytes that may further potentiate neurogenic inflammation. Enzymatic degradation limits the physiological effects of tachykinins but may be impaired by respiratory infection or other factors. It is possible that neuropeptide-containing sensory nerves play an important role in mediating airway responses in human disease because of their sensitivity to noxious compounds and physical stimuli and their potent effects on airway function.

III. CELLS INVOLVED IN INFLAMMATION

Various cells are associated with the inflammatory events that are characteristic of atopic allergy and asthma. Although eosinophil infiltration is a feature of asthmatic airways, there is also an increase in the number of neutrophils and mononuclear cells (10). Even mild asthmatics show degranulation of mast cells, infiltration of eosinophils, and an increase in mononuclear cells in airway mucosal biopsies. Accumulation of lymphocytes at the sites of inflammation is a characteristic of all allergic disorders including atopic asthma, rhinitis, and dermatitis. In addition, T cells, eosinophils, mast cells, basophils, mononuclear phagocytes, and platelets must all be considered, particularly as their mediators have potential for contributing directly to the features of bronchial asthma. A comparison of the cell counts in the submucosa of biopsies taken from asthmatic subjects compared with those from normal subjects is shown in Figure 2.

The identification of cell surface markers and their subsequent use in identifying cell subsets and also in detecting cell activation has been important in the study of the inflammatory response. Cells may be labeled with specific cell surface determinant antibodies and separated using fluorescence-activated cell-sorting (FACS) analysis. Alternatively, in situ hybridization may be used to identify cell subpopulations in tissues obtained by biopsy or in cytospin preparations of cells.

A. T Lymphocytes

A striking feature of asthma is the intense infiltration of bronchial mucosa with eosinophils, macrophages, and lymphocytes. The accumulation of mononuclear cells at the site of chronic inflammation is dependent on a number of factors, including the adherence of lymphocytes to vascular endothelial cells, the production of chemotactic factors, and increased permeability of the endothelium.

The relationship between T cells and allergic inflammation was studied by Frew et al. (11), who showed that there was a significant infiltration by CD3$^+$/CD4$^+$ T cells and also evidence of T-cell activation in the allergen-induced late-phase skin reaction in atopic subjects. Activated T cells were also detected in the blood of subjects with acute severe asthma and there was evidence of increased eosinophil infiltration and activation. In a more recent study, the T-cell response to anti-CD2, -CD3, or -CD28 monoclonal antibodies was measured in atopic subjects and subjects who had undergone immunotherapy. The T-cell response to anti-CD2 monoclonal antibodies in subjects who had undergone immunotherapy was normal, although IL-2 production and the proliferative response in T cells stimulated via CD3 was impaired. Costimulation with anti-CD28 monoclonal antibodies restored both IL-2 production and proliferative response in all tested patients. The response to CD28-mediated stimulation was more pronounced in atopic than in normal subjects, appeared to have a major role in T-cell proliferation of atopic subjects, and may provide a suitable model for analyzing CD3/CD28 interactions in the regulation of IL-2 expression (12).

There is an increased expression of the cell surface markers CD25, HLA-DR, and VLA-1 on T cells recovered by BAL (13), and in bronchial biopsies from subjects with asthma, there are increased numbers of CD$^+$ cells (14,15). These data suggest that activation of T cells may have a role in the pathogenesis of asthma. Furthermore, by in situ hybridization it has been shown that there are increased numbers of cells that are positive for IL-2, IL-3, IL-4, IL-5, and GM-CSF mRNA in BALF from atopic asthmatic compared with control subjects, but with no differences in IFN-γ mRNA expression (16).

The activation of CD4$^+$ T cells plays an important role in allergic inflammation and is dependent on the recognition of allergen-derived peptides in association with major histocompatibility complex class II gene products. In a study by Damle and Doyle (17), T cells were separated into CD4$^+$ (helper/inducer), CD8$^+$ (cytotoxic/suppressor), CD29$^+$ CD45RA$^-$ CD45RO$^+$ (memory), and CD29A$^-$ CD45RA$^+$ CD45RO$^-$ (naïve) T-cell subsets. The subsets were stimulated with phytohemagglutinin (PHA) and phorbol myristate acetate (PMA) and their adherence to endothelial cells was examined. All subpopulations showed increased adherence to endothelial cells, although resting memory T cells showed greater adherence than naïve T cells. Activated memory T cells also increased endothelial permeability to albumin.

Walker et al. (18) compared the activation of lymphocyte subpopulations and cytokine production in the peripheral blood and BALF of asthmatic subjects. Allergic asthmatic subjects had increased numbers of T cells positive for the markers CD4 and IL-2R in both peripheral blood and BALF. T-cell activation was closely correlated with numbers of low-affinity IgE receptor (CD23)-bearing B cells. In contrast, in nonallergic asthmatic subjects, both CD4$^+$ and

CD8$^+$ T cells from blood and BALF had increased expression of IL-2R, HLA-DR, and VLA-1. In the nonallergic asthmatic subjects, CD8$^+$ T cells were decreased in blood but increased in BALF. Cytokine levels were determined in BALF and supernatants from purified peripheral blood T cells and enriched BAL lymphocyte preparations. Allergic asthmatic subjects were characterized by increased levels of IL-4 and IL-5, and this elevated IL-4 contributed to the raised IgE levels found in these allergic subjects. Nonallergic asthmatic subjects had raised levels of IL-2 and IL-5. The close correlation of IL-5 levels with eosinophilia suggested that IL-5 is responsible for the characteristic eosinophilia of asthma.

It has been suggested that IL-2 may be a contributory factor in T-cell activation. Support for this suggestion was provided by a study in which T cells of atopic subjects were found to secrete low quantities of IL-2 and to express low amounts of Tac antigen. Addition of recombinant IL-2 to cultures restored the T-cell proliferative response and Tac antigen expression. This effect was specific to IL-2 and the investigators concluded that T cells of atopic patients have a defect in CD2 and CD3 pathways of activation, relying on impairment of IL-2 production without involving IL-2 responsiveness or other lymphokine defects (19).

B. Mast Cells

Mast cells comprise between 0.25 and 0.5% of the total lymphocyte population recovered by BAL from normal subjects (20). They are found throughout the respiratory tract and in large numbers in the walls of the alveoli and airways and are characterized by the presence of high-affinity receptors for the Fc portion of IgE (Fc$_\varepsilon$R1). The cytoplasm of mast cells is filled with granules containing preformed mediators including histamine. As a direct consequence of cell activation and gene transcription, a family of interleukins and cytokines including interleukins-4, -5, and -6 and TNF-α (21,22) and lipid mediators such as leukotriene C$_4$, prostaglandin, and PAF are produced. A review of the mediators and enzymes released by mast cells has recently been presented (23, 24).

Studies of allergic asthma show a direct link between mast cell degranulation, neutrophil and eosinophil influxes into the lung, and worsening pulmonary function and airway reactivity. It has been shown that prevention of mast cell degranulation attenuates the early and late asthmatic responses and decreases the eosinophils found in BALF of allergic asthmatics (25,26). Mast cell degranulation occurs when antibodies on the cell surface are crosslinked either by specific antigen or by corresponding divalent anti-immunoglobulin or by antibodies to the Fc$_\varepsilon$R. This crosslinking causes activation of intracellular signaling.

More mast cells are found in BALF of asthmatics than nonasthmatic subjects (27) and mast cells from asthmatic subjects exhibit greater spontaneous and stimulated anti-IgE histamine release (28). Many studies suggest that exposure of sensitive subjects to antigen leads to mast cell degranulation and the subsequent lung inflammatory response (25,26,29–32). The influx of neutrophils into inflammatory sites results from the release of chemoattractants from mast cells among others. The role of mast cells in asthma has been reviewed in some detail (33,34).

C. Eosinophils

Eosinophils are cells of granulocyte lineage that are generated in the bone marrow and represent a small proportion of the total lymphocyte population in normal subjects. Recruitment of eosinophils from the blood to tissues initially involves their adherence to endothelial cells and subsequent migration into inflamed tissues. Normal endothelial cells can interact with inflammatory cells to mediate their adherence properties but these are enhanced by inflammatory cytokines that induce increased expression of specialized adhesion molecules, e.g., ICAM-1, ECAM-1, and VCAM.

There is evidence that during diapedesis, granulocytes interact with epithelial and endothelial cells to produce regionally secreted mediators that upregulate the responsiveness of adjacent airway smooth muscle and/or cause luminal edema, thus augmenting the effect of constrictor stimuli. Most evidence suggests that the eosinophil is the most important granulocyte in these responses and that eosinophilic infiltration and activation may account for the unique, spasmodic, and cyclic nature of hyperreactive airways.

Eosinophils, through their ability to generate an array of potent mediators, are thought to be the major effector cells in a number of conditions, including parasitic infection, asthma, and other allergic diseases. The production and release of eosinophils is modulated by cytokines (35). Eosinophils have been shown to be present in bronchial biopsies, BAL fluid, and peripheral blood of patients with mild to moderate asthma (36). Activated eosinophils are believed to be the major contributors to the chronic inflammatory sequelae of asthma, although the mechanism of eosinophil activation and prolonged survival in vivo is unknown. In a later study by Djukanovic et al. (37), the numbers of eosinophils in bronchial biopsies were greatest in asthmatic subjects, low or absent in the normal, and intermediate in the nonasthmatic atopic subjects. In both atopic groups, eosinophils showed ultrastructural features of degranulation. Additionally, the collagen layer was thickest in the asthmatics, intermediate in the atopic nonasthmatic subjects, and thinnest in the normal individuals. The results suggested that airways eosinophilia and degranulation of eosinophils and mast cells, as well as increased subepithelial collagen deposition, are features of atopy in general and that the degree of change may determine the clinical expression of this immune disorder.

The cytoplasmic granules of eosinophils contain a number of basic proteins including eosinophil cationic protein (ECP) and major basic protein (MBP). These are released on activation and degranulation of eosinophils and can damage the upper and lower respiratory epithelium. Release of PAF at inflammatory sites can alter vascular permeability, affect eosinophil chemotaxis, and stimulate the release of leukotrienes and MBP by eosinophils. During status asthmaticus, mast cells and eosinophils are activated and release arachidonic acid–derived inflammatory mediators such as the sulfidopeptide leukotrienes. These metabolites, particularly LTC_4, are present in BAL from asthmatic patients, and it has been demonstrated that alveolar macrophages recovered by BAL and purified by adherence are able to transform LTC_4 into its metabolite LTE_4. In asthmatic subjects with severe local inflammation, alveolar macrophages that were incubated in the presence of LTC_4 were shown to generate LTB_4 and 5-HETE, which remained within the cells (38). The role of leukotrienes in the inflammatory response is discussed later.

Eosinophils from sputum, nasal polyps, and BAL samples from asthmatic subjects have increased levels of CD11b expression compared to their blood eosinophils. Tissue eosinophils were shown to express ICAM-1 and HLA-DR whereas blood eosinophils did not (39). This shows that the eosinophils in the inflammatory response are activated and have an increased ability to bind to endothelial cells via ICAM-1 and to present antigen in the context of HLA-DR. The mechanism of eosinophil adhesion in allergic inflammation has recently been reviewed (40).

The mechanism by which eosinophils accumulate at inflammatory sites is unknown, although one possible mechanism is the adhesion of eosinophils to the vascular endothelium. In a study by Walsh et al. (41), human eosinophils but not neutrophils were shown to constitutively express alpha 4 beta 1 (CD49d/CD29). Eosinophils, and not neutrophils, specifically adhered to COS cells transfected with vascular adhesion molecule-1 in a CD49d/CD29-dependent manner, and eosinophil adhesion to IL-1-stimulated human umbilical vascular endothelial cells was significantly inhibited by a monoclonal antibody specific to CD49d/CD29. Inhibition of resting and PAF-stimulated eosinophil adhesion was observed. These data suggested that the CD49d/CD29/ vascular adhesion molecule-1 adhesion pathway may be involved specifically in the migration of eosinophils into sites of eosinophilic inflammation.

Recent studies have suggested that airway inflammation in atopic asthma is characterized by T-cell activation and local eosinophilia. This may also apply to nonatopic asthma, as shown in a study by Marini et al. (42) in which the cytokine mRNA profile and activation status of inflammatory cells in the BALF of nonallergic subjects with symptomatic asthma and nonallergic healthy control subjects were compared. The asthmatic subjects had an increased number of inflammatory cells in their BALF, including activated eosinophils and activated T cells. There was an increased production of the cytokines IL-5, GM-CSF, IL-1, and IL-6 in the airways of subjects with nonatopic asymptomatic asthma, which may contribute to the persistence of inflammation by inducing the local activation of eosinophils (IL-5, GM-CSF) and promoting T-cell activation and proliferation (IL-1, IL-6).

PAF-acether is a phospholipid mediator formed by a variety of cells including eosinophils, macrophages, platelets, neutrophils, and vascular endothelial cells. Its biosynthesis involves the acetylation of a precursor released from membrane phospholipids by activated phospholipase A_2. PAF-acether activates most inflammatory cells and induces a variety of in vivo effects related to inflammation, such as airway edema, eosinophil accumulation in the airway, and bronchial hyperresponsiveness. In the guinea pig lung, these effects have been shown to include acute bronchoconstriction and bronchopulmonary hyperreactivity, accompanied by platelet, eosinophil, and macrophage activation and their recruitment into the lung parenchyma and airways. However, the precise role of PAF in asthma has yet to be established. To evaluate the effect of PAF on leukocyte-dependent inflammation, purified populations of human blood eosinophils and neutrophils were isolated from the same subject. The two granulocyte populations were then incubated with PAF, and superoxide anion (O_2^-) generation was measured by reduction of cytochrome C in a microassay system. Both granulocyte cell types generated O_2^- when they were incubated with PAF. However, the generation of O_2^- was greater with eosinophils than neutrophils. When the effect of PAF on intracellular calcium concentration was measured, similar increases in the intracellular calcium were shown. Furthermore, when similar experiments were conducted in the presence of an extracellular calcium chelator, there was partial suppression in both the cellular calcium and O_2^- generation induced by PAF; this suggested that full expression of eosinophil generation of O_2^- by PAF requires both intracellular mobilization and a transmembrane influx of Ca^{2+}. PAF was shown to stimulate leukocyte O_2^- generation but this response was greater in the eosinophils than in the neutrophils (43).

The role of eosinophils in the pathogenesis of asthma has been reviewed by Seminario and Gleich (44).

D. Neutrophils

Neutrophils comprise over 90% of the circulating granulocytes in the peripheral blood. They possess two forms of intracellular granules, namely lysosomes containing acid hydrolases and specific granules containing lactoferrin. The precise role of the neutrophil in the pathophysiology of bronchial asthma is not conclusive, although some investigators report their presence in BALF, and biopsies taken post allergen challenge from asthmatic subjects and others have demonstrated chemotaxis of neutrophils toward mediators released during the inflammatory process.

To test whether neutrophils infiltrate and degranulate in areas of chronic respiratory allergic inflammation, tissue specimens from patients with fatal asthma, chronic sinusitis, and nasal polyposis were examined for the presence of elastase and major basic protein. Neutrophil infiltration and extracellular elastase deposition in association with damage to respiratory epithelium were found in few of the specimens examined. In contrast, eosinophil infiltration and extracellular MBP deposition were generally marked in the majority of specimens. The results suggest that the neutrophil does not usually infiltrate tissues showing allergic inflammation (45). The presence of increased numbers of neutrophils in the BALF and biopsies of asthmatic subjects has been a subject of some debate. However, some of these differences may be attributed to the time of sampling post allergen challenge. In one study (31), BAL performed 4 hr post challenge showed an increase in both neutrophils and eosinophils, although at 24 hr post challenge, the numbers of neutrophils had decreased but the eosinophils remained elevated. However, in another study, bronchial biopsies performed in mild asthmatic subjects post allergen challenge showed little evidence of neutrophilic infiltration (25). Bronchial biopsies provide information about local infiltration of the bronchial mucosa but are not able to provide much information with respect to the dynamic changes that occur during an inflammatory response.

Neutrophils at the sites of inflammation may contribute to tissue damage by releasing lysosomal enzymes and toxic oxygen radicals. Reactive oxygen species (ROS) may be generated by several inflammatory cells that participate in airway inflammation and their production may be increased in asthma. Oxygen metabolites may contribute to the epithelial damage that is characteristic of asthmatic airway and may activate cells such as mast cells in the airway mucosa. They may also cause bronchoconstriction and mucus secretion, have effects on airway vasculature, and increase airway responsiveness. The effects of antiasthma drugs on airway inflammation or antioxidative actions due to the inhibition of O_2^- generation were investigated by Kato et al. (46). The results of this study suggested these drugs may be beneficial in the treatment of airway inflammation caused by O_2^- generation in bronchial asthma.

E. Monocytes and Macrophages

In normal and asthmatic individuals, alveolar macrophages are the predominant inflammatory cells in the airways (47). In normal subjects, it has been shown that alveolar macrophages are a heterogeneous cell population. When the density of alveolar macrophages from asthmatic patients and normal subjects was compared, macrophages recovered from asthmatic patients were shown to be of lower density than those from normal subjects (48). The low-density alveolar macrophages from both the asthmatic and the normal subjects appeared to have the morphological characteristics of activated cells. The functional activity of the alveolar macrophage fractions of asthmatic and control subjects was assessed and there was no difference between the fractions of asthmatic or control subjects with regard to oxygen species release, suggesting that this is a normal function of the macrophage. However, thromboxane B_2 (TxB$_2$) generation was increased in low-density alveolar macrophages from asthmatic subjects when compared with the same fractions of normal subjects. The hypodense cells produced less TxB$_2$ than did cells of higher density in both asthmatic and normal subjects.

Capron et al. (49) showed the existence of Fcε receptors (Fc$_\varepsilon$R) on macrophages by implicating the role of IgE antibodies in the macrophage-dependent cytotoxic killing of *Schistosoma mansoni* larvae. The Fc$_\varepsilon$R expressed on the surface of macrophages is similar to that found on lymphocytes and platelets and is referred to as the Fc$_\varepsilon$RII/CD23. This differs from the Fc$_\varepsilon$R expressed on the surface of mast cells and basophils, which is known as the Fc$_\varepsilon$RI. Between 5 and 10% of peripheral blood mononuclear cells and lung macrophages from normal subjects express Fc$_\varepsilon$RII (50–52). This proportion is increased in atopic subjects compared with normal individuals (52), and up to 20% of alveolar macrophages in mild atopic asthmatic subjects express Fc$_\varepsilon$RII (51). It has been suggested that Fc$_\varepsilon$RII has multiple functions as a membrane-bound or soluble molecule, a function in B-cell growth and differentiation, and a role in the effector phase of IgE-mediated immunity. To study further the function of the soluble Fc$_\varepsilon$RII/CD23 (sFC$_\varepsilon$RII), the recombinant receptor was produced and was shown to competitively block the IgE binding of eosinophils, monocytes, and basophils and could inhibit the IgE-mediated function of effector cells such as monocytes. These findings suggested that sFc$_\varepsilon$RII could competitively regulate the function of effector cells in IgE-mediated immunity and that the recombinant sFc$_\varepsilon$RII could be applied clinically for the control of allergic reactions (53).

F. Cell Interactions

In the previous sections, the relative involvements of T cells, neutrophils, mast cells, macrophages, and eosinophils have been discussed briefly. However, the interactions between these cells may be of particular significance in the inflammatory response involved in asthma and atopy since it is clear that mediators released by some cell regulate the function of others (Fig. 3). The acute symptoms of allergy and asthma such as sneezing, bronchospasm, and urticaria are

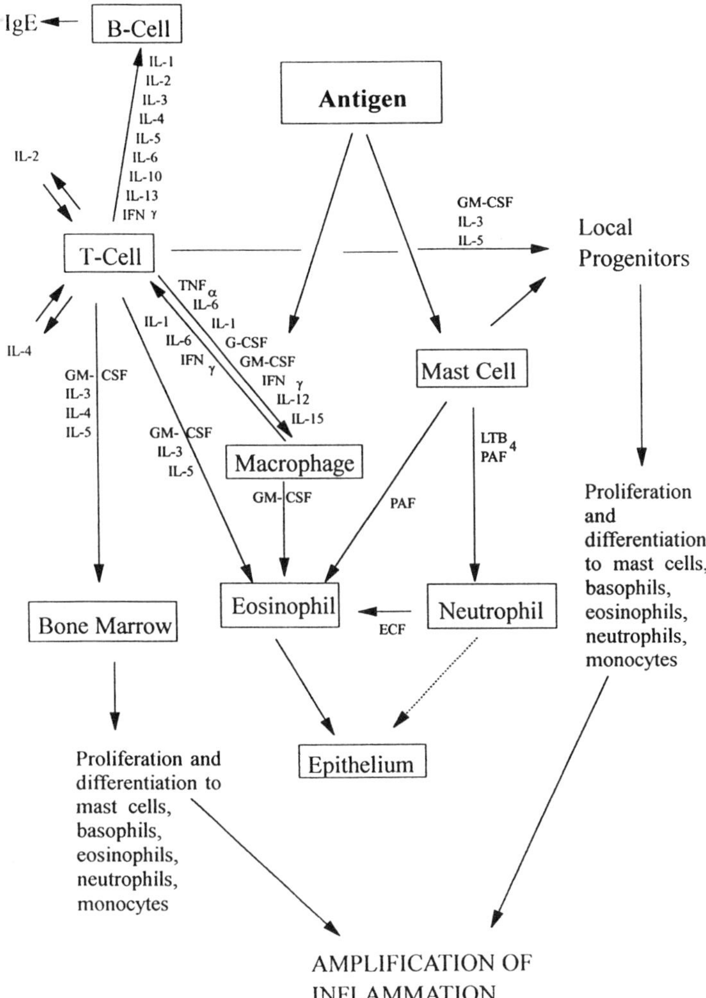

FIGURE 3 Schematic representation of the mediators released from inflammatory cells and their influence on other cells involved in the inflammatory process.

believed to be largely the result of mediator release from mast cells whereas chronic symptoms (the result of allergic inflammation) can be explained on the basis of eosinophil-mediated tissue damage. In humans, specialized T cells, possibly the human equivalent of the murine TH2 subset, predominate in allergy and produce IL-4 and IL-5. IL-5 potentiates the terminal differentiation and activation of the eosinophil. Basic proteins together with PAF and leuk-otrienes secreted by eosinophils produce chronic wheeze and bronchial irritability and might also be involved in permanent nasal blockage in chronic rhinitis. PAF can induce clinical and pathological features seen in the airways of asthmatic subjects, including edema, eosinophil accumulation, and bronchial hyperresponsiveness; PAF is a potent chemoattractant and can activate eosinophils via specific surface receptors. Major basic protein appears to cause direct, noncytotoxic stimulation of epithelial secretion that up-regulates nonspecifically the response of airway smooth muscle to contractile stimuli. A review of the interactions between macrophages and granulocytes in asthma has been published (54).

IV. CHEMICAL MEDIATORS

Cellular communication and control through the release of mediators is important in the regulation of the inflammatory response. Three main classes of chemical mediators control this response: histamine, cytokines, and leukotrienes.

A. Histamine

The mechanism of acute inflammation involves the initial release of histamine and 5-HT from mast cells and circulating basophils followed by the release of kinins and prostaglandins. The response to histamine comprises vasodilatation involving H1 and H2 receptors (55–57), increased microvascular permeability, and edema.

Histamine is a naturally occurring amine stored in the body following formation by decarboxylation of histidine, a naturally occurring amino acid. Studies that have detected histamine at the site of inflammation have shown that histamine release in inflammation is transient and comprises one of the factors of acute rather than chronic inflammation. An important feature of the inflammatory response to histamine is that the increased microvascular permeability component is self-limiting and rapidly reverses even when the microcirculation remains exposed to histamine. The acute inflammatory response to histamine comprise vasodilatation, an increase in microvascular permeability, and edema formation. The release of histamine and 5-HT during acute inflammation controls vascular permeability. The initial transient arteriolar constriction is followed by prolonged vasodilatation, which is associated with increased vascular permeability and increased blood flow. The initial dilatation is an axomal reflex after which histamine acts on the smooth muscle. Initial increased flow is dependent on the available histamine in the immediate area. Kinins are small peptides that increase vascular permeability and have a role in the maintenance of vascular permeability in the later stages of acute inflammation and also act as neutrophil chemotactic agents.

B. Cytokines

Cytokines are soluble proteins that have a major regulatory role in the immune and inflammatory systems and to a large extent mediate interactions between immune and inflammatory cells. They bind to specific receptors on the cell surface of target cells and are associated with intracellular signal transduction and second-messenger pathways. They have a variety of functions including promotion of cell growth, differentiation, and activation. In addition to the stimulation of lymphocytes, macrophages, and eosinophils, they stimulate the production of arachidonic acid metabolites such as prostaglandins and leukotrienes and are therefore important in both acute and chronic inflammation. Some cytokines are constitutively expressed, e.g., G-CSF, IL-6, others are stored in cytoplasmic granules, e.g., GM-CSF, TGF-β, PDGF, or as membrane proteins, e.g., TNF-α, IL-1β, TGF-α, or are complexed with cell surface binding proteins, e.g., IL-8, TGF-β. However, the majority of cytokines are only produced in response to stimuli such as infection, inflammatory mediators, and mechanical injury.

The nomenclature surrounding the cytokine proteins is complex and, in general, uninformative with respect to the structure and function of the cytokines. However, they may be subdivided into families showing sequence homology at the amino acid and sequence levels. This has recently been described in some detail by Callard and Gearing (58). Cytokines may also be loosely classified according to their primary function, into chemotactic cytokines, those which affect cell growth and differentiation, and those involved in the regulation of the inflammatory process. This is illustrated in Table 1, which also includes the chromosomal assignment of the cytokines where known. A schematic representation of the production of some of the cytokines involved in the regulation of the inflammatory response is presented in Figure 3, which also illustrates the synergism involved in the inflammatory process. The primary functions of the major cytokines are described in Table 2. Cytokines which are now thought to be important in the regulation of the asthmatic and allergic responses are discussed more fully in other chapters.

1. Regulation of the Inflammatory Response by Cytokines

As previously discussed, the eosinophil is a cell commonly found during the inflammatory process. It has been shown that the cytokines IL-3, IL-5, and GM-CSF increase the survival of eosinophils in culture and enhance eosinophil mediator generation and consequently toxicity (59,60). IL-5 is a selective eosinophil chemotaxin, whereas GM-CSF is a chemoattractant for eosinophils

TABLE 1　Grouping of Cytokines into Families According to Their Main Functions: Sources and Target Cells of the Major Cytokines Currently Known

Cytokine	Secreted by	Target cells	Chromosomal location
Chemotactic cytokines			
IL-5	Mast cells, T cells, eosinophils	Eosinophils	5q23–31
IL-8	Monocytes, lymphocytes	Neutrophils	4q12
MCP	Monocytes, T cells, fibroblasts, endothelial cells	Monocytes, basophils	17q11–12
RANTES	T cells, macrophages	Monocytes, T cells, eosinophils	17q11–21
Cytokines that affect cell growth and differentiation			
IL-1	Monocytes, macrophages, T cells, B cells	B cells, T cells, monocytes	2q12–21
IL-2	T cells	T cells, B cells, monocytes, macrophages	4q26–27
IL-3	Activated T cells, mast cells, eosinophils	Eosinophils, neutrophils, basophils, mast cells	5q23
IL-4	T cells, mast cells	B cells, T cells, monocytes, endothelial cells	5q31
IL-5	Mast cells, T cells, eosinophils	Eosinophils	5q23–31
IL-7	Bone marrow	B cells, T cells	8q12
IL-9	IL-2-activated T cells	T cells	5q31
IL-11	IL-1-stimulated fibroblasts, bone marrow	Macrophage progenitor cells	19q13
IL-12	B cells, monocytes, macrophages	T cells	Not known
IL-14	T cells	B cells	Not known
IL-15	Peripheral blood mononuclear cells	See IL-2	Not known
EGF	Monocytes	Epithelial cells	4q25
G-CSF	Macrophages, fibroblasts	Neutrophils	17q21–22
GM-CSF	T cells, macrophages	Granulocytes, monocytes, T cells	5q21–32
IFN-γ	CD4, CD8 T cells	T cells, B cells	12q24
PDGF	Platelets, macrophages, endothelial cells	Connective tissue cells	4q11–12
TGF-β1–3	Platelets, nucleated cells	Majority of cell types	19q13, 1q41, 14q24
TNF	Activated monocytes, macrophages, B cells, T cells	Majority of nucleated cells	6p21

TABLE 1 Continued

Cytokine	Secreted by	Target cells	Chromosomal location
Cytokines involved in regulation of the inflammatory process			
IL-1	Monocytes, macrophages, T cells, B cells	B cells, T cells, monocytes, macrophages	2q12–21
IL-6	B cells, T cells, monocytes	B cells, macrophages	7p21
IL-8	Monocytes, lymphocytes	Neutrophils	4q12
IL-10	CD4, CD8 T cells	T cells, monocytes	1
IL-13	Activated T cells	Monocytes	5q31
PDGF	Platelets, macrophages, endothelial cells	Connective tissue cells	4q11–12
TNF	T cells, B cells	Majority of nucleated cells	6p21

and neutrophils (61). GM-CSF production is increased in subjects with asthma when compared to normal subjects, and the culture media taken from mononuclear cells of asthmatic subjects has been shown to stimulate the proliferation and survival of eosinophils, an activity that can be partially inhibited by anti-GM-CSF antibodies (62). The expression of IL-5 and GM-CSF by eosinophils at sites of allergic inflammation in asthmatics may be an important autocrine pathway, maintaining the viability and effector function of the recruited eosinophils. Using in situ hybridization with ^{35}S-labeled mRNA probes, Broide et al. (63) studied the expression of IL-5 and GM-CSF mRNA in BAL eosinophils derived from asthmatic subjects before and after endobronchial allergen challenge which induced a significant airway eosinophilia. Following allergen challenge, the eosinophils expressed IL-5 and GM-CSF mRNA. Double mRNA labeling experiments with an IL-5 RNA probe and a GM-CSF RNA probe demonstrated that individual eosinophils expressed one of four cytokine mRNA profiles (IL-5 only, GM-CSF only, IL-5 and GM-CSF, or neither IL-5 nor GM-CSF). These results are in agreement with those presented in a study of the cytokine levels found in the BALF and supernatants from purified peripheral blood T cells and BAL lymphocytes from asthmatic subjects by Walker et al. (18). Allergic asthmatic subjects had increased levels of IL-4 and IL-5 and nonallergic asthmatic subjects had increased levels of IL-2 and IL-5. These data demonstrate the importance of these cytokines in the maintenance of eosinophils at inflammatory sites and also illustrate the synergy between cytokines in the regulatory processes.

TABLE 2 Function of the Major Cytokines Involved in Cell Growth and Differentiation and the Inflammatory Response

Cytokine	Main functions
Cytokines that affect cell growth and differentiation	
IL-1	Activates T cells, initiates cellular transcription of many genes
IL-2	T-cell proliferation, also stimulates B-cell, monocyte, and macrophage growth and differentiation
IL-3	Stimulates formation and differentiation of eosinophils, neutrophils, basophils, monocytes, and mast cells
IL-4	T-cell activation, promotes B-cell growth and differentiation, promotes immunoglobulin class switch, growth factor with IL-3
IL-5	Stimulates growth and differentiation of eosinophils and basophils, activates eosinophils and prolongs their survival
IL-7	Progenitor B-cell differentiation, proliferation, and stimulation of mature T cells
IL-9	Promotes growth and differentiation of T cells, enhances mast cell growth
IL-11	Growth factor for many cells, is related to IL-6, has synergistic actions with IL-3
IL-12	Induces IFN-γ production, costimulates lymphocyte proliferation, induces the differentiation of TH1 T-cell subset
IL-14	Induces proliferation of activated B cells, inhibits immunoglobulin synthesis
IL-15	Stimulates CTLL proliferation
EGF	Stimulates growth of epithelial cells
G-CSF	Stimulates growth and differentiation of granulocyte stem cells, activates neutrophils and eosinophils
GM-CSF	Stimulates growth and differentiation of haemopoietic stem cells, activates mature granulocytes
IFN-γ	Inhibits B-cell differentiation, activates growth and differentiation of T cells, B cells, macrophages, and endothelial cells
PDGF	Mitogen for connective tissue and glial cells, important in wound healing, may also act as chemoattractant for fibroblasts, monocytes, and neutrophils
TGF-β1–3	Switch factor for IgA, involved in tissue remodeling, wound repair, and development, inhibits cell growth
TNF	Mediator of inflammation, regulates growth and differentiation of a wide variety of cell types, may be selectively toxic for some cells
Cytokines involved in the regulation of the inflammatory process	
IL-1	Activates T cells, initiate cellular transcription of many genes
IL-6	B-cell growth and differentiation, stimulates transcription and synthesis of many genes of proinflammatory proteins in acute-phase response

TABLE 2 Continued

Cytokine	Main functions
IL-8	Neutrophil chemotaxin, cofactor in granulocyte differentiation
IL-10	Inhibits synthesis of cytokines from TH1-type T cells, enhances expression of MHC II on B cells, cofactor in mast cell growth and differentiation, T-cell growth factor
IL-13	Inhibits production of inflammatory cytokines in vitro, prolongs survival of human monocytes, and increases surface expression of MHC class II and CD23
PDGF	Mitogen for connective tissue and glial cells, important in wound healing, and may also act as chemoattractant for fibroblasts, monocytes, and neutrophils
TNF	Mediator of inflammation, regulates growth and differentiation of a wide variety of cell types, may be selectively toxic for some cells

Cultured human bronchial epithelial cells constitutively produce GM-CSF. Increased levels of immunoreactive and biologically active IL-1 have been identified in the airway secretions of asthmatic patients, together with an increase in GM-CSF. In vivo, asthmatic airway epithelium expresses significantly greater quantities of GM-CSF (64) (Fig. 4a and 4b). In a study by Marini et al. (65), the ability of IL-1 to bind to specific receptors on bronchial epithelial cells and promote GM-CSF synthesis and release was investigated. Bronchial epithelial cells possessed specific single-class surface receptors for recombinant IL-1. The addition of exogenous IL-1 led to a dose-dependent increase in the accumulation of GM-CSF mRNA and release of immunoreactive GM-CSF to the culture medium. The release of IL-1 in the bronchial mucosa during allergic and nonallergic responses may lead to enhanced GM-CSF synthesis and release by epithelial cells, thus promoting inflammation of the airways. The techniques of in situ hybridization to localize the mRNA and immunoassay to determine levels of secretion were used to determine whether GM-CSF was present in the airways of asthmatic subjects who had airway eosinophilia after endobronchial allergen challenge. Levels of immunoreactive GM-CSF increased significantly 24 hr after endobronchial allergen stimulation. The cellular source of BAL GM-CSF, as determined by in situ hybridization and immunoperoxidase staining, was derived predominantly from UCHL-1-positive BAL lymphocytes, as well as from a smaller population of alveolar macrophages. Before local endobronchial allergen challenge, less than 1% of lymphocytes and alveolar macrophages recovered by BAL expressed GM-CSF mRNA, whereas after allergen stimulation 92.6% of lymphocytes and 17.5%

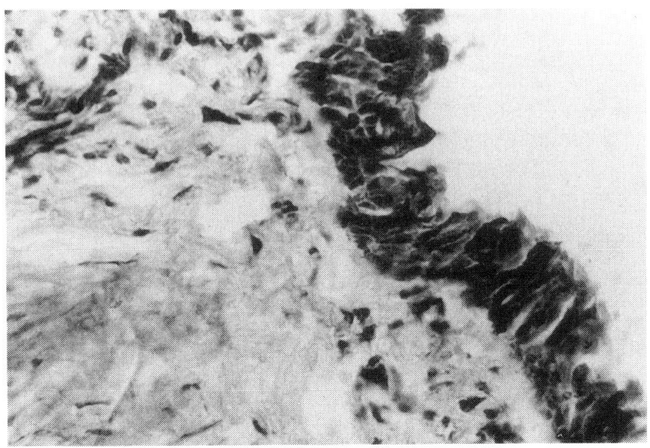

(a)

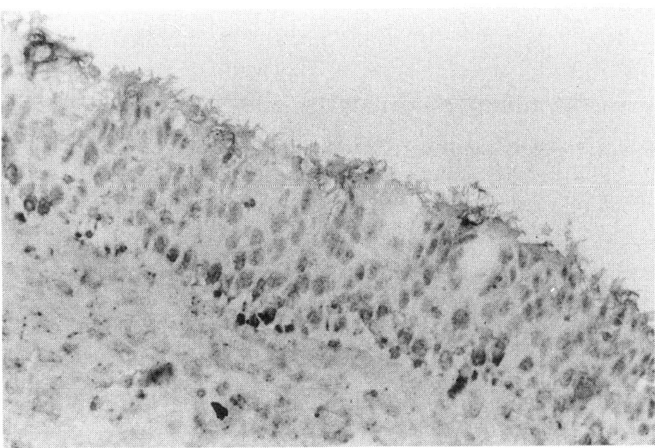

(b)

FIGURE 4   (a) Bronchial biopsy of an asthmatic subject stained for GM-CSF by a polyclonal goat antibody using the avidin-biotin complex (ABC) immunoperoxidase method. The epithelium shows intense staining by the reaction product. Staining can also be seen in the cellular infiltrate present in the submucosa. (b) Bronchial biopsy from a control subject stained by the same method. The epithelium and submucosa show only weak staining. (From Ref. 64.)

of alveolar macrophages expressed GM-CSF mRNA. This study provided evidence that in an experimental model of allergen-induced asthma, activation of the immune and inflammatory response (BAL lymphocyte and alveolar macrophage production of GM-CSF) was temporally associated with an inflammatory cell influx of eosinophils into the airway (66).

An important consequence of macrophage activation is the synthesis and secretion of cytokines including IL-1 and TNF. These are important proinflammatory cytokines that activate other inflammatory cells and are capable of initiating cellular gene transcription. Alveolar macrophages from normal subjects and subjects with pneumonia, pulmonary lymphoma, and idiopathic pulmonary fibrosis have been shown to express mRNA for IL-1β and TGF-β. Alveolar macrophages from some normal subjects also contained mRNA for insulin-like growth factor-1 (ILGF-1). A majority of subjects with lung disease also produced one or more additional growth factors, e.g., EGF, TGF, IL-1β, and PDGF (67). A recent study showed that interleukin-1 receptor antagonist (IL-1ra), a natural inhibitor of IL-1 released by macrophages, inhibited PGE_2. Pretreatment of purified human peripheral monocytes with IL-1ra at different concentrations inhibited the generation of LTB_4 released after treatment with calcium ionophore, in a dose-dependent manner. The authors suggested that the inhibition of LTB_4 synthesis indicated that this glycoprotein plays a modulatory role in immunity and inflammation (68). In a study of the inflammatory response induced by IL-1β in the guinea pig respiratory system, injection of IL-1β into the plural spaces resulted in a dose-dependent inflammatory response, as shown by the formation of pleural exudate and the recruitment of leukocytes. The tracheas and parenchymal strips isolated from guinea pigs exposed to IL-1β showed increased contractile activity of histamine. These results provide evidence for a possible role of IL-1β in airway inflammation and bronchial hyperreactivity (69).

As previously discussed, the initiation and activation of the inflammatory response is mediated by cell-cell communication, which is dependent upon the release of cytokines. One of the earliest cytokines to be released is TNF-α, which has important roles in the mediation of both acute and chronic inflammation, including up-regulation of adhesion molecule expression, induction of IL-1 and IL-6, and activation of chemokines. The importance of TNF-α in atopic allergic inflammation was suggested by a study by Ying et al. (70) in which in situ hybridization was used to identify messenger RNA for TNF-α in cells infiltrating allergen-induced late-phase reaction (LPR) of the skin and nose of atopic subjects. The number of TNF-α mRNA-positive cells in BAL from atopic asthmatic and normal subjects was determined. Twenty-four hours after local allergen challenge, 12/14 skin biopsies and 9/10 nasal biopsies had positive hybridization signals for TNF-α mRNA whereas only 4/14 and 2/10 biopsies were positive in the relevant diluent controls. Compared with diluent sites, significantly increased numbers of cells expressing mRNA for TNF-α were observed in the LPR of skin and nose. All BAL from asthmatics and from normal volunteers had cells showing positive hybridization signals for TNF mRNA but these were at increased frequency in asthmatics.

Differential hybridization has been used to identify several primary response genes induced by TNF in human umbilical vein endothelial (HUVE) cells. One of these cDNA, B94, detected a rapidly and transiently induced 4-kb transcript in TNF-treated HUVE. Other proinflammatory stimuli including IL-1β and LPS also induced B94 mRNA expression. Nuclear run-on experiments demonstrated that TNF induction of B94 transcript occurred primarily at the level of transcriptional activation. B94 was shown to be a single-copy gene that is evolutionarily conserved and is located on chromosome 14q32 (71).

Atopy is associated with elevated serum levels of allergen-specific IgE, which is preferentially induced by the T-cell-derived lymphokine IL-4 and is suppressed by IFN and prostaglandins. Panels of house dust mite–specific T-lymphocyte clones (TLC) from atopic and nonatopic individuals were established. TLC from house dust mite allergic patients produced IL-4 but not IFN-τ whereas TLC from a nonatopic individual produced IFN-τ and only in some cases small amounts of IL-4. *Candida albicans* and tetanus toxoid–specific TLC established from one of the atopic donors also produced IFN-τ without IL-4, suggesting that the atopic state is characterized by a defective accumulation of IL-4-producing CD4$^+$ T cells into the allergen-specific T-cell repertoires (72). However, this has yet to be confirmed.

Recently, using cDNA subtraction libraries from peripheral blood mononuclear cells and using the inducibility of lymphokine messenger RNAs by anti-CD28 as a screening criterion, the effects on inflammation of a new cytokine, IL-13, have been reported by Minty et al. (73). Recombinant IL-13 inhibits inflammatory LPS-induced cytokine production in human peripheral blood monocytes and has actions that are synergistic with IL-2 in the regulation of IFN-γ synthesis in granular lymphocytes.

Polymorphisms have been demonstrated for some of the cytokines discussed above and are shown in Tables 1 and 2. It is possible that polymorphisms within the gene encoding the cytokines, their promoter regions, or their receptors contribute to a genetic predisposition for the development of excessive inflammation. The analysis of cytokines can now be undertaken at the DNA, RNA, and protein level using the techniques of restriction fragment length polymorphism (RFLP) analysis, microsatellite analysis, PCR, in situ hybridization, and enzyme-linked immunosorbant assay (ELISA). The majority of these techniques have been well described in the literature. Recently, a study of the analysis of mRNA for cytokines by PCR has been published (74).

In general, in situ hybridization has been used to establish the chromosomal location of a number of the cytokine genes, and gene mapping by either RFLP, microsatellites, or chromosome mapping has been used to locate the genes more accurately and also to identify polymorphisms within the genes. The human IL-4 gene has been shown to be located at chromosome 5q23.3–31.2 (75). Pulse-field gel electrophoresis was used to define the linkage between IL-3, IL-5, and GM-CSF and IL-4. This was confirmed by the results of a study by Le Beau et al. (76) in which IL-4 and IL-5 were mapped by in situ hybridization to chromosome 5q23–31. Again by in situ hybridization the gene for human IL-7 has been mapped to chromosome 8q12–q13 (77). The genomic sequence of IL-11 has been isolated and by in situ hybridization has been shown to be located on chromosome 19 (78). The structure of the interferon alpha/beta receptor gene has been proposed by Lutfalla et al. (79) and has been physically mapped to chromosome 21 and more specifically to the region 21q22.1. The TNF gene is located in close proximity to the HLA-B locus and is situated on the short arm of chromosome 6; its structure has been analyzed by Spriggs et al. (80) and polymorphisms identified (81).

C. Leukotrienes

Arachidonic acid is released by the action of PLA_2 on cell membrane phospholipids. It is then metabolized either by the cyclooxygenase or by the lipoxygenase pathways. Metabolism of arachidonic acid by cyclooxygenase can be stimulated by mechanical, chemical, or immunological challenge and leads to the formation of prostaglandins and thromboxane (Fig. 5). Oxidative metabolism of arachidonic acid is increased in inflamed tissues. Prostaglandins are polyunsaturated long-chain fatty acid derivatives that have a large number of pharmacological effects mainly involved in acute inflammation. There are three major lipoxygenase pathways in mammalian tissue, i.e., 5-, 12-, and 15-lipoxygenases (82–84), resulting in the production of leukotrienes. The recent progress in the identification of active metabolites from this metabolic pathway has been reviewed (85).

It has been suggested that leukotrienes have a role in many inflammatory conditions in humans including psoriasis, allergic asthma, rheumatoid arthritis, and myocardial infarction. The pharmacological actions of the leukotrienes and their cell sources provide strong evidence that they should contribute to allergic airway disease. Another potential role of leukotrienes is in nonrespiratory inflammatory diseases such as inflammatory bowel disease, rheumatoid arthritis, and psoriasis. Therefore, the role of leukotrienes in inflammation may not be limited to the respiratory system but may be more universal in their ability to cause tissue injury. Consequently, studies that have shown benefit from inhibition of leukotriene synthesis and antagonism of the LTD_4 receptor

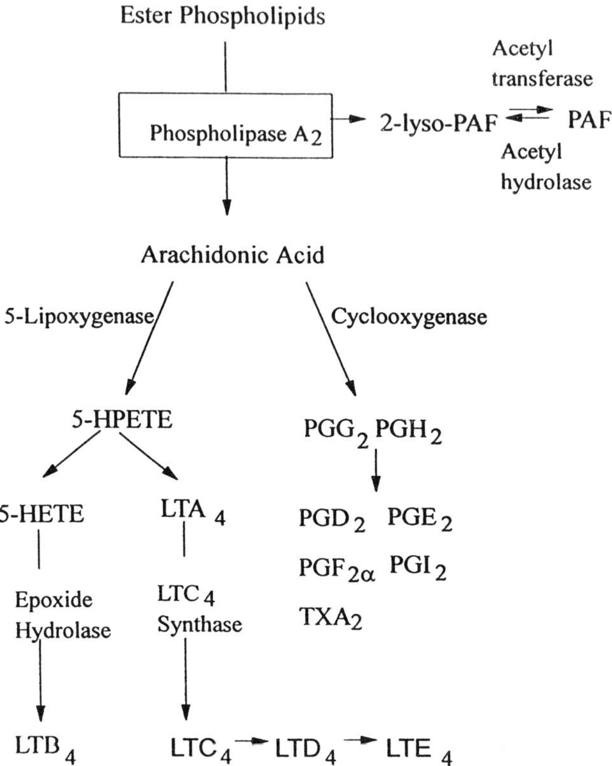

FIGURE 5 Schematic representation of the metabolism of arachidonic acid by the 5-lipoxygenase and cyclooxygenase pathways.

in respiratory diseases are suggestive that such an approach will also be beneficial in other inflammatory diseases.

Thromboxane A_2 (TxA_2), which is produced by the metabolism of arachidonic acid through the cyclooxygenase pathway, is a potent bronchial smooth muscle spasmogen in vitro, which has been implicated in airway inflammation and in the genesis of bronchial hyperresponsiveness in asthma. The urinary excretion of a variety of TxA_2 and prostacyclin metabolites was measured in patients with severe asthma and in atopic subjects after bronchial antigen challenge. The urinary excretion of all thromboxane-derived products was markedly increased in a number of patients with severe acute asthma compared with that in a nonsmoking control population. Urinary prostacyclin metabolites were also significantly raised in acute asthma. In contrast, after inhaled allergen challenge in atopic volunteers, which caused significant bronchoconstriction, urinary excretion of thromboxane-derived products was not significantly elevated (86), suggesting that TxA_2 is an important inflammatory mediator in asthma.

Bronchial asthma is characterized by inflammation and hyperresponsiveness of the airways. The possibility that leukotrienes may contribute to the pathogenesis of the inflammatory component of bronchial asthma is suggested by the properties of these lipid mediators, the preferential capacity of inflammatory cells to generate leukotrienes, and the presence of leukotrienes in the airways of asthmatic subjects (87). In addition, leukotrienes have been detected in BAL of asthmatic subjects at rest (88,89) and following BAL with allergen and isocapnic hyperventilation (90).

The sulfidopeptide leukotrienes are potent bronchoconstrictor agonists when inhaled and it has been shown that the airways of asthmatic subjects are hyperresponsive to leukotrienes and to other bronchoconstrictor agonists. Although the airways of asthmatic subjects are relatively less responsive to LTC_4 and LTD_4 than to histamine or methacholine, they demonstrate a marked and selective hyperresponsiveness to LTE_4, suggesting a possibly unique role for this mediator in the pathogenesis of airways hyperresponsiveness. The capacity of the sulphidopeptide leukotrienes to increase the airways responsiveness of normal subjects to methacholine and of asthmatic subjects to histamine is further evidence for a role for these substances in the pathogenesis of bronchial asthma (91).

Leukotriene B_4 (LTB_4) is involved in both inflammation and chemotaxis although it is not clear whether it acts directly or indirectly by stimulating the release of chemotactic and inflammatory cytokines. LTB_4 is a potent chemotactic agent for leukocytes, stimulates chemokinesis, degranulation, and aggregation of leukocytes and it induces neutrophil-dependent increased microvascular permeability. Leukotrienes C_4, D_4, and E_4 are bronchoconstrictors and potent mediators of microvascular tone and permeability. The contribution of leukotrienes to inflammatory process is likely to be a global phenomenon, and the introduction of leukotriene antagonists and 5-lipoxygenase inhibitors may represent new forms of treatment for many inflammatory diseases. The LTB_4 receptor has not been characterized in human eosinophils although Ng et al. (92) reported a functional high-affinity receptor for LTB_4 on guinea pig eosinophils. It was suggested by these workers that guinea pig eosinophil membranes expressed only a high-affinity LTB_4 receptor population.

It has recently been shown that LTB_4 induces the synthesis of IL-6 by monocytes through transcriptional regulation of the IL-6 gene (93). Activation of the IL-6 promoter by LTB_4 was associated with the accumulation of the respective transcripts and resulted in the synthesis of functional IL-6 protein. When human monocytes were cultured in the presence of LTB_4, significant stimulation of the production of IL-6 was observed by Rola-Pleszczynski and Stankova (94). Nanomolar concentrations of LTB_4 were optimal and the LTB_4 activity could be blocked by an LTB_4 receptor antagonist. LTB_4 induced an accumulation of IL-6 messenger RNA (mRNA) in treated monocytes with a dose response similar to that of IL-6 protein production. The half-life of IL-6 mRNA was extended in LTB_4-treated monocytes and the nuclear transcription of IL-6 mRNA was increased fivefold in LTB_4-treated cells. Cyclohexamide pretreatment of cells before exposure to LTB_4 resulted in superinduced IL-6 message expression, but partially inhibited the effect of LTB_4 on IL-6 mRNA accumulation, suggesting that newly synthesized proteins may be involved in the transcriptional activation of the IL-6 gene by LTB_4. This may constitute an important mechanism through which rapidly produced mediators may modulate the subsequent production of regulatory growth-promoting cytokines.

The vascular and cellular responses resulting from inflammatory injury are controlled by several classes of chemical mediators. These mediators act together to amplify the inflammatory response. Neurogenic inflammation due to release of neuropeptides from sensory nerves has been demonstrated in the airways of several species and may contribute to the inflammatory response in asthmatic airways. Substance P and neurokinin A released from airway sensory nerves may cause bronchoconstriction, vasodilatation, plasma exudation, and mucus secretion, whereas calcitonin may contribute to hyperemia of inflammation. Airway epithelial damage in asthma exposes sensory nerves that may become sensitized by inflammatory products so that neuropeptides are released via a local reflex trigger such as bradykinin resulting in exaggerated inflammation. The effects of tachykinins may be amplified by the loss of the major degrading enzyme neutral endopeptidase from epithelial cells.

V. CELL ADHESION MOLECULES

The role of adhesion molecules in inflammation is reviewed by Montefort and Holgate (95) and the functional role of adhesion molecules in inflammation has been reviewed by Canonica et al. (96). A series of cell adhesion molecules mediate interactions between vascular endothelium and leukocyte cell surfaces. Three major families of adhesion molecules have been identified and contribute to this process; integrins, selectins, and immunoglobulin-like receptors.

Integrins are heterodimers consisting of an $\alpha\beta$ subunit (noncovalently associated), an extracellular ligand binding site, and an intracellular portion linked to the cytoskeleton (97). These are subdivided into families according to the associated β subunit (98). LFA-1 (CD11a/CD18) is a β_2 integrin that is found on all leukocyte populations including eosinophils and binds to ICAM-1 and ICAM-2 (99,100). Adherence between LFA-1 and ICAM-1 depends on leukocyte activation transiently increasing LFA-1 binding activity. The β_2 integrin MAC-1 (CD11b/CD18) binds to ICAM-1 and is confined to monocytes, eosinophils, and PMNs (98,100). VLA-4 (CD49d/CD29) is a β_1 integrin that is expressed on eosinophils, monocytes, and memory T cells (CD45RA-) and whose endothelial cell ligand is VCAM-1. The selectins are glycoproteins that are characterized by an N-terminal lectin-like domain, an epidermal growth factor region, and a series of proteins with structural similarities to those involved in complement activation. Three major selectins have been identified: E-selectin, P-selectin, and L-selectin. P- and E-selectin act as ligand for neutrophils and eosinophils, monocytes, and memory T cells (101–105). The members of the immunoglobulin gene superfamily consist of single-chain molecules with a variable number of immunoglobulin-like extracellular domains. ICAM-1 (106), ICAM-2 (107), and VCAM (108) are members of this group. ICAM-1 is constitutively expressed on isolated human umbilical vein endothelial cells (HUVECs) and on normal endothelium in vivo. VCAM-1 is absent from unstimulated vascular endothelium but is up-regulated by a number of cytokines including IL-1 and TNF-α (108).

The adhesion of eosinophils and neutrophils to HUVECs stimulated with IL-1, TNF, and LPS was shown by Kyan-Aung et al. (109). These investigators showed that ELAM-1 and ICAM-1 were involved in the adhesion of eosinophils and polymorphonuclear leukocytes to endothelial cells stimulated with TNF. ELAM-1 and ICAM were expressed with greater intensity in antigen-challenged biopsies, which suggests that these molecules may be involved in granulocyte recruitment in vivo. The authors established similarities between the mechanisms of neutrophil and eosinophil adhesion to cytokine-stimulated eosinophils, which suggested that leukocyte-endothelial cell adhesion may be responsible for the selective accumulation of eosinophils at the sites of allergic inflammation.

The up-regulation of endothelial cell adhesion molecules, specifically E-selectin and ICAM-1, is responsible for the recruitment of leukocytes in the late-phase asthmatic response while recruitment of T cells and their subsequent activation contributes to the ongoing inflammatory response of asthma. Inflammation, metastasis, and ischemia all require lymphocyte or leukocyte cell recognition and adherence to endothelial counterreceptors such as intercellular adhesion molecule-1 (ICAM-1). ICAM-1 is a glycoprotein expressed by endothelial cells activated by cytokines. The lymphocyte-function-associated antigen (LFA-1) is an integrin expressed by activated white blood cells. Together, this receptor-ligand pair is responsible, at least in part, for the localization of neutrophils at sites of inflammation. Novel inhibitors of inflammation may result from mapping of the receptor for ICAM-1, LFA-1, on lymphocytes. Constructs of recombinant soluble ICAM-1 cDNA in baculovirus were designed by Cobb et al. (110). Relatively high expressions of two soluble forms of ICAM-1 were produced and isolated. These proteins were shown to promote the adherence of HL-60 cells and Molt-4 cells and to inhibit cell adherence to purified intact ICAM-1 isolated from K562 cells.

Human CD11b/CD18 (complement receptor type 3) is a member of the β2 integrin subfamily, which also includes the heterodimers CD11a/CD18 and CD11c/CD18. The CD11 molecules and the common β2 subunit CD18 are the products of different genes that exhibit distinct, though overlapping, patterns of tissue- and development-specific expression. The expression of CD11b and CD11c is almost exclusively restricted to cells of the myeloid lineage; however, that of CD11a and CD18 is panleukocytic. The promoter region of the CD11b gene has been cloned and characterized by Shelley and Arnaout (111). A single transcription initiation site was identified and the region extending 242 base pairs upstream and 71 base pairs downstream of this site was shown to be sufficient to direct tissue-, cell-, and development-specific expression in vitro, which mimics that of the CD11b gene in vivo.

The importance of the adhesion of leukocytes to the microvascular endothelium is demonstrated by subjects who are deficient in the expression of the CD18 family of adhesion molecules. Subjects with leukocyte adhesion molecule deficiency have structural defects in CD18, which prevents heterodimer formation and normal cell surface expression of these receptors and can result in life-threatening bacterial infections. Abnormal CD18 cDNA clones were isolated from an individual with partial deficiency, using the polymerase chain reaction to amplify the B-cell-derived cDNA. Sequence analysis of these clones revealed two mutant alleles, one containing an insertion and the other containing a nucleotide transition. cDNA clones, which represented a maternal allele, contained a 12-base-pair insertion resulting in an in-frame addition of four amino acids. The in-frame insertion arose by a single nucleotide transversion in the 3′ terminus of an intron, resulting in the generation of an aberrant splice acceptor site. Other cDNA clones contained a nucleotide transition that was not present in either parent and that resulted in a substitution. To determine the functional importance of these changes, cDNA encoding a normal alpha chain (CD11b) was cotransfected into COS cells with CD18 cDNAs encoding for wild-type CD18, the maternal mutant allele, or CD18 containing a substitution. Immunostaining of transfectants with anti-CD18 monoclonal antibodies revealed no cell surface expression of the maternal mutant CD18 and 22% surface expression of substituted CD18. Both the insertion and the substitution mutants occurred in an extracellular region of CD18 that is highly conserved among beta integrins, supporting a role for this region in heterodimer formation (112).

VI. OTHER MEDIATORS OF THE INFLAMMATORY RESPONSE

A. Complement System

Inflammation and phagocytosis are highly complex events involving many humoral and cellular factors with complement components playing a key role. Complement is a series of proteins that can react together to trigger cell function, aid in the recognition of invading pathogens, and regulate the phagocytic process via interactions with specific cell surface receptors. Complement stimulates phagocytosis of bacteria and dead cells, destroys bacterial cell walls and causes lysis, and increases vasodilatation, vascular permeability, and neutrophil migration. Complement is active if bacteria are present whether or not they are causing inflammation. There is a high frequency of allelic variation in complement proteins. The major functions of complement are to resist infection against bacteria and to prevent immune complex disease. The complement system of blood plasma and extravascular tissue fluid plays an important role in many immune defense reactions. Activation of the complement system promotes acute inflammation, recruitment of leukocytes, and the killing of pathogens by phagocytosis, lysis, or the release of toxic products. The central event in complement activation is cleavage of C3 with the liberation of C3a and its metabolite, C3a des Arg. Similarly, activation of the fifth complement component results in the formation of C5a and C5a des Arg. C3a and C5a release histamine and stimulate smooth muscle contraction. The C5-derived peptides have potent effects on leukocytes in vitro and promote the interaction between neutrophils and endothelial cells in vivo that leads to neutrophil accumulation and edema formation.

The complement system stimulates macrophages to digest bacteria, and certain complement complexes can destroy bacterial cell walls and are vasoactive. There are three pathways to the complement system of activation: the alternative pathways A and B and the classic pathway. The alternative pathway A is only activated through factor XII and the alternative pathway B reacts mainly to bacterial cell walls or viruses (polysaccharide coats). The classic pathway, however, is dependent on recognition of antibody-antigen complexes. Macrophages in the blood recognize this complex and trigger active complement formation.

B. Heat Shock Proteins

Exposure to elevated temperatures and a variety of other types of cellular injury, including oxidative injury, induces immediate and transient pathological response—the heat shock response. Under stressful conditions, such as the local release of mediator including leukotrienes, reactive oxygen species such as superoxide anions (O_2^-), hydroxyl radicals ($\cdot OH$), or hydrogen peroxide

(H_2O_2), and cytokines, the selective activation of heat shock genes leads to the synthesis of heat shock (heat stress) proteins (HSPs). These are named according to their molecular weight and are classified into families.

As previously discussed, inflammatory cells recruited to the sites of injury release cytokines and reactive oxygen species (ROS). Cytokines and ROS have the potential to regulate the expression of HSPs that have the ability to project cells and tissues from the deleterious effects of inflammation. The regulation of HSPs is discussed in two recent reviews (113,114).

From the data presented in this chapter, the importance of the contribution of molecular biological techniques to the analysis of the inflammatory response is apparent. The comparatively recent progress in methodology, which includes sequencing, in situ hybridization, PCR analysis, and the use of subtraction libraries, will be vital in establishing the basis of the genetic control of the inflammatory response. New inflammatory mediators such as cytokines have recently been identified, characterized, and localized to specific chromosomal regions using such techniques. In addition, it may be possible to characterize the receptors for inflammatory mediators and identify the precise mechanism of cell-cell communication that controls the inflammatory response.

REFERENCES

1. Stiffel C, Ibanez OM, Ribeiro OG, Decreusefond C, Mouton D, Siqueira M, Biozzi G. Genetics of acute inflammation: inflammatory reactions in inbred lines of mice and in their interline crosses. Exp Clin Immunogenet 1990; 7(4):221–233.
2. Ibanez OM, Stiffel C, Ribeiro OG, Cabrera WK, Massa S, de Franco M, Sant'Anna OA, Decreusefond C, Mouton D, Siqueira M, et al. Genetics of nonspecific immunity. I. Bidirectional selective breeding of lines of mice endowed with maximal or minimal inflammatory responsiveness. Eur J Immunol 1992; 22(10):2555–2563.
3. Demoly P, Basset-Seguin N, Chanez P, Campbell AM, Gauthier-Rouviere C, Godard P, Michel FB, Bousquet J. c-*fos* proto-oncogene expression in bronchial biopsies of asthmatics. Am J Respir Cell Mol Biol 1992; 7(2):128–133.
4. Kazmierowski JA, Gallin JI, Reynolds HY. Mechanism for the inflammatory response in primate lungs. J Clin Invest 1977; 59:273–281.
5. Kirby JG, Hargreave FE, Gleich GS, O'Byrne PM. Bronchoalveolar cell profiles of asthmatic and nonasthmatic subjects. Am Rev Respir Dis 1987; 136:379–383.
6. Beasley R, Roche WR, Roberts JA, Holgate ST. Cellular events in the bronchi in mild asthma and after bronchial provocation. Am Rev Respir Dis 1989; 139:806–817.
7. Poston RN, Chanez P, Lacoste JY, Litchfield T, Lee TH, Bousquet J. Immunohistochemical characterisation of the cellular infiltration in asthmatic bronchil. Am Rev Respir Dis 1992; 145:918–921.
8. Poulter LW, Norris A, Power C, Condez A, Burnes H, Schmekel B, Burke C. T-cell dominated inflammatory reactions in the bronchioles of astymptomatic asthmatics are also present in the nasal mucosa. Postgrad Med J 1992; 67(790):747–753.

9. Bentley AM, Meng Q, Robinson DS, Hamid Q, Kay AB, Durham SR. Increases in activated T lymphocytes, eosinophils, and cytokine mRNA expression for interleukin-5 and granulocyte macrophage colony-stimulating factor in bronchial biopsies after allergen inhalation challenge in atopic asthmatics. Am J Respir Cell Mol Biol 1993; 8(1):35–42.

10. Dunnill MS, Massarella GR, Anderson JA. A comparison of the quantitative anatomy of the bronchi in normal subjects in status asthmaticus in chronic bronchitis and emphysema. Thorax 1969; 24:176.

11. Frew AJ, Corrigan CJ, Maestrelli P, Tsai JJ, Kurihara K, O'Hehir RE, Hartnell A, Cromwell O, Kay AB. T lymphocytes in allergen-induced late-phase reactions and asthma. Int Arch Allergy Appl Immunol 1989; 88(1-2):63–67.

12. Romano MF, Turco MC, Stanziola A, Giarrusso PC, Petrella A, Tassone P, Van Lier R, Venuta S, Formisano S. Defect of interleukin-2 production and T cell proliferation in atopic patients: restoring ability of the CD28-mediated activation pathway. Cell Immunol 1993; 148(2):455–463.

13. Wilson JW, Djukanovic R, Howarth PH, Holgate ST. Lymphocyte activation in bronchoalveolar lavage and peripheral blood in atopic asthma. Am Rev Respir Dis 1992; 145:958–960.

14. Azzawi M, Bradley B, Jeffrey K, Frew AJ, Wardlaw AJ, Knowles G, Assoufi B, Collins JV, Durham S, Kay AB. Identification of activated T lymphocytes and eosinophils in bronchial biopsies in stable atopic asthma. Am Rev Respir Dis 1990; 142:1407–1413.

15. Bentley AB, Menz G, Storz C, Robinson DS, Bradley B, Jeffrey PK, Durham SR, Kay AB. Identification of T lymphocytes, macrophages and activated eosinophils in the bronchial mucosa in intrinsic asthma: relationship to symptoms and bronchial responsiveness. Am Rev Respir Dis 1992; 146:500–506.

16. Robinson DS, Hamid Q, Ying S, Tsicopoulos A, Barkans J, Bentley AM, Corrigan C, Durham SR, Kay AB. Evidence for a predominant TH2 type bronchoalveolar lavage T lymphocyte population in atopic asthma. N Engl J Med 1992; 326:298–304.

17. Damle NK, Doyle LV. Ability of human T lymphocytes to adhere to vascular endothelial cells and to augment endothelial permeability to macromolecules is linked to their state of post-thymic maturation. J Immunol 1990; 144(4):1233–1240.

18. Walker C, Bode E, Boer L, Hansel TT, Blaser K, Virchow JC Jr. Allergic and nonallergic asthmatics have distinct patterns of T-cell activation and cytokine production in peripheral blood and bronchoalveolar lavage. Am Rev Respir Dis 1992; 146(1):109–115.

19. Romano MF, Valerio B, Turco MC, Spadaro G, Venuta S, Formisano S. Defect of CD2- and CD3-mediated activation pathways in T cells of atopic patients: role of interleukin 2. Cell Immunol 1992; 139(1):91–97.

20. Flint KC, Leung KB, Pearce FL, Hudspith BN, Brostoff J, Johnston NM. Human mast cells recovered by bronchoalveolar lavage: their morphology, histamine release and the effects of sodium cromoglycate. Clin Sci 1985; 68:427–432.

21. Bradding P, Feather IH, Wilson S, Bardin PG, Heusser CH, Holgate ST, Howarth PH. Immunolocalisation of cytokines in the nasal mucosa and perennial rhinitis

subjects: the mast cell as a source of IL-4, IL-5 and IL-6 in human allergic mucosal inflammation. J Immunol 1993; 151:3853–3865.

22. Galli SJ, Gordon JR, Wershil BK. Cytokine production by mast cells and basophils. Curr Opin Immunol 1991; 3:865–872.

23. Wasserman SI. Mast cells and airway inflammation in asthma. Am J Respir Crit Care Med 1994; 150:s39–41.

24. Bittleman DB, Casale TB. Allergic models and cytokines. Am J Respir Crit Care Med 1994; 150:s72–76.

25. Beasley R, Roche WR, Roberts JA, Holgate ST. Cellular events in the bronchi in mild asthma and after bronchial provocation. Am Rev Respir Dis 1989; 139:806–817.

26. Casale TB, Wood D, Richarson HB, Zehr B, Zavala D, Hunninghake GW. Direct evidence of a role for mast cells in the pathogenesis of antigen-induced broncho-constriction. J Clin Invest 1987; 80:1507–1511.

27. Agius RM, Howarth PH, Robinson C, Holgate ST. Human bronchoalveolar mast cells and their mediators. In: Kay AB, ed. Asthma: Clinical Pharmacology and Therapeutic Progress. Oxford: Blackwell Scientific, 1986:274–285.

28. Flint KC, Leung KBP, Hudspith BN, Brostoff J, Pearce FL, McJohnson N. Bron-choalveolar mast cells in extrinsic asthma: a mechanism for mutation of antigen specific bronchoconstriction. Br Med J 1985; 291:923–926.

29. Metzger WJ, Richerson HB, Worden K, Monick M, Hunninghake GW. Bronchial lavage of allergic asthmatic patients following allergen bronchoprovocation. Chest 1986; 89:477–483.

30. Diaz P, Gonzalez MC, Galleguillos FR, Ancic P, Cromwell O, Shepherd D, Dur-ham SR, Gleich GJ, Kay AB. Leukocytes and mediators in bronchoalveolar lavage during allergen-induced late-phase asthmatic reaction. Am Rev Respir Dis 1989; 139:1383–1389.

31. Metzger WJ, Zaval D, Richarson HB, Moseley P, Iwamota P, Monick M, Sjoerd-sma K, Hunninghake GW. Local allergen challenge and bronchoalveolar lavage of allergic asthmatic lungs. Am Rev Respir Dis 1987; 135:433–440.

32. Holgate ST, Twentyman OP, Rafferty P, Beasley R, Hutson PA, Robinson C, Church MK. Primary and secondary effector cells in the pathogenesis of bronchial asthma. Int Arch Allergy Appl Immunol 1987; 82:498–506.

33. Arm JP, Lee TH. The pathobiology of bronchial asthma. Adv Immunol 1992; 51:323–382.

34. Marshall JS, Bienenstock J. The role of mast cells in inflammatory reaction of the airways, skin and intestine. Curr Opin Immunol 1994; 6:853–859.

35. Schall TJ, Bacon KB. Chemokines, leukocyte trafficking and inflammation. Cur-rent Opin Immunol 1994; 6:865–873.

36. Bousquet J, Chanez P, Lacoste JY, Barneon G, Gharanian N, Enander I, Venge P, Ahlstedt S, Simony-Lafontaine J, Godard P, et al. Eosinophilic inflammation in asthma. N Engl J Med 1990; 323:1033–1039.

37. Djukanovic R, Lai CK, Wilson JW, Britten KM, Wilson SJ, Roche WR, H. HP, Holgate ST. Bronchial mucosal manifestations of atopy: a comparison of markers of inflammation between atopic asthmatics, atopic nonasthmatics and healthy con-trols. Eur Respir J 1992; 5(5):538–544.

38. Chavis C, Godard P, Michel FB, Crastes de Paulet A, Damon M. Sulfidopeptide leukotrienes contribute to human alveolar macrophage activation in asthma. Prostaglandins Leukot Essent Fatty Acids 1991; 42(2):95–100.

39. Walker C, Rihs S, Braun RK, Betz S, Bruijnzeel PL. Increased expression of CD11b and functional changes in eosinophilia after migration across endothelial cells monolayers. J Immunol 1993; 159(9):4061–4071.

40. Wardlaw AJ, Symon FS, Walsh GM. Eosinophil adhesion in allergic inflammation. J Allergy Clin Immunol 1994; 94 (6 pt 2):1163–1171.

41. Walsh GM, Mermod JJ, Hartnell A, Kay AB, Wardlaw AJ. Human eosinophil, but not neutrophil, adherence to IL-1-stimulated human umbilical vascular endothelial cells is alpha 4 beta 1 (very late antigen-4) dependent. J Immunol 1991; 146(10): 3419–3423.

42. Marini M, Avoni E, Hollemborg J, Mattoli S. Cytokine mRNA profile and cell activation in bronchoalveolar lavage fluid from nonatopic patients with symptomatic asthma. Chest 1992; 102(3):661–669.

43. Zoratti EM, Sedgwick JB, Vrtis RR, Busse WW. The effect of platelet-activating factor on the generation of superoxide anion in human eosinophils and neutrophils. J Allergy Clin Immunol 1991; 88(5):749–758.

44. Seminario M-C, Gleich GJ. The role of eosinophils in the pathogenesis of asthma. Curr Opin Immunol 1994; 6:860–864.

45. Fujisawa T, Kephart GM, Gray BH, Gleich GJ. The neutrophil and chronic allergic inflammation: immunochemical localization of neutrophil elastase. Am Rev Respir Dis 1990; 141(3):689–697.

46. Kato M, Morikawa A, Kimura H, Shimizu T, Nakano M, Kuroume T. Effects of anti-asthma drugs on superoxide anion generation from human polymorphonuclear leukocytes or hypoxanthine-xanthine oxidase system. Int Arch Allergy Appl Immunol 1991; 96(2):128–133.

47. Balter MS, Eschenbacher WL, Peters-Golden M. Arachidonic acid metabolism in cultured alveolar macrophages from normal, atopic and asthmatic subjects. Am Rev Respir Dis 1988; 138:1134–1142.

48. Chanez P, Bousquet J, Couret I, Cornillac L, Barneon G, Vic P, Michel FB, Godard P. Increased numbers of hypodense alveolar macrophages in patients with bronchial asthma. Am Rev Respir Dis 1991; 144(4):923–930.

49. Capron A, Dessaint JP, Rousseau R, Capron M, Bazin H. Specific IgE antibodies in immune adherence of normal macrophages to *Schistosoma mansoni* schistosomules. Nature 1975; 253:474–475.

50. Melewicz FM, Kline LE, Cohen AB, Spiegelberg HL. Characterisation of IgE receptors for IgE on human alveolar macrophages. Clin Exp Immunol 1982; 49: 364–370.

51. Joseph M, Tonnel AB, Torpier G, Capron A, Arnoux B, Benveniste J. Involvement of immunoglobulin E in the secretory processes of alveolar macrophages from asthmatic patients. J Clin Invest 1983; 71:221–230.

52. Spiegelberg HL. Structure and function of Fc receptors for IgE on lymphocytes, monocytes and macrophages. Adv Immunol 1984; 35:61–88.

53. Kikutani H, Yokota A, Uchibayashi N, Yukawa K, Tanaka T, Sugiyama K, Barsumian EL, Suemura M, Kishimoto T. Structure and function of Fc epsilon receptor

II (Fc epsilon RII/CD23): a point of contact between the effector phase of allergy and B cell differentiation. Ciba Found Symp 1989; 147:31–35.

54. Wilkinson JR, Lane SJ, Lee TH. Interactions between macrophages and granulocytes in bronchial asthma. In: Wong PYK, Serhan CN, eds. Cell-Cell Interactions in the Release of Inflammatory Mediators. New York: Plenum Press, 1991:269–279.

55. Black JW, Owen DAA, Parsons ME. An analysis of the depressor responses to histamine in the cat and dog: involvement of both H1- and H2-receptors. Br J Pharmacol 1975; 64:319–324.

56. Owen DAA, Poy E, Woodward DF. Evaluation of the role of histamine H1 and H2 receptors in cutaneous inflammation in the guinea-pig produced by histamine and mast cell degranulation. Br J Pharmacol 1980; 69:615–623.

57. Levi R, Owen DAA, Trzeciakowski J. Actions of histamine on the heart and vasculature. In: Ganellin CR, Parsons PA, eds. Pharmacology of Histamine Receptors. Bristol: Wright, 1982:236– 297.

58. Callard R, Gearing A. The Cytokine Facts Book. London: Academic Press, 1994.

59. Tai P-C, Sun L, Spry CJF. Effects of IL-5, granulocyte/macrophage colony stimulating factor (GM-CSF) and IL-3 on the survival of human blood eosinophils in vitro. Clin Exp Immunol 1991; 85:312–316.

60. Fabian I, Kletter Y, Mor S, Geller-Bernstein C, Ben-Yaakov M, Volovitz B, Golde DW. Activation of human eosinophil and neutrophil functions by haematopoietic growth factors: comparisons of IL-1, IL-3, IL-5 and GM-CSF. Br J Haematol 1992; 80(2):137–143.

61. Wang JM, Rambaldi A, Biondi A, Chen ZG, Sanderson CJ, Mantovani A. Recombinant human interleukin 5 is a selective eosinophil chemoattractant. Eur J Immunol 1989; 19(4):701–705.

62. Burke LA, Hallsworth MP, Litchfield TM, Davidson R, Lee TH. Identification of the major activity derived from cultured human peripheral blood mononuclear cells, which enhances eosinophil viability, as granulocyte-macrophage colony-stimulating factor (GM-CSF). J Allergy Clin Immunol 1991; 88:226–235.

63. Broide DH, Paine MM, Firestein GS. Eosinophils express interleukin 5 and granulocyte macrophage-colony-stimulating factor mRNA at sites of allergic inflammation in asthmatics. J Clin Invest 1992; 90(4):1414–1424.

64. Sousa AR, Poston RN, Lane SJ, Nakhosteen JA, Lee TH. Detection of GM-CSF in asthmatic bronchial epithelium and decrease by inhaled corticosteroids. Am Rev Respir Dis 1993; 147:1557–1561.

65. Marini M, Soloperto M, Mezzetti M, Fasoli A, Mattoli S. Interleukin-1 binds to specific receptors on human bronchial epithelial cells and upregulates granulocyte/macrophage colony-stimulating factor synthesis and release. Am J Respir Cell Mol Biol 1991; 4(6):519–524.

66. Broide DH, Firestein GS. Endobronchial allergen challenge in asthma: demonstration of cellular source of granulocyte macrophage colony-stimulating factor by in situ hybridization. J Clin Invest 1991; 88(3):1048–1053.

67. Adolff CH, Golden JA, Kennedy PW, Goetzl EJ, Turck CW. Polymerase chain reaction amplification of messages for growth factors in cells from human bronchoalveolar lavage fluids. Inflammation 1991; 15(4):259–268.

68. Conti P, Panara MR, Barbacane RC, Reale M, Bongrazio M, Dempsey RA. Inhibition of leukotriene B4 (LTB4) by recombinant interleukin-1 receptor antagonist (IL-1RA) on human monocytes. Agents Actions 1992; Spec No:C93–C95.

69. Hernandez A, Omini C, Daffonchio L. Interleukin-1 beta: a possible mediator of lung inflammation and airway hyperreactivity. Pharmacol Res 1991; 24(4):385–393.

70. Ying S, Robinson DS, Varney V, Meng Q, Tsicopoulos A, Moqbel R, Durham SR, Kay AB, Hamid Q. TNF alpha mRNA expression in allergic inflammation. Clin Exp Allergy 1991; 21(6):745–750.

71. Sarma V, Wolf FW, Marks RM, Shows TB, Dixit VM. Cloning of a novel tumor necrosis factor-alpha-inducible primary response gene that is differentially expressed in development and capillary tube-like formation in vitro. J Immunol 1992; 148(10):3302–3312.

72. Kapsenberg ML, Wierenga EA, Bos JD, Jansen HM. Aberrant T cell regulation of IgE production in atopy. Eur Respir J 1991; supplement 13:27s–30s.

73. Minty A, Chalon P, Derocq JM, Dumont X, Guillemot JC, Kaghad M, Labit C, Leplatois P, Liauzun P, Miloux B. Interleukin-13 is a new human lymphokine regulating inflammatory and immune responses. Nature 1993; 362(6417):248–250.

74. Doi S, Gemou-Engesaeth V, Kay AB, Corrigan CJ. Polymerase chain reaction quantification of cytokine messenger RNA in peripheral blood mononuclear cells of patients with acute exacerbation of asthma: effect of glucocorticoid therapy. Clin Exp Allergy 1994; 24:854–867.

75. van Leeuwen BH, Martinson ME, Webb GC, Young IG. Molecular organization of the cytokine gene cluster, involving the human IL-3, IL-4, IL-5 and GM-CSF genes, on human chromosome 5. Blood 1989; 73(5):1142–1148.

76. Le Beau MM, Lemons RS, Espinosa R III, Larson RA, Arai N, Rowley JD. Interleukin-4 and interleukin-5 map to human chromosome 5 in a region encoding growth factors and receptors and are deleted in myeloid leukemias with a del (5q). Blood 1989; 73(3):647–650.

77. Sutherland GR, Baker E, Fernandez KE, Callen DF, Goodwin RG, Lupton S, Namen AE, Shannon MF, Vadas MA. The gene for human interleukin 7 (IL-7) is at 8q13-13. Hum Genet 1989; 82(4):371–372.

78. McKinley D, Wu Q, Yang-Feng T, Yang YC. Genomic sequence and chromosomal location of human interleukin-11 gene (IL-11). Genomics 1992; 13(3):814–819.

79. Lutfalla G, Gardiner K, Proudhon D, Vielh E, Uze G. The structure of the human interferon alpha/beta receptor gene. J Biol Chem 1992; 267(4):2802–2809.

80. Spriggs DR, Deutsch S, Kufe DW. Genomic structure, induction, and production of TNF-alpha. Immunol Series 1992; 56:3–34.

81. Udalova IA, Nedospasov SA, Webb GC, Chaplin DD, Turetskaya RL. Highly informative typing of the human TNF locus using six adjacent polymorphic markers. Genomics 1993; 16:180–186.

82. Borgeat P, Samuelsson B. Metabolism of arachidonic acid in polymorphonuclear leukocytes; structural analysis of novel hydroxylated compounds. J Biol Chem 1979; 254:7865–7868.

83. Hamberg M, Samuelsson B. Prostaglandin endoperoxides: novel transformations of arachidonic acid in human platelets. Proc Natl Acad Sci USA 1974; 71:3400–3444.

84. Borgeat P, Samuelsson B. Arachidonic acid metabolism in polymorphonuclear leukocytes; effects of ionophore A23187. Proc Natl Acad Sci USA 1979; 76:2148–2152.

85. Lee TH. Lipoxin A_4, a novel anti-inflammatory molecule? Thorax 1995; 50:111–112.

86. Taylor IK, Ward PS, O'Shaughnessy KM, Dollery CT, Black P, Barrow SE, W. TG, Fuller RW. Thromboxane A2 biosynthesis in acute asthma and after antigen challenge. Am Rev Respir Dis 1991; 143(1):119–125.

87. Lee TH, Arm J. Leukotrienes. Allergy Proc 1991; 12(3):139–142.

88. Lam S, Chan H, Le Riche JC. Release of leukotrienes in patients with bronchial asthma. J Allergy Clin Immunol 1988; 81:711–717.

89. Wardlaw AJ, Hay H, Cromwell O, Collins JV, Kay AB. Leukotrienes, LTC4 and LTB_4, in bronchoalveolar lavage in bronchial asthma and other respiratory diseases. J Allergy Clin Immunol 1989; 84:19–26.

90. Wenzel SE, Larsen GL, Johnston K, Voelkel NF, Westoctt JY. Elevated levels of leukotriene C4 in bronchoalveolar lavage fluid from atopic asthmatics after endobronchial allergen challenge. Am Rev Respir Dis 1990; 142:112–119.

91. Lee TH, O'Hickey SP, Jacques C, Hawksworth RJ, Arm JP, Christie P, Spur BW, Crea AE. Sulphidopeptide leukotrienes in asthma. Adv Prostaglandin Thromboxane Leukotriene Res 1991; 21A:415–419.

92. Ng CF, Sun FF, Taylor BM, Wolin MS, Wong PY. Functional properties of guinea pig eosinophil leukotriene B4 receptor. J Immunol 1991; 147(9):3096–3103.

93. Brach MA, de Vos S, Arnold C, Gruss HJ, Mertelsmann R, Herrmann F. Leukotriene B4 transcriptionally activates interleukin-6 expression involving NK-chi B and NF-IL6. Eur J Immunol 1992; 22(10):2705–2711.

94. Rola-Pleszczynski M, Stankova J. Leukotriene B4 enhances interleukin-6 (IL-6) production and IL-6 messenger RNA accumulation in human monocytes in vitro: transcriptional and posttranscriptional mechanisms. Blood 1992; 80(4):1004–1011.

95. Montefort S, Holgate ST. Adhesion molecules and their role in inflammation. Respir Med 1991; 85:91–99.

96. Canonica GW, Ciprandi G, Buscaglia S, Pesce G, Banasico M. Adhesion molecules of allergic inflammation: recent insights into functional roles. Allergy 1994; 49: 135–141.

97. Kishomoto TK, Larson RS, Corbi AL, Dustin ML, Staunton DE, Springer TA. The leukocyte integrins: LFA-1, MAC-1 and p150,95. Adv Immunol 1989; 46: 149–182.

98. Larson RS, Springer TA. Structure and function of the leukocyte integrins. Immunol Rev 1990; 114:181–217.

99. Staunton DE, Marlin SD, Stratowa C, Dustin ML, Springer TA. Primary structure of ICAM-1 demonstrates interaction between members of the immunoglobulin and integrin supergene families. Cell 1988; 52:925–933.

100. Diamond MS, Staunton DE, Martin SD, Springer TA. Binding of the integrin Mac-1 (CD11b/CD18) to the third immunoglobulin-like domain of ICAM-1 (CD45) and its regulation by glycosylation. Cell 1991; 65:961–971.

101. Geng J-G, Bevilacqua MP, Moore KL, McIntyre TM, Prescott SM, Kim JM, Bliss GA, Zimmerman GA, McEver RP. Rapid neutrophil adhesion to activated endothelium mediated by GMP-140. Nature 1990; 343:757–760.
102. Bevilacqua MP, Prober JS, Mendrick DL, Cotran RS, Gimbrone MA. Identification of an inducible endothelial-leukocyte adhesion molecule. Proc Natl Acad Sci USA 1987; 84:9238–9248.
103. Bevilacqua MP, Stengelin S, Gimbrone MAJ, Seed B. Endothelial leukocyte adhesion molecule 1: an inducible receptor for neutrophils related to complement regulatory proteins and lectins. Science 1989; 243:1160–1163.
104. Kuijpers TW, Hakkert BC, Hoogerwerf H, Leeuwenberg JFM, Roos D. Role of endothelial leukocyte adhesion molecule-1 and platelet-activating factor in neutrophil adherence to IL-1 prestimulated endothelial cells. J Immunol 1991; 147: 1369–1376.
105. Shimizu Y, Shaw S, Graber N, Gopal TV, Horgan KJ, Van Seventer GA, Newman W. Activation-independent binding of human memory T cells to adhesion molecule ELAM-1. Nature 1991; 349:799–802.
106. Rothlein R, Dustin ML, Marlin SD, Springer TA. A human intercellular adhesion molecule (ICAM-1) distinct from LFA-1. J Immunol 1986; 137:1270–1274.
107. Staunton DE, Dustin ML, Springer TA. Functional cloning ICAM-2, a cell adhesion ligand for LFA-1 homologous to ICAM-1. Nature 1989; 339:61–63.
108. Osborn L, Hession C, Tizard R, Vassallo C, Luhowskyj S, Chi-Rosso G, Lobb R. Direct expression cloning of vascular cell adhesion molecule-1, a cytokine-induced endothelial protein that binds to lymphocytes. Cell 1989; 59:1203–1211.
109. Kyan-Aung U, Haskard DO, Poston RN, Thornhill MH, Lee TH. Endothelial leukocyte adhesion molecule-1 and intercellular adhesion molecule-1 mediate the adhesion of eosinophils to endothelial cells in vitro and are expressed by endothelium in allergic cutaneous inflammation in vivo. J Immunol 1991; 146(2): 521–528.
110. Cobb RR, Dubins JS, Warner J, Molony L. Functional expression of soluble ICAM-1 by baculovirus-infected Sf9 cells. Biochem Biophys Res Commun 1992; 185(3):1022–1033.
111. Shelley CS, Arnaout MA. The promoter of the CD11b gene directs myeloid-specific and developmentally regulated expression. Proc Natl Acad Sci USA 1991; 88(23):10525–10529.
112. Nelson C, Rabb H, Arnaout MA. Genetic cause of leukocyte adhesion molecule deficiency: abnormal splicing and a missense mutation in a conserved region of CD18 impair cell surface expression of beta 2 integrins. J Biol Chem 1992; 267(5): 3351–3357.
113. Polla BS, Perin M, Pizurki L. Regulation and functions of stress proteins in allergy and inflammation. Clin Exp Allergy 1993; 23:548–556.
114. Jacquier-Sarlin MR, Fuller K, Dinh-Xuan AT, Richard MJ, Polla BS. Protective effects of hsp70 in inflammation. Experientia 1994; 50(11–12):1031–1038.

12

Ventilation, Dynamics, and Gas Exchange

Göran Hedenstierna

University Hospital
Uppsala, Sweden

I. INTRODUCTION

Asthma is characterized by episodic airways obstruction. Major clinical manifestations of asthma such as wheezing, breathlessness, and tightness of the chest are due to airway narrowing. A functional evaluation of the airways can be made by spirometry with the recording of air flow and lung volumes as well as by lung mechanics tests with the recording of airway resistance. Since airway obstruction will affect the distribution of inspired gas in the lungs, ventilation-perfusion inequality or mismatch will ensue. This causes a gas exchange impairment signified by impaired arterial oxygenation, sometimes with hypoxemia, and, when respiratory work is overwhelmingly increased, retention of CO_2. Surprisingly, there is no or only poor correlation between spirometric or mechanics indices and gas exchange impairment. This has made it obvious that different functional disturbances have different pathophysiological backgrounds and that lung function impairment in asthma is more complex than previously understood. The well-established facts on lung function in asthma as well as recent advances, some still under debate, will be dealt with in this chapter.

II. MECHANICS OF THE LUNG

A. Airway Resistance

The primary mechanical abnormality during an asthma attack is an increase in the resistance of the airways. There are several techniques to measure the resistance. Basically, the driving force (alveolar minus mouth pressure) and flow rate must be measured. This can be achieved by body plethysmography, which enables the assessment of alveolar pressure during panting against an occluded mouthpiece (1). In theory, forced oscillation techniques in which an oscillating pressure (2) is superimposed on the pressure generated by gas flow, and interrupter techniques (3) in which gas flow is briefly halted by a shutter at the mouth to allow a pressure equilibration between mouth and alveoli, can be used. In practice, the accuracy is limited. Finally, the driving force can be measured as pleural minus mouth pressure, with pleural pressure substituted for esophageal pressure (4) obtained by a balloon catheter. The latter technique gives both airway and lung tissue resistance. Whatever technique is used, resistance is increased from normal values of 1–2 cm $H_2O \times L^{-1} \times s^{-1}$ to 4–6 cm in moderate asthma and as much as 10–20 cm $H_2O \times L^{-1} \times s^{-1}$ in severe asthma (5,6). Such an increase in resistance will produce a heavy burden on the respiratory muscles, which will be dealt with later. Severe narrowing of the airways may also cause gas trapping and an increase in FRC and residual volume (7,8).

The airway narrowing is in general caused by bronchial smooth muscle contraction, which may range from the glottis (9) to the peripheral airway (10). The fast response, sometimes with complete recovery of expiratory flow rates, to β-stimulators indicates that bronchial tone is a major determinant of the resistance in these cases. In addition, during recent years it has become obvious that asthma is an inflammatory disease with airway secretions, mucosal swelling, and even adventitial edema. These morphological changes will also have an effect on airway narrowing and the resistance to gas flow (11). Thus, as shown in Figure 1, excessive airway narrowing can be caused by (1) increased bronchial muscle strength and contractility, (2) an increase in submucosal thickness that will augment the effect of smooth muscle contraction, and (3) decreased elastic load by the surrounding lung tissue on the bronchial smooth muscles. This latter mechanism is based on the hypothesis that interstitial or adventitial edema may unlink the forces that tend to keep the airway open (surrounding lung tissue) from forces that cause bronchoconstriction (bronchial smooth muscle, surface tension of the bronchial wall) (12). Paré (13) made morphometric measurements of the airway wall in an attempt to quantify the importance of these three mechanisms on airway narrowing. Data on the thickness of the adventitia, smooth muscle layer of the airways, and the mucosal layer from 15 asthmatic and 15 nonasthmatic subjects were entered into

NORMAL

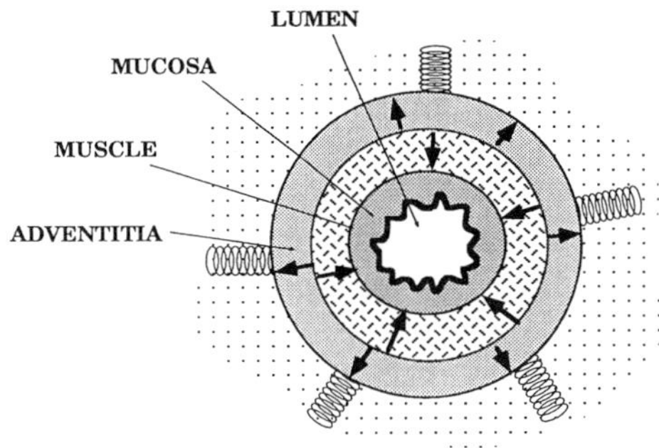

ASTHMATIC

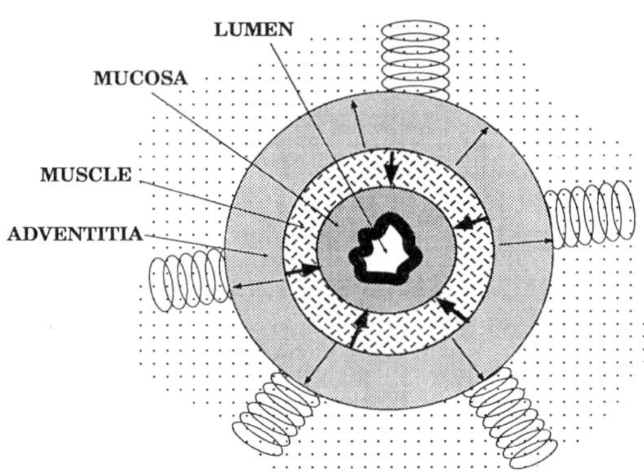

FIGURE 1 Schematic drawing of forces that act on the airway wall. There is a balance between forces acting inward, reducing the airway lumen, and forces that tend to open up the airway. The inward forces are the tone of the bronchial smooth muscle and the surface tension of the mucosa. The outwardly acting forces are exerted by the surrounding lung tissue as a consequence of interdependence between different lung regions. Excessive narrowing of the airway for the asthmatic is illustrated in the lower panel. This can be the effect of an increased submucosal layer due to edema, both by reducing the airway lumen and by exaggerating the airway narrowing by smooth muscle contraction. Increased smooth muscle layer and/or increased strength/contractility can also contribute to narrowing of the airway lumen. Finally, an adventitial edema reduces or unlinks the external load exerted by the lung tissue on the bronchial smooth muscle, enabling indefinite contraction.

a computer model of the tracheobronchial tree. Dose-response curves of airway resistance versus a bronchoconstricting agent were simulated. The bronchial muscle was allowed to shorten as a response to the bronchoconstrictor, until the tension generated in the muscle was equal and opposite to the stress developed in the surrounding lung tissue. The analysis suggested that increased muscle strength due to hypertrophy and hyperplasia of the airway smooth muscle is the most important factor in causing excessive airway narrowing in asthma. However, swelling and edema also contribute to excessive narrowing; some clinical and experimental data seem to support this. Thus, a decrease in dietary salt intake reduces the airway response to a bronchoconstrictor (14), and inhaled furosemide improves asthma (15). Some preliminary data are also available from a rabbit study. Thus, nebulization with saline augmented the response to a succeeding nebulization with histamine so that lung resistance increased 2.5 times more for a given dose of histamine than when histamine had been given alone (16).

Airway hyperreactivity and dose-response curves during challenge tests are the subject of another chapter and will not be dealt with here. It should, however, be mentioned that the unlinking hypothesis described above offers an explanation why the airways of patients with severe asthma can contract indefinitely, compared to airways in normal subjects in whom airway provocation tests result in a dose-response curve that reaches a plateau (17).

It has also been reported that some asthmatic patients have an increased compliance, i.e., loss of lung elastic recoil pressure (18). The reason is not clear but it seems unlikely that it is caused by real loss of elastic tissue.

B. Work of Breathing

The increased airway resistance and increased ventilatory demand because of ventilation-perfusion mismatch (see below) increase the work of breathing. This raises the load on the inspiratory muscles and is the most likely cause of the dyspnea. Good correlations between the plural (esophageal) pressure swings and the degree of dyspnea have been shown (19,20). To reduce the work of breathing, ventilation under these circumstances should be with low flow rates (low respiratory frequency and large tidal volume) (21), but the asthmatic often shows a pattern of rapid, shallow breathing. This breathing pattern may signal additional factors that interfere with ordinary breathing. Hyperinflation of the lungs may be one such factor (7,8), making deep inspirations difficult because of the less compliant lung at higher lung volume. The hyperinflation will also make the respiratory muscles, in particular the diaphragm, less efficient by shortening the muscle fibers (22), and possibly more vulnerable to muscle fatigue (23).

III. SPIROMETRY

The expiratory flow-volume curve is determined by the recoil pressure of the lung and the mechanical properties of the airways. The respiratory muscles have little influence on the shape of the flow-volume curve, contributing to the peak flow at the beginning of expiration (24). Since asthma causes airway narrowing and sometimes also reduced recoil pressure of the lung, the flow-volume curve is affected in most patients (25). There may be complete remission of the asthma with all tests of pulmonary function being normal. However, this is rare even in spasmodic asthma. More common is the finding of measurable defects in pulmonary function despite the fact that the patient is completely asymptomatic.

In patients with only mild disease the earliest sign may be reduced midexpiratory flows (FEF_{50}, FEF_{75}, FEF_{25-75}) whereas peak expiratory flow and the FEV_1 are normal (25) (Fig. 2) (spirometric symbols are explained in Table 1). Prompt reversibility of airway obstruction by a bronchodilator, as evidenced by at least 15–20% improvement of expiratory flows, should also be seen in the asthmatic (26). The greater sensitivity to mild airway obstruction, at least

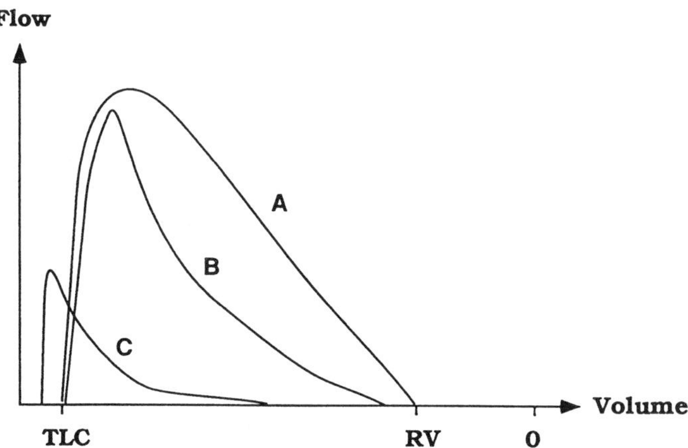

FIGURE 2 Expiratory flow-volume curves. (A) Normal subject: note the peak flow early during expiration and the almost linear decrease in flow rate during the continuing expiration. (B) Mild asthma: note the almost maintained peak flow but more rapid decrease in flow rate during the continuing expiration. Also, expiration ceases earlier than in the normal subject (increased residual volume). (C) Severe asthma: note the decrease in peak flow and the dramatic decrease in expiratory flow rate, as well as the leftward shift of the curve, indicating increased TLC and considerably increased RV.

TABLE 1 Spirometric Symbols Used in the Text

TLC:	total lung capacity, the gas volume in the lungs after a maximum inspiration.
VC:	vital capacity, a maximum breath, i.e., the volume difference between end-inspiration and end-expiration.
RV:	residual volume, the volume of gas that remains in the lungs after a maximum expiration.
FRC:	functional residual capacity, the volume of gas in the lungs after an ordinary expiration to "resting level."
FEV_1:	forced expired volume in 1 sec, the maximum volume that can be expired in 1 sec.
FEV%:	FEV_1 divided by VC times 100.
FEF_{50}:	forced expiratory flow at 50% of the vital capacity.
FEF_{75}:	forced expiratory flow at 75% expired VC.
FEF_{25-75}:	mean forced expiratory flow between 25 and 75% expired VC.
Phase III:	the slope of the alveolar plateau of the nitrogen washout curve, expressed as % N_2 per liter expired gas.
CV:	closing volume, the volume above RV at which airways begin to close during an expiration.

in theory, by recording mid and late expiratory flow is because of the decreasing lung volume during expiration that will also reduce airway caliber. This will enhance the effect of secretions, edema, and bronchoconstriction on the airway lumen. On the other hand, the reproducibility of the flow variables is poorer than that of vital capacity and FEV_1 (27).

With increasing severity of the disease, the FEV_1 is reduced as is also the forced vital capacity.

As mentioned earlier, air trapping and increased FRC can be seen in more severe asthma (7,8). Even total lung capacity can be increased above normal, sometimes by as much as 1 L or more.

The increased TLC is a consequence of the enlarged RV whereas vital capacity is mostly reduced. Relief of the airway obstruction by, for example, β-stimulators can prompt a rapid increase in VC paralleled by a decrease in RV (7). As might be expected, there is a relationship between the increase in airway resistance and the degree of hyperinflation. However, the airway resistance can be doubled before any trapping of gas (increase in FRC) can be seen (28).

IV. AIRWAY CLOSURE AND VENTILATION DISTRIBUTION

That airways may close in dependent lung regions (e.g., basal lung units with the subject in an upright position) during a deep expiration was proposed for the first time by Milic-Emili et al. in 1966 (29). Evidence of such closure was later presented (30,31). The volume above RV at which airways begin to close during an expiration, the closing volume (CV), has subsequently been the subject of many studies in health and disease. CV increases with age, an effect of loss of elastic tissue with aging (32), but is independent of body position (32). CV is increased in chronic bronchitis (33) due to inflammatory changes in distal airways, making them less resistant to external compression. CV is often increased in asthma (33), although varying results have been obtained (34).

Many studies have analyzed the distribution of inspired gas in health and lung disease. Multiple-breath washout techniques have shown that the efficiency of the ventilation in terms of ventilation/lung volume ratios is impaired in asthma, with longer washout times than in the normal subject (35,36). The assessment of CV also allows an analysis of the ventilation distribution by recording the slope of the alveolar plateau (phase III) (37). More details of the technique are given in Figure 3. In obstructive lung disease the slope of phase III increases, and it is often held that the slope of the alveolar plateau is a better discriminator of airway dysfunction than any other lung function variable (37,38). However, some disagreement about how to interpret the single-breath nitrogen washout test in a mild asthmatic may have emerged from the varying results obtained by giving the patient a β-agonist aerosol. This often results in a reduced CV whereas phase III may vary in both directions (39). This may be a consequence of other factors than airflow obstruction influencing the slope of the nitrogen plateau. One factor that has become more obvious during recent years is regional differences in lung compliance (40); another is the volume of the lung acini in which diffusive gas mixing takes place (41).

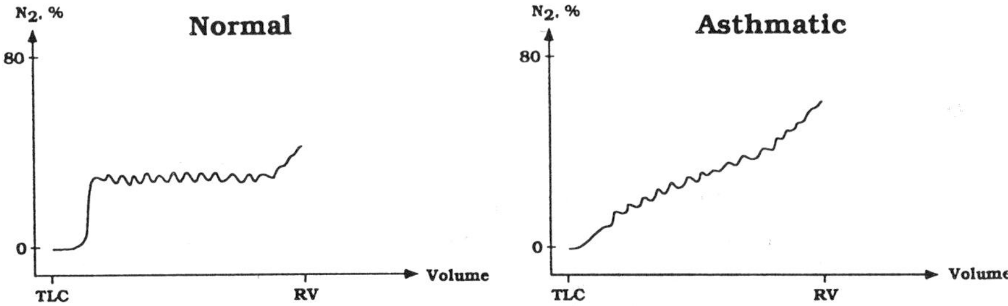

FIGURE 3 Single-breath nitrogen washout curves. Normal subject: note the almost horizontal alveolar plateau (phase III) and the distinct inflection point, indicating onset of airway closure. The expired volume from the inflection point to RV corresponds to CV. Asthmatic subject: note the much steeper phase III and the insidious inflection point, making it difficult to determine where airway closure begins.

The spatial distribution of ventilation, assessed by isotope techniques, has demonstrated considerable regional variation in gas distribution. It has also been demonstrated that one lung unit may be autonomous in the sense that it can react with bronchospasm when subjected to an allergen via a bronchospirometric catheter whereas the remaining, nonexposed lung does not react (42).

V. LUNG PERFUSION

Cardiac output, and thus total pulmonary perfusion, is often increased during asthma, possibly an effect of treatment with adrenergic agonists and an endogenous increase in sympathetic tone. The pulmonary vascular pressures are only little increased in mild or moderate asthma, but more so in extreme cases as status asthmaticus (43). The perfusion distribution, as assessed by isotope techniques, is also affected. This may be due in part to hypoxic pulmonary vasoconstriction, diverting blood flow away from poorly ventilated lung regions (44). There is also evidence of reduced perfusion of lung regions that are still ventilated. One possible explanation is hyperinflation with persisting ventilation and impediment of blood flow by compression of alveolar capillaries by the expanded alveoli (45).

VI. VENTILATION PERFUSION RELATIONSHIP

The gas exchange, or, more explicitly, the arterial oxygenation and the elimination of CO_2 from the blood, is dependent primarily on the ventilation-perfusion relationship ($\dot{V}_A/\dot{Q}$). It will also depend on the cardiac output in relation to the metabolic demand and there are additional minor influences from the hemoglobin content and the oxygen dissociation curve of the blood. The two latter mechanisms will not be dealt with further in this chapter.

A. Blood Gas Analysis

The recording of arterial oxygen tension (PaO_2) and carbon dioxide tension ($PaCO_2$) will tell whether there is hypoxemia and CO_2 retention. In the mild and moderate asthmatic no hypoxemia may be seen, despite certain or even considerable $\dot{V}_A/\dot{Q}$ mismatch (as will be discussed below). This can be explained by increased cardiac output that raises venous PO_2 and reduces the effect of a $\dot{V}_A/\dot{Q}$ mismatch (46). In more severe asthma PaO_2 may drop to dangerously low levels (47). Death in an asthmatic attack has been attributed to hypoxemia in some cases but may equally well be caused by arrhythmia and cardiac arrest due to acidosis and abuse of adrenergic drugs (48). CO_2 retention is rare in mild and moderate asthma (49). This is because the impaired CO_2 removal caused by a $\dot{V}_A/\dot{Q}$ mismatch can be compensated for by an increase in the minute ventilation. However important the blood gas analysis may be, it does not offer much explanation as to what has caused a hypoxemia and a CO_2 retention. Knowledge of the $\dot{V}_A/\dot{Q}$ distribution may guide in the understanding of underlying mechanisms. The next section will deal with multicompartmental analysis of the ventilation and perfusion distribution.

B. Three-Compartment Analysis

A three-compartment analysis can be made by the recording of the O_2 and CO_2 content in arterial and mixed venous blood and mixed expired gas (50). This enables the calculation of one compartment that is perfused but not ventilated (venous admixture), one compartment that is ventilated but not perfused (dead space), and an ideal compartment that is both ventilated and perfused. However, venous admixture in this three-compartment model includes not only perfusion of nonventilated lung tissue (true pulmonary shunt), but also regions that are poorly ventilated or perfused in excess of their ventilation (low $\dot{V}_A/\dot{Q}$ regions). Similarly, the dead space compartment includes not only true dead space (airways and nonperfused alveoli) but also regions that are ventilated well in excess of their perfusion (high $\dot{V}_A/\dot{Q}$ regions). Using the three-compartment model, asthmatics have been shown to have an increased dead space ventilation and increased venous admixture (increase in "shunt") (51). It has also been shown that adrenergic agonists may decrease the airway resistance without a concomitant improvement in PaO_2; on the contrary, venous admixture may increase and PaO_2 deteriorate further (52,53). Oxygen breathing may also worsen the $\dot{V}_A/\dot{Q}$ distribution as shown by an increase in physiological dead space and venous admixture (54). This may be an effect of attenuated hypoxic pulmonary vasoconstriction.

C. Multicompartment Analysis

By using more than two gases with different solubilities in blood, a better resolution can be obtained, allowing a truly multicompartmental analysis. This can be achieved by multiple inert gas elimination. Fahri made a pioneering work on inert gas elimination for the assessment of ventilation and gas exchange (55). Based on this work, the multiple inert gas elimination technique was introduced in 1974 by Wagner, West, and Saltzman (56,57). Ventilation and blood flow may be allocated to a number of hypothetical compartments (e.g., 50) ranging from shunt ($\dot{V}_A/\dot{Q} = 0$) over compartments with low, normal, and high $\dot{V}_A/\dot{Q}$ ratios to dead space ($\dot{V}_A/\dot{Q}$ = infinity). The procedure is based on measurement of the retention and elimination of several (usually six) "inert" gases (gases obeying Henry's law, i.e., showing a linear relationship between partial pressure and concentration in blood) with different solubilities in blood. The resulting $\dot{V}_A/\dot{Q}$ distribution will depend on both vertical and nongravitational distributions of ventilation of blood flow but does not allow any spatial analysis. The $\dot{V}_A/\dot{Q}$ distribution may rather be considered a fingerprint of the lungs' ability to transfer gas between alveoli and capillary blood. The more important variables that can be derived by the multiple inert gas elimination technique are listed in Table 2. The $\dot{V}_A/\dot{Q}$ distribution in a normal subject is shown in Figure 4, left upper panel.

Soon after its introduction in 1974, the multiple inert gas elimination technique was used in experimental asthma in a canine model and subsequently in human asthmatics. Some rather unexpected observations were made. Thus, when anesthetized dogs were exposed to nebulized *Ascaris* and other bronchoirritants, a bimodal $\dot{V}_A/\dot{Q}$ distribution developed with the new mode appearing in the low $\dot{V}_A/\dot{Q}$ region (58). The new low $\dot{V}_A/\dot{Q}$ mode was often distinctly separated from the ordinary mode centered around a $\dot{V}_A/\dot{Q}$ ratio of 1. The other unexpected finding was that no shunt developed, contrary to the generally held opinion that asthma causes shunt. That this was not a finding that was limited to the dog became apparent when the inert gas technique was applied in human asthmatics. Thus, in patients with asthma a bimodal $\dot{V}_A/\dot{Q}$ distribution was again obtained, similarly to the provocation results in dogs. About a quarter of the total blood flow went to lung units with $\dot{V}_A/\dot{Q}$ ratios in the region of 0.1. Again, there was no blood flow to unventilated units; i.e., there was no shunt (59). Even more unexpected may be the fact that also in severe asthma, requiring hospitalization, no or only minor shunt was seen (mean shunt 1.1% in 10 patients with a mean PaO_2 of 55 mmHg on admission) (60). Examples of $\dot{V}_A/\dot{Q}$ distributions in asthma and other lung diseases are shown in Figure 4.

TABLE 2 Variables That Can Be Derived from Multiple Inert Gas Elimination Data

V_{mean}:	the mean $\dot{V}_A/\dot{Q}$ ratio of the ventilation distribution.
Q_{mean}:	the mean $\dot{V}_A/\dot{Q}$ ratio of the perfusion distribution.
Log SDV:	the logarithmic standard deviation of the ventilation distribution around V_{mean}.
Log SDQ:	the logarithmic standard deviation of the perfusion distribution around Q_{mean}.
Shunt:	perfusion of lung regions with $\dot{V}_A/\dot{Q} < 0.005$.
Low $\dot{V}_A/\dot{Q}$:	perfusion of lung regions with $0.005 < \dot{V}_A/\dot{Q} < 0.1$.
Normal $\dot{V}_A/\dot{Q}$:	perfusion of lung regions with $0.1 < \dot{V}_A/\dot{Q} < 10$.
High $\dot{V}_A/\dot{Q}$:	ventilation of lung regions with $10 < \dot{V}_A/\dot{Q} < 100$.
Dead space:	ventilation of lung regions with $\dot{V}_A/\dot{Q} > 100$.

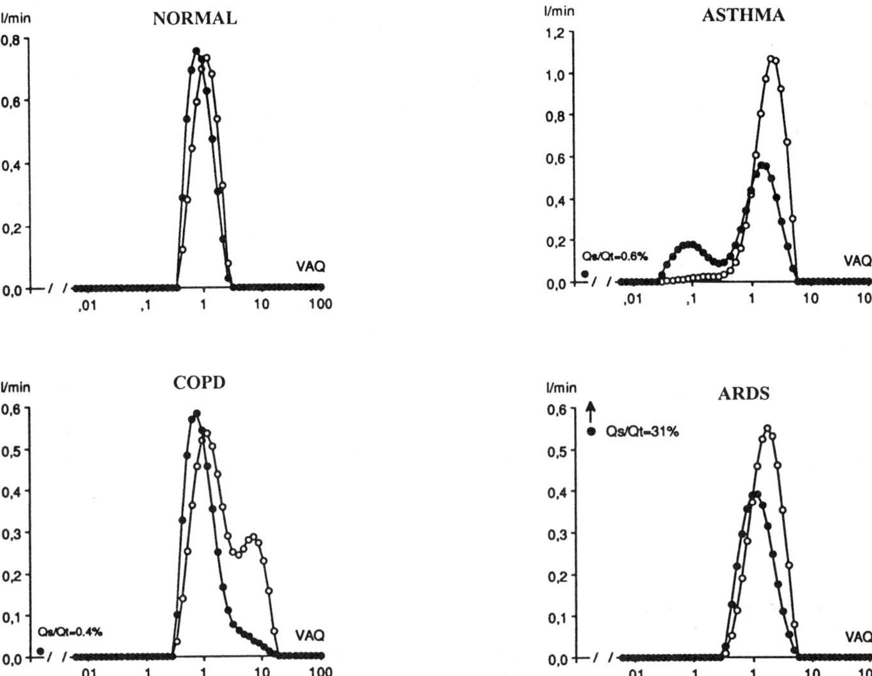

FIGURE 4 Ventilation-perfusion distribution by multiple inert gas elimination technique. O: Ventilation, ● : Perfusion. (Left upper panel) $\dot{V}_A/\dot{Q}$ in a normal subject. Note the good match between ventilation and blood flow with unimodal distributions of both. The modes are centered on a $\dot{V}_A/\dot{Q}$ ratio of 1. (Right upper panel) $\dot{V}_A/\dot{Q}$ in an asthmatic patient with moderately severe disease. Note the much broader $\dot{V}_A/\dot{Q}$ distribution (increased log SDQ) and the bimodal pattern with an additional low $\dot{V}_A/\dot{Q}$ mode, centered on a ratio of approximately 0.1. For further details see text. (Left lower panel) $\dot{V}_A/\dot{Q}$ distribution in a patient with chronic obstructive pulmonary disease (COPD). Note the broad distribution with both normal and high $\dot{V}_A/\dot{Q}$ regions, resulting in both normal $\dot{V}_A/\dot{Q}$ and dead space–like (high $\dot{V}_A/\dot{Q}$) effects. (Right lower panel) $\dot{V}_A/\dot{Q}$ in a patient with acute respiratory failure, adult respiratory distress syndrome (ARDS). Note the unimodal, although broader than normal, $\dot{V}_A/\dot{Q}$ distribution. There is also a very large shunt, which is not seen in asthma and COPD.

D. Mechanisms of Bimodal $\dot{V}_A/\dot{Q}$ Distribution

The findings of mucus plugging, airway wall edema, and bronchoconstriction to the point that complete closure of airways occurs, all of which are recurrent in severe asthma, do not fit with the absence of shunt. However, a possible mechanism may be that lung units behind completely occluded airways are still ventilated via collateral channels between bronchioli and alveoli (58,59). The dog has been shown to have large collateral ventilation (61,62) and morphological studies suggest that collateral ventilation is also a possibility in humans (63). When, on the other hand, the pig is challenged with methacholine, a large shunt develops, but no perfusion of low $\dot{V}_A/\dot{Q}$ regions (64). The pig has well-developed interlobar and lobular septa that prevent any collateral ventilation (65). Thus, the different $\dot{V}_A/\dot{Q}$ patterns in dog and human compared to the pig support the hypothesis that collateral ventilation is the cause of the distinct low $\dot{V}_A/\dot{Q}$ mode (Fig. 5). This was further analyzed in dog experiments by Lee et al. (66). Beads were inserted via bronchoscopy until the PaO_2 fell by 20 mmHg, or below 70 mmHg. Occlusion of small airways by beads 1.6 mm in diameter resulted in a mild increase in the dispersion of $\dot{V}_A/\dot{Q}$, and with 2.4 mm beads the dispersion increased further. By contrast, dogs given large beads (4.8 mm) showed a bimodal distribution of $\dot{V}_A/\dot{Q}$. The authors suggested that the bimodal distribution seen in asthma is compatible with complete obstruction of some airways and that the levels of obstruction may affect the pattern of

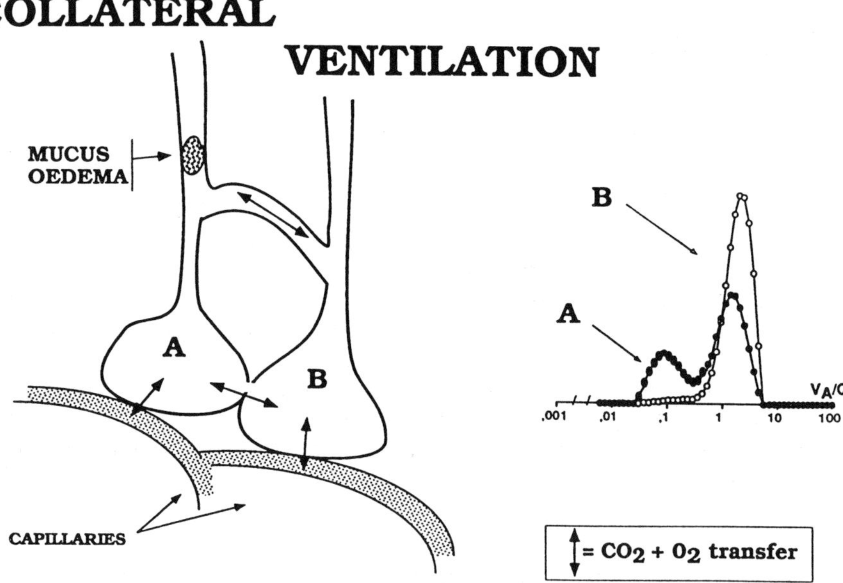

FIGURE 5 Schematic drawing of the morphological and functional basis of a low $\dot{V}_A/\dot{Q}$ mode, but not shunt, in asthma. Note the mucus plugging in distal airways and the continuing ventilation of subtended lung units via collaterals. This so-called parasitic ventilation results in the distinct low $\dot{V}_A/\dot{Q}$ mode.

$\dot{V}_A/\dot{Q}$ distribution. To test the possible influence of peripheral airway edema and mucus on the $\dot{V}_A/\dot{Q}$ distribution, a rabbit model was used for different provocation tests (67,68). The physiological opportunity for collateral ventilation has been shown in the rabbit similar to that in human and dog (63). In initial experiments the $\dot{V}_A/\dot{Q}$ distributions in the rabbit were studied under normal conditions and after airway provocation tests with inhaled methacholine. Baseline data showed a unimodal $\dot{V}_A/\dot{Q}$ distribution centered upon a ratio of 1 with no or only minor shunt (67). Inhaled methacholine resulted in a bimodal $\dot{V}_A/\dot{Q}$ distribution with the new mode centered around the $\dot{V}_A/\dot{Q}$ of 0.1 (Fig. 6, lower left panel). No increase in shunt was seen. The findings were thus much the same as in adult asthma.

In a subsequent study (68), airway wall edema and mucus were simulated by nebulization of isotonic saline in the rabbit model. The nebulizer produced saline droplets with a mass median diameter of 3 μm, and tests with a tracer

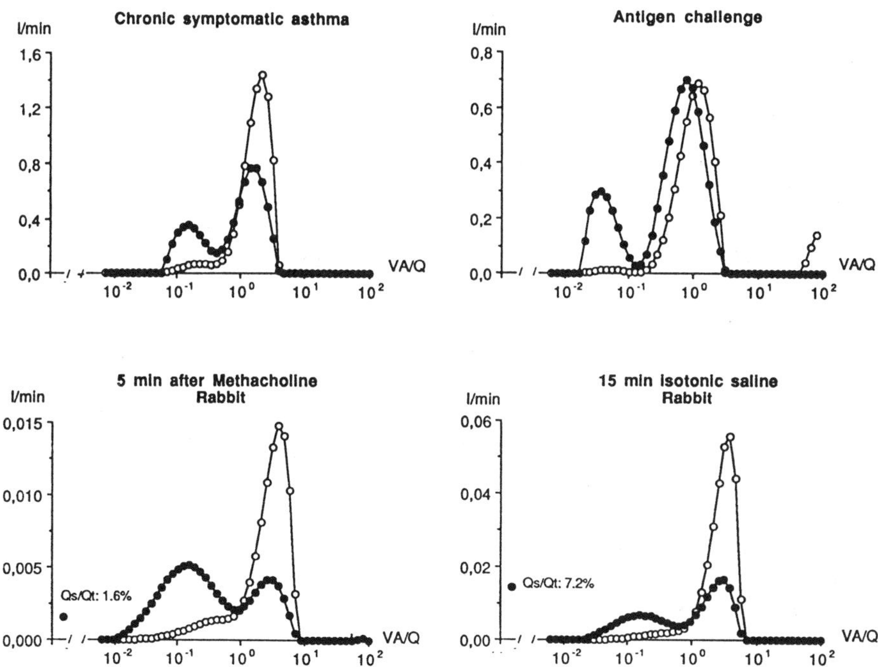

FIGURE 6 Ventilation-perfusion distributions in a patient with chronic stable asthma (left upper panel), allergic asthma (right upper panel), a rabbit after a bronchial challenge with methacholine (left lower panel), and a rabbit after nebulization of isotonic saline (right lower panel). Note the similarity between all four recordings.

aerosol (Evans blue dye) showed that the droplets deposited mainly in peripheral airways, approximately 85% of the total deposited fluid. Despite several milliliters of nebulized fluid, as little as 0.15 ml was retained in the lung. The interesting observation was that this peripheral deposition resulted in a bimodal $\dot{V}_A/\dot{Q}$ distribution, again with the additional mode in low $\dot{V}_A/\dot{Q}$ regions. Shunt, on the other hand, increased very little for the first 10 min, but on a continued nebulization of saline it continued to increase. Thus, the early $\dot{V}_A/\dot{Q}$ disturbance was again very similar to what can be seen in adult asthma (Fig. 6, lower right panel). Simultaneous recordings of the mechanics of the respiratory systems showed no measurable changes in the resistance, whereas compliance fell in parallel with increasing shunt. These findings taken together support the theory that gas exchange impairment in asthma is related to events in small airways, possibly mucus secretion and/or mucosal edema.

VII. $\dot{V}_A/\dot{Q}$ UNDER DIFFERENT ASTHMA CONDITIONS

So far, descriptions have been made of $\dot{V}_A/\dot{Q}$ in severe asthma in adults, and in patients who have required hospitalization. This section will deal with the gas exchange abnormalities that can be seen in other groups with asthma.

A. Chronic, Stable Asthma

In 26 stable symptomatic asthmatics with a mean FEV% of 79% of predicted and FEF_{75} of 43% of predicted, bimodal distributions with an additional low $\dot{V}_A/\dot{Q}$ mode were seen in one-third of all measurements (69). The logarithmic standard deviation of the perfusion distribution (log SDQ) averaged 0.74, thus above the upper limit of the normal (0.60), and in only five patients was mean log SDQ less than 0.6. Thus, the $\dot{V}_A/\dot{Q}$ abnormality in these outclinic patients in stable condition was essentially the same as in more severe asthma (Fig. 6, upper left panel). Moreover, the patients were followed once a week for 9 consecutive weeks. During this period, bimodal $\dot{V}_A/\dot{Q}$ distributions were observed at some point in 24 of 26 subjects and log SDQ exceeded 0.60 in every patient in 2 weeks or more. Finally, arterial PO_2 measured three times in each subject was inversely related to log SDQ but only 60% of the variance was explained by a $\dot{V}_A/\dot{Q}$ mismatch. The remaining variation must therefore be attributed to other factors such as variation in mixed venous PO_2 and oxygen uptake (see below). Thus, most asthmatics with moderate, stable disease have a $\dot{V}_A/\dot{Q}$ mismatch. This mismatch is due mainly to development of low $\dot{V}_A/\dot{Q}$ areas and is variable both between patients and over time.

B. Allergic Asthma

Patients studied after an allergen challenge (70) developed the same $\dot{V}_A/\dot{Q}$ mismatch as patients exposed to methacholine challenge (59) or studied during a stable chronic asthma (69). Thus, in a rather young group of patients with allergic asthma (mean age 26 years) spirometry as well as the $\dot{V}_A/\dot{Q}$ distribution were normal prior to challenge (70). Immediately after challenge FEV_1 fell from mean 3.9 to 2.3 L, $PaO2$ from 13.1 to 9.5 kPa, and a $\dot{V}_A/\dot{Q}$ mismatch developed with an increasing mean log SDQ from 0.35 to 0.73. Bimodal $\dot{V}_A/\dot{Q}$ distribution appeared in some patients (Fig. 6, upper right panel). No or minimal shunt was seen. Thirty minutes after challenge the spirometric variables had improved significantly whereas the gas exchange impairment remained. A near-normalization was noticed at the recording 2.5 hr after challenge. Five of eight patients developed a late-phase reaction as shown by recordings 5 hr after challenge with deterioration in spirometry and gas exchange. These findings are in line with previous observations that the amount of $\dot{V}_A/\dot{Q}$ inequality is increased after bronchial challenge with antigen (71). However, the mismatch seems to be somewhat less marked with less frequent bimodality of the $\dot{V}_A/\dot{Q}$ distribution. Wagner and co-workers also found that nebulization with a β-stimulator caused a rapid return of the $\dot{V}_A/\dot{Q}$ toward normal in the patients with antigen-induced asthma (71), contrary to the persisting mismatch after such nebulization in patients with spontaneous asthma (59). These small qualitative and quantitative differences between spontaneous and antigen-induced asthma raise the question whether the gas exchange abnormalities induced by antigen challenge are not, or less, associated with secretions or mucosal edema whereas those in spontaneous asthma probably are.

C. Exercise-Induced Asthma

An early report on worsened lung function during exercise-induced asthma (EIA) was presented in 1966 by McNeill and co-workers (72). They found a fall in FEV_1, an increase in airway resistance, and impairment of gas distribution after 8 min of exercise. Peak effects were seen 15 min after termination of the exercise test. The observations have been confirmed in many other studies although only a fraction of the asthmatics showed an impairment of function during or after exercise; some even improved during the exercise test (73). The causative mechanism of EIA is not clear and this section will deal only with more recent observations on the $\dot{V}_A/\dot{Q}$ relationship during exercise.

Young and co-workers (74) studied six asthmatic subjects during exercise. Prior to the test all subjects had unimodal $\dot{V}_A/\dot{Q}$ distributions and only one had a clearly increased log SDQ, above 0.60. All had normal PaO_2. An 8-min treadmill exercise test to attain a heart rate of 160 beats/min caused a 20% or greater decrease in peak expiratory flow and/or FEV_1 in all subjects 10–20 min after termination of exercise. The $\dot{V}_A/\dot{Q}$ distribution broadened in all subjects (increased log SDQ) from mean 0.54 to 1.02, and two subjects developed a bimodal distribution. PaO_2 fells in all subjects. All $\dot{V}_A/\dot{Q}$ distributions returned to baseline configuration within the hour, usually before the spirometric indices had returned to baseline values. This time discrepancy may appear surprising in view of the fact that antigen asthma caused the opposite pattern—spirometric induces returning faster to baseline than the $\dot{V}_A/\dot{Q}$ relationship (70). However, the major feature is that exercise-induced gas exchange abnormality shows the same pattern as in other types of asthma, i.e., broadened $\dot{V}_A/\dot{Q}$ distribution and sometimes bimodality.

D. Asthma in Childhood

Children with asthma often display signs of bronchial obstruction on spirometry, even during symptom-free periods (75). Since children usually have a shorter history of asthma than adult asthmatics and usually are nonsmokers, one might anticipate that they have less intractable airway changes than adults and that bronchial obstructions would be more reversible, either spontaneously or by bronchodilators. Arterial oxygenation appears to be less affected in childhood asthma (76). Gas distribution studies using multiple-breath nitrogen washout technique (77) showed less efficient gas mixing with slowly ventilated compartments in asthmatic children.

The application of the multiple inert gas elimination technique in children with asthma was made in a couple of studies during exercise and after histamine provocation (78,79). Thus in 11 children with a history of EIA a unimodal distribution of $\dot{V}_A/\dot{Q}$ was seen before the test. The exercise test provoked asthma in seven children who all developed a broader $\dot{V}_A/\dot{Q}$ (increased log SDQ) and six of these displayed a bimodal distribution. The pattern was different from that of adult asthmatics in that the additional mode was located within high $\dot{V}_A/\dot{Q}$ regions (Fig. 7). The magnitude of this mode correlated to the reduction in FEV_1 and PaO_2. It was hypothesized that the high $\dot{V}_A/\dot{Q}$ mode reflects hyperinflated regions that by check valve mechanisms can be subjected to increased alveolar pressure. Support for the hypothesis can be obtained from studies with positive end-expiratory pressure ventilation, which has been shown to create an additional high $\dot{V}_A/\dot{Q}$ mode in animal experiments (80) as well as in human studies (81). This might be attributable to the development of a zone 1 (alveolar pressure exceeding pulmonary capillary pressure). In this zone there is no capillary blood flow but a small corner vessel blood flow that may take part in gas exchange and cause the high mode. There are also earlier reports on hyperinflation and reduced regional perfusion during an asthmatic attack. Mishkin and Wagner (45) found focal areas of decreased pulmonary blood flow and proposed two explanations—increased intra-alveolar pressure, impeding blood flow, and/or regional hypoventilation, leading to hypoxic vasoconstriction.

In the other study on childhood asthma, histamine inhalation provocation was done in five children (79). Again, unimodal distributions of ventilation

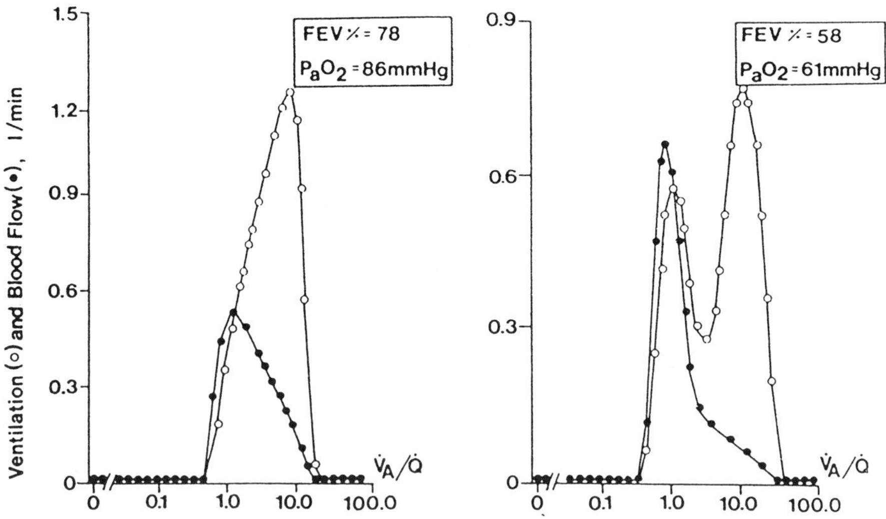

FIGURE 7 $\dot{V}_A/\dot{Q}$ distributions in a 13-year-old boy with asthma, prior to (left) and 10 min after (right) a bicycle ergometer exercise. Note the unimodal, somewhat broad $\dot{V}_A/\dot{Q}$ distribution prior to the test and the bimodal distribution after exercise, with high $\dot{V}_A/\dot{Q}$ regions. This pattern is thus different from that seen in adult asthma (see Figs. 4 and 6). (From Ref. 78, with permission by the editor of *American Review of Respiratory Diseases*.)

of perfusion were seen during baseline. The histamine provocation caused bimodal distribution in all children, again with the additional mode within high $\dot{V}_A/\dot{Q}$ regions. The high $\dot{V}_A/\dot{Q}$ mode correlated inversely with FEV$_1$. Thus the findings after histamine provocation were the same as in EIA in children, and different from what has been seen in adult asthmatics.

VIII. RELATIONSHIPS BETWEEN SYMPTOMS SPIROMETRY AND GAS EXCHANGE

It might be assumed that dyspnea, spirometric indices, and gas exchange impairment vary together, so that worsening in one variable is accompanied by a similar worsening in the other. However, this is not the case. When a group of adult patients ($n = 26$) was followed for 9 weeks (see also above), no or only poor correlations were obtained between symptoms, spirometry, and $\dot{V}_A/\dot{Q}$ (82). In particular, the presence of abnormal gas exchange could not be predicted from symptoms or spirometric values. The findings suggest that spirometric and gas exchange abnormalities in asthma are caused by different pathophysiological events. Thus, spirometry may be more affected by bronchial contraction in upper airways whereas gas exchange impairment is an effect of peripheral airway edema and secretions.

A similar dissociation between spirometry and $\dot{V}_A/\dot{Q}$ inequality was seen in patients with acute severe asthma requiring hospitalization (60). In this study both clinical and spirometric improvement were noted in all patients after hospitalization but there was simultaneous improvement in $\dot{V}_A/\dot{Q}$ in only one patient. Also, an extreme of this dissociation between spirometry and gas exchange is the frequent effect of β-agonist administration with worsening of the $\dot{V}_A/\dot{Q}$ relationship simultaneously with reduced airways obstruction (59,83). In the latter case the adrenergic drug presumably acts via pulmonary vasodilation, increasing blood flow more than ventilation in certain regions. By this means, a low $\dot{V}_A/\dot{Q}$ mode may increase in size during bronchodilation (53,59). Animal data also support this conclusion. Thus Rodriquez-Roisin and co-workers (84) gave different α- and β-agonists to dogs that had developed airway obstruction after methacholine provocations. Epinephrine (α), isoproterenol ($\beta1$), and salbutamol ($\beta2$) caused similar bronchial relaxation but had different effects on pulmonary vessels and perfusion of low $\dot{V}_A/\dot{Q}$. The drug that had the most powerful vasodilatory action (isoproterenol) produced the largest increase of low $\dot{V}_A/\dot{Q}$ ratios, salbutamol caused less mismatch although of certain duration, and epinephrine a small increase in the mismatch (as for salbutamol) but of short duration.

IX. GENETIC INFLUENCE

This section will deal with the limited knowledge we have of genetic influence on pulmonary function.

The normal interindividual variability of expiratory flow rate was proposed by Green et al. (85) to be due to the geometry of the airways but independent of the size of the lung. They hypothesized that the variability of the expiratory flow rates had an embryological basis, reflecting disproportionate but physiologically normal growth of the airways and parenchyma within the lung. This was tested by Man and Zamel (86) and more recently by Redline et al. (87). They found that the variability of the expiratory flow rate was much smaller among monozygote twins, who have similar embryological constitution, than in heterozygote twins. This was further evidence that there is a genetic influence on respiratory function. Studies on airway responsiveness have also shown a smaller intrapair variation in homozygote twins than in nonidentical twins (88,89).

A large number of studies have utilized methods of airway responsiveness to help establish a genetic link to asthma. Since airway responsiveness is dealt with elsewhere, only a few comments will be made on the genetic influence. Townley et al. (90) proposed that airway hyperresponsiveness has a genetic basis, after the demonstration of reactive airways in relatives to asthmatics but not in families without an asthma/allergy family history. Longo et al. (91) measured airway responsiveness to inhaled carbacholine in nonasthmatic parents of asthmatics, nonasthmatic controls, and current symptomatic asthmatics. They found that 50% of parents of asthmatics had hyperreactive airways but only 10% of the controls. They concluded that the findings indicate an autosomal dominant pattern of inheritance. Similar observations were made by Bruderman et al. (92), who, in agreement with Townley et al. (90) and Longo et al. (91), observed a bimodal distribution of the response to a bronchoconstrictor in parents of asthmatics.

Higgins and Keller (93) found significant correlation between spirometry (FEV_1) in first-degree relatives and between parents and children. Moreover, they found that chronic bronchitis, asthma, and allergic rhinitis were more common when a parent had the same condition. These observations may be taken as indirect evidence for genetic factors in the development of various pulmonary disorders.

Exercise tests were used as an airway challenge by Konig and Godfrey, who also made skin tests in 65 first-degree relatives of asthmatic children (94). As many as 43% had a positive response. However, there was no control group in the study.

It can thus be summarized that there is evidence of a genetic influence on the respiratory function. There are also a large number of studies that support the view that the ventilatory impairment in asthma has an embryological basis.

X. CONCLUSION

The major functional impairment in asthma is increased resistance to respiratory gas flow. This causes an increased work of breathing that may be appreciated as dyspnea. Another consequence of the increased airway resistance is impeded expiratory gas flow that can also be measured as a reduced FEV_1 or FEV%. In more severe cases the airway obstruction may increase the resting lung volume (FRC), as well as residual volume, and reduce vital capacity. The airway dysfunction causes an uneven distribution of inspired gas and premature closure of airways (increased closing volume). Uneven gas distribution results in a ventilation-perfusion mismatch with subsequent impairment of the oxygenation of blood. In severe asthma, overwhelming respiratory work may cause hypoventilation, which, together with $\dot{V}_A/\dot{Q}$ mismatch, causes CO_2 retention. The $\dot{V}_A/\dot{Q}$ mismatch, as evidenced by multiple inert gas elimination technique, is typically characterized by bimodal distribution of blood flow. The additional, low $\dot{V}_A/\dot{Q}$ mode may be explained by collateral ventilation behind completely closed airways. Interestingly, the $\dot{V}_A/\dot{Q}$ pattern is different in childhood asthma as compared to adult. Thus, the child does not show a low $\dot{V}_A/\dot{Q}$ mode, but an additional high $\dot{V}_A/\dot{Q}$ mode, presumably due to regional hyperinflation with impediment of perfusion. Finally, the variation in spirometric and lung mechanics variables in a particular patient is not paralleled by similar variation in gas exchange. Thus, improvement in a spirometric variable may be accompanied by deterioration in gas exchange. This finding suggests that there are different pathophysiological mechanisms behind impairment in spirometry and gas exchange. Most likely, the measurements of airway resistance and spirometry reflect phenomena in larger airways, whereas gas exchange and ventilation-perfusion matching describe phenomena in small airways. It has thus become obvious that pulmonary dysfunction in asthma is more complex than was earlier thought. We still do not have a full picture of the excessive airway narrowing in asthma and its causes, and the pathophysiology of asthma is still a challenge to the scientist. By combining physiological knowledge with the rapid advances in morphological techniques and microbiology, a more complete picture of the airway dysfunction in asthma may finally be obtained.

ACKNOWLEDGMENT

This study was supported by a grant from the Swedish Heart and Lung Fund.

REFERENCES

1. DuBois AB, Botelho SY, Comroe JH. A new method of measuring airway resistance in man using a body plethysmograph. J Clin Invest 1956; 35:327–335.
2. Aronsson H, Solymar L, Dempsey J, Bjure J, Olsson T, Bake B. A modified forced oscillation technique for measurements of respiratory resistance. J Appl Physiol 1977; 42(4):650–655.
3. Jackson AC, Milhorn HT, Norman JR. A reevaluation of the interrupter technique for airway resistance measurement. J Appl Physiol 1974; 36(2):264–268.
4. Mead J, Whittenberger JL. Physical properties of human lungs measured during spontaneous respiration. J Appl Physiol 1953; 5:779–787.
5. Pattle RE, Claireaux AE, Davis PA, Cameron AH. Inability to form a lung-lining film as a cause of the respiratory-distress syndrome in the newborn. Lancet 1962; 2:469.
6. Fairbairn AS, Fletcher CM, Tinker CM, Wood CH. A comparison of spirometric and peak expiratory flow measurements in men with and without chronic bronchitis. Thorax 1962; 17:168.
7. Woolcock AJ, Read J. Improvement in bronchial asthma not reflected in forced expiratory volume. Lancet 1965; 2:1323–1325.
8. Meisner P, Hugh-Jones P. Pulmonary function in bronchial asthma. Br Med J 1968; 1:470–475.

9. Colett PW, Brancatisano T, Engel LA. Changes in the glottic aperture during bronchial asthma. Am Rev Respir Dis 1983; 128:719–723.

10. Despas P, LeRoux M, Macklem PT. Site of airway obstruction in asthma as determined by measuring maximal expiratory flow breathing air and helium-oxygen mixture. J Clin Invest 1972; 51:3235–3243.

11. James AL, Paré PD, Hogg JC. The mechanics of airway narrowing in asthma. Am Rev Respir Dis 1989; 139:242–246.

12. Macklem PT. A hypothesis linking bronchial hyperreactivity and airway inflammation: implications for therapy. Ann Allergy 1990; 64:113–119.

13. Paré PD. Hyperplasia and hypertrophy of airway smooth muscle in asthma the cause of airway hyperresponsiveness? Eur Respir J 1993; 6(17):228.

14. Burney PGJ, Nield JE, Twort CHC, Chinn S, Jones TD, Mitchell WD, Bateman C, Cameron IR. Effect of changing dietary sodium on the airway response to histamine. Thorax 1989; 44:36–41.

15. Bianco S, Pieroni MG, Refini RM, Rottoli L, Sestini P. Protective effect of inhaled furosemide on allergen-induced early and late asthmatic reactions. N Engl J Med 1989; 321:1069–1073.

16. Högman M, Almirall J, Arnberg H, Hedenstierna G. Aerosol challenge in a rabbit asthma model. Eur Respir J 1993; 6(17):597.

17. Woolcock AJ, Salome CM, Yan K. The shape of the dose-response curve to histamine in asthmatic and normal subjects. Am Rev Respir Dis 1984; 130:71–75.

18. Woolcock AJ, Read J. The static elastic properties of the lungs in asthma. Am Rev Respir Dis 1968; 98:788–794.

19. Marshall R, Stone RW, Christie RV. The relationship of dyspnea to respiratory effort in normal subjects, mitral stenosis and emphysema. Clin Sci 1954; 13:625–631.

20. Cockcroft A, Adams L. Measurement and mechanism of breathlessness. Clin Respir Physiol 1986; 22:85–92.

21. Otis AB. The work of breathing. In: Fenn WO, Rahn H, eds. Handbook of Physiology. Section 3: Respiration. Vol I. Washington, DC: American Physiology Society, 1964:463.

22. Loring SH, Mead J, Griscom NT. Dependence of diaphragmatic length on lung volume and thoracoabdominal configuration. J Appl Physiol 1985; 59:1961–1970.

23. Begin P, Grassino A. Inspiratory muscle dysfunction and chronic hypercapnia in chronic obstructive pulmonary disease. Am Rev Respir Dis 1991; 143:905–912.

24. Mead J, Turner JM, Macklem PT, Little JB. Significance of the relationship between lung recoil and maximum expiratory flow. J Appl Physiol 1967; 22(1):95–108.

25. McFadden ER Jr. Asthma: airway dynamics, cardiac function and clinical correlates. In: Middleton E Jr, Reed CE, Ellis EF, eds. Allergy Principles and Practice, 2d ed, St. Louis: CV Mosby, 1983:843–862.

26. Falliers CJ. Acute effects of albuterol aerosol in reversible obstructive airway disease. Ann Allergy 1981; 47:387.

27. Clement J, Woestijne KP. Variability of maximum expiratory flow-volume curves and effort independency. J Appl Physiol 1971; 31(1):55–62.

28. Petit JM, Melon J, Milic-Emili J. Application pratique de la technique de l'interruption du courant aérien dans les tests de provocation. Int Arch Allergy Appl Immunol 1960; 16:141.

29. Milic-Emili J, Henderson JAM, Dolovich MB, Trop D, Kaneko K. Regional distribution of inspired gas in the lung. J Appl Physiol 1966; 21:749–759.

30. Engel LA, Grassino A, Anthonisen NR. Demonstration of airway closure in man. J Appl Physiol 1975; 38(6):1117–1125.

31. Burger EJ, Macklem P. Airway closure: demonstration by breathing 100% O_2 at low lung volumes and by N_2 washout. J Appl Physiol 1968; 25:139–148.

32. Leblanc P, Ruff F, Milic-Emili J. Effects of age and body position on "airway closure" in man. J Appl Physiol 1970; 28(4):448–451.

33. McCarthy DS, Spencere R, Greene R, Milic-Emili J. Measurement of "closing volume" as a simple and sensitive test for early detection of small airway disease. Am J Med 1972; 52:757–753.

34. Abboud RT, Morton JW. Comparisons of maximal mid-expiratory flow volume curves, and nitrogen closing volumes in patients with mild airway obstruction. Am Rev Respir Dis 1975; 111:405.

35. Prowse K, Cumming G. Effects of lung volume and disease on the lung nitrogen decay curve. J Appl Physiol 1973; 34(1):23–33.

36. Martin CJ, Tsunoda S, Young AC. Lung emptying patterns in diffuse obstructive pulmonary syndromes. Respir Physiol 1974; 21:157–168.

37. Buist AS, Ross BB. Quantitative analysis of the alveolar plateau in the diagnosis of early airway obstruction. Am Rev Respir Dis 1973; 108:1078–1087.

38. Hedenström H, Malmberg P. Optimal combinations of lung function tests in the detection of various types of early lung disease. Eur J Respir Dis 1987; 71:273–285.

39. Siegler D, Fukuchi Y, Engel L. Influence of bronchomotor tone on ventilation distribution and airway closure in asymptomatic asthma. Am Rev Respir Dis 1976; 114:123.

40. Niu Shan-fu, Sixt R, Bake B. Non-uniform lung elastic properties and the slope of the alveolar plateau. Bull Eur Physiopathol Respir 1987; 23:163–169.

41. Neufeld GR, Schwardt JD, Gobran SR, Baumgardner JE, Schreiner MS, Aukburg SJ, Scherer PW. Modelling steady state pulmonary elimination of He, SF_6 and CO_2: effect of morphometry. Respir Physiol 1992; 88:257–275.

42. Arborelius M, Ekvall B, Jernérus R, Lundin G, Svanberg L. Unilateral provoked bronchial asthma in man. J Clin Invest 1962; 41:1236.

43. Williams MH, Zohman LR. Cardiopulmonary function in bronchial asthma: a comparison with chronic pulmonary emphysema. Am Rev Respir Dis 1960; 81:173.

44. Novey HS, Wilson AF, Surprenant EL, Bennett LR. Early ventilation-perfusion changes in asthma. J Allergy 1979; 46:221–230.

45. Mishkin F, Wagner HN. Regional abnormalities in pulmonary arterial blood flow during asthmatic attacks. Radiology 1967; 88:142–144.

46. West JB. Ventilation-perfusion relationships. Am Rev Respir Dis 1977; 116:919–943.

47. McFadden ER, Lyons HA. Arterial blood gas tensions in asthma. N Engl J Med 1968; 278:1027–1032.
48. Benatar SR. Fatal asthma. N Engl J Med 1986; 314(7):423–429.
49. Palmer KNV, Diament ML. Dynamic and static lung volumes and blood-gas tensions in bronchial asthma. Lancet 1969; 1:591–593.
50. Riley RL, Cournand A. "Ideal" alveolar air and the analysis of ventilation-perfusion relationships in the lungs. J Appl Physiol 1949; 1:825–847.
51. Field GB. The effects of posture, oxygen, isoproterenol and atropine on ventilation-perfusion relationships in the lung in asthma. Clin Sci 1967; 32:279–288.
52. Palmer KNV, Diament ML. Effect of aerosol isoprenaline on blood-gas tensions in severe bronchial asthma. Lancet 1967; 2:1532–1533.
53. Ballester E, Reyes A, Roca J, Guitart R, Wagner PD, Rodriguez-Roisin R. Ventilation-perfusion mismatching in acute severe asthma: effects of salbutamol and 100% oxygen. Thorax 1989; 44:258–267.
54. Valabhji P. Gas exchange in the acute and asymptomatic phases of asthma breathing air and oxygen. Clin Sci 1968; 34:431–440.
55. Fahri LE. Elimination of inert gas by the lung. Respir Physiol 1967; 3:1–11.
56. Wagner PD, Saltzman HA, West JB. Measurement of continuous distribution of ventilation-perfusion ratios: theory. J Appl Physiol 1974; 36(5):588–599.
57. West JB, Wagner PD. Ventilation-perfusion relationships. In: Crystal RG, West JB, eds. The Lung, Scientific Foundations. New York: Raven Press, 1991:1289–1305.
58. Rubinfeld AR, Wagner PD, West JB. Gas exchange during experimental canine asthma. Am Rev Respir Dis 1978; 118:525–536.
59. Wagner PD, Dantzker DR, Iacovoni VE, Tomlin WC, West JB. Ventilation-perfusion inequality in asymptomatic asthma. Am Rev Respir Dis 1978; 118:511–524.
60. Roca J, Ramis LI, Rodriguez-Roisin R, Ballester E, Montserrat JM, Wagner PD. Serial relationships between ventilation-perfusion inequality and spirometry in acute severe asthma requiring hospitalization. Am Rev Respir Dis 1988; 137:1055–1061.
61. Macklin CC. Pulmonic alveolar vents. J Anat 1935; 69:188–193.
62. Martin HB. Respiratory bronchioles as the pathway for collateral ventilation. J Appl Physiol 1966; 21:1443–1447.
63. Van Allen CM, Lindskog GE, Richter HG. Collateral respiration: transfer of air collaterally between pulmonary lobules. J Clin Invest 1931; 10:559–590.
64. Kubo S, Tomioka S, Kapitan K, Wagner PD. Effects of methacholine (MCH) inflation on pulmonary gas exchange in pigs. Fed Proc 1985; 44(5):1383.
65. Sylvester JT, Menkes HA, Stitik F. Lung volumes and interdependence in the pig. J Appl Physiol 1975; 38:395–401.
66. Lee Li-Na, Ueno O, Wagner PD, West JB. Pulmonary gas exchange after multiple airway occlusion by beads in the dog. Am Rev Respir Dis 1989; 140:1216–1221.
67. Lagerstrand L, Hedenstierna G. Gas-exchange impairment: its correlation to lung mechanics in acute airway obstruction (studies on a rabbit asthma model). Clin Physiol 1990; 10:363–380.
68. Lagerstrand L, Dahlbäck M, Hedenstierna G. Gas exchange during simulated airway secretion in the anaesthetized rabbit. Eur Respir J 1992; 5:1215–1222.

69. Wagner PD, Hedenstierna G, Bylin G. Ventilation-perfusion inequality in chronic asthma. Am Rev Respir Dis 1987; 136:605–612.

70. Lagerstrand L, Larsson K, Ihre E, Zetterström O, Hedenstierna G. Pulmonary gas exchange response following allergen challenge in patients with allergic asthma. Eur Respir J 1992; 5:1176–1183.

71. Wagner PD, Ramsdell JW, Incavdo GA, Rubinfeldt AR, Young IH. Gas exchange following bronchial challenge with antigen in patients with extrinsic asthma. Am Rev Respir Dis 1978; 117(Suppl):409.

72. McNeill RS, Nairn JR, Millar JS, Ingram CG. Exercise-induced asthma. Q J Med 1966; 35:55–67.

73. Irnell L, Swartling S. Maximal expiratory flow at rest and during muscular work in patients with bronchial asthma. Scand J Respir Dis 1966; 47:103–113.

74. Young IH, Corte P, Schoeffel RE. Pattern and time course of ventilation-perfusion inequality in exercise-induced asthma. Am Rev Respir Dis 1982; 125:304–311.

75. Engström I. Respiratory studies in children. XI. Mechanics of breathing, lung volumes and ventilatory capacity in asthmatic children from attack to symptomfree status. Acta Paediatr Scand 1964; (Suppl):155.

76. Graff-Lonnevig V, Bevegård S, Eriksson BO. Ventilation and pulmonary gas exchange at rest and during exercise in boys with bronchial asthma. J Respir Dis 1980; 61:357–366.

77. Ledbetter MK, Bruck E, Fahri LE. Perfusion of the underventilated compartment of the lungs in asthmatic children. J Clin Invest 1964; 43:2233–2240.

78. Freyschuss U, Hedlin G, Hedenstierna G. Ventilation-perfusion relationships during exercise-induced asthma in children. Am Rev Respir Dis 1984; 130:888– 894.

79. Hedlin G, Freyschuss U, Hedenstierna G. Histamine induced asthma in children: effects on the ventilatin-perfusion relationships. Clin Physiol 1985; 5:19–34.

80. Dueck R, Wagner PD, West JB. Effects of positive end-expiratory pressure on gas exchange in dogs with normal and edmatous lungs. Anesthesiology 1977; 47:359.

81. Hedenstierna G, White FC, Mazzone R, Wagner PD. Redistribution of pulmonary blood flow in the dog with PEEP ventilation. J Appl Physiol 1979; 46:278–287.

82. Lagerstand L, Bylin G, Hedenstierna G, Wagner PD. Relationships among gas exchange spirometry and symptoms in asthma. Eur J Med 1992; 1(3):145–152.

83. Tai E, Read J. Response of blood gas tensions to aminophylline and isopenalin in patients with asthma. Thorax 1967; 22:543–550.

84. Rodriguez-Roisin R, Bencowitz HZ, Ziegler MG, Wagner PD. Gas exchange response to bronchodilators following methacholine challenge in dogs. Am Rev Respir Dis 1984; 130:617–626.

85. Green M, Mead J, Turner JM. Variability of maximum expiratory flow volume curves. J Appl Physiol 1974; 37:67–74.

86. Man P, Zamel N. Genetic influence on normal variability of maximum expiratory flow-volume curves. J Appl Physiol 1976; 41(6):874–877.

87. Redline S, Tishler PV, Lewitter FI, Tager IB, Munoz A, Speizer FE. Assessment of genetic and nongenetic influences on pulmonary function. Am Rev Respir Dis 1987; 135:217–222.

88. Hopp RJ, Bewtra AK, Watt GD, Nair NM, Townley RG. Genetic analysis of allergic disease in twins. J Allergy Clin Immunol 1984; 73:265–270.

89. Falliers CJ, de A Cardoso RR, Bane HN, Coffey R, Middleton E Jr. Discordant allergic manifestations in monozygotic twins: genetic identity versus clinical, physiologic and biochemical differences. J Allergy 1971; 47:207–219.
90. Townley RG, Bewtra AK, Nair NM, Brodkey FD, Watt GD, Burke KM. Methacholine inhalation challenge studies. J Allergy Clin Immunol 1979; 64(2):569–574.
91. Longo G, Strinati R, Poli F, Fumi F. Genetic factors in nonspecific bronchial hyperreactivity. Am J Dis Child 1989; 141:331–334.
92. Bruderman I, Cohen R, Schachor J, Horowitz I. Bronchial response to methacholine in parents of asthmatic children. Chest 1987; 91(2):210–213.
93. Higgins M, Keller J. Familial occurrence of chronic respiratory disease and familial resemblance in ventilatory capacity. J Chronic Dis 1975; 28:239–251.
94. Konig P, Godfrey S. Exercise-induced bronchial lability in monozygotic (identical) and dizygotic (nonidentical) twins. J Allergy Clin Immunol 1974; 54:280–287.

13

Bronchial Hyperresponsiveness and Regulation of Total Serum IgE Levels

Eugene R. Bleecker

University of Maryland School of Medicine
Baltimore, Maryland

Deborah A. Meyers

Center for Medical Genetics
Johns Hopkins University School of Medicine
Baltimore, Maryland

I. INTRODUCTION

Asthma, an episodic obstructive pulmonary disease, is thought to be initiated by genetic factors that interact with environmental or other exposures to produce the clinical manifestations of this disorder. Susceptibility to this complex genetic disorder is not inherited in a simple Mendelian fashion since more than one gene appears to be involved in the development of asthma. Clinical expression of this disorder is clearly influenced by environmental exposure to allergens, air pollutants (cigarette smoke, ozone, etc.), and infectious agents (viruses). Because of the recent worldwide increase in the prevalence and severity of asthma (1), its etiology and pathophysiology are under intensive study. Thus, the investigation of the underlying genetic mechanisms that are responsible for susceptibility to asthma as well as to closely associated phenotypes such as bronchial hyperresponsiveness and allergic responses that include elevated total serum IgE levels will improve our understanding of the factors that lead to the development and progression of this disorder. This approach will ultimately lead to improved therapies and new methods for disease identification (2).

One of the principal obstacles to studying the genetics of asthma is the lack of a uniform definition of this disorder that includes the following clinical spectrum found in asthma: symptomatic asthma as well as mild or intermittent asthma and the early or presymptomatic stages of disease development in susceptible individuals (3,4). Characterization of intermediate phenotypes that either precede or represent risk factors for the development of asthma is another useful approach for genetic studies of this disease (2,5). For bronchial hyperresponsiveness this approach permits inclusion potentially of a larger group of individuals who may have the genetic predisposition but have not fully developed all of the clinical findings found in asthma (2). An additional compounding issue related to the definition of the asthma phenotype is that there is considerable heterogeneity in the presentation of this disease. There may be differences in the genetic factors that are responsible for susceptibility to asthma in a young child with clear allergic triggers when compared to an older patient with a history of cigarette smoking and a syndrome best characterized as chronic obstructive pulmonary disease (COPD) with "asthmatic" bronchitis (6). These issues have been recognized and, in fact, led to the development of the "Dutch hypothesis," which emphasizes the similarities between asthma and COPD as well as the important role of allergy and bronchial inflammation in their development (7,8). Important national and international differences in the definition of asthma must be recognized in the design and interpretation of genetic studies in this complex disease.

In addition, the definition of asthma has changed dramatically throughout the years (9–13). Recently, inflammation has become the central feature of most definitions of asthma; however, there is no readily available validated marker of airways inflammation that can be used to differentiate asthma from closely related conditions such as allergic rhinitis (12). Furthermore, clinical asthma can be a variable disease process over time; childhood asthma may appear to resolve only to develop later in life (14,15). In older individuals, asthma may be accompanied by a fixed or irreversible airflow obstruction (16–20). These patients often present with a history of cigarette smoking and episodic wheezing especially associated with infectious triggers. Asthma severity may be altered by medications and may be worsened by exposure to environmental stimuli. Studies in asthmatics at specific time points may show variability of some in the physiological markers depending on disease activity and current therapy. The level of bronchial hyperresponsiveness may change

TABLE 1 Potential Phenotypes in Allergy and Asthma

Allergic parameters
   Total serum IgE
   Specific IgE levels
   Specific allergen skin tests
Bronchial hyperresponsiveness
Asthma
   Prior physician diagnosis
   Asthma symptoms
   Assessments of asthma severity
Pulmonary function test results
   Assessment of airflow obstruction
   Bronchodilator reversibility
   Peak expiratory flow rates
Analysis of interrelationship of allergic and asthmatic phenotypes

depending on exposure to environmental triggers and the effects of therapeutic interventions (21–23). Thus, there is a wide spectrum of specific phenotypic manifestations among individuals with asthma. Potential phenotypes associated with asthma and allergy that can be used in genetic studies are listed in Table 1.

II. BRONCHIAL HYPERRESPONSIVENESS

Because of the complexity in developing a uniform definition of asthma, investigators have begun to study individual physiological characteristics that are closely associated with the development and progression of asthma, such as bronchial hyperresponsiveness (BHR) and elevated total serum IgE levels, both components of the asthma phenotype that can be objectively measured. BHR is the most common physiological abnormality associated with bronchial asthma (24–27). While this increased bronchoconstrictor response to a variety of immunological, biochemical, and physical agents is found in virtually all individuals with asthma, many patients with other obstructive airways disease, such as COPD or cystic fibrosis, also have BHR (28–30). In addition, there are individuals with BHR who are asymptomatic or allergic but do not have a history of asthma symptoms (27,31–35). Thus, this response is a sensitive physiological measure that is not always specific for asthma. It is a useful parameter to study because airways responsiveness is an objective measurement that can be readily measured using pharmacological, physical, or allergen challenge methods (28,36).

A. Mechanism of BHR

The mechanisms responsible for BHR in asthma include genetic predisposition and the effects of environmental exposures to inflammatory stimuli in the airways of susceptible individuals (5,28,29). BHR is a trait that can be measured objectively either as a qualitative (positive or negative) or as a quantitative [slope, provocative dose (PD), or provocative concentration (PC)] measure in most individuals (37–42). The advantage of this latter approach is that phenotypic information is then available on the majority of individuals within a family or population. The limitation inherent in the use of BHR as a marker for asthma is that it is found in other conditions and, therefore, may not always reflect genetic susceptibility to asthma. It is important to note that there are several different methods for assessing BHR that may produce different results. Responses to methacholine and histamine tend to be similar (36,43), but responses to exercise and inhalation challenge with allergic stimuli may be less sensitive (36,44). Possibly, the results from adenosine challenge may be more specific for asthma and related to disease severity (45,46). Also, the use of physical stimuli that include exercise, hyperventilation with cold air, or inhalation of hypo- or hypertonic solutions should be considered.

Several factors are related to BHR in asthma. These include geometrical factors related to airway caliber, the role of autonomic neural pathways, and the degree of bronchial inflammation (12,28,47). There are important links between markers of inflammation and BHR in asthma based on studies using investigative bronchoscopic techniques to demonstrate migration or activation of inflammatory cellular elements in the airways under baseline conditions (48,49) or after allergen exposure in allergic asthmatics (50,51). Allergen exposure in sensitive asthmatics is a well-recognized mechanism that leads to increases in BHR (21,52). Release of biochemical mediators that include mast cell products or regulatory cytokines by inflammatory cells in the airways could provide a local mechanism to amplify or modulate inflammatory responses in the airways (53–56). Significant elevations of certain cytokines have been shown in bronchoalveolar lavage of airways (TNF, GM-CSF, IL-1, IL-2, IL-3, IL-5, and IL-6) of asthmatics (57–62). Other studies have evaluated mucosal biopsies obtained from patients with asthma demonstrating accumulation of inflammatory cells including eosinophils, lymphocytes, and mast cells (55,56,63,64). Immunohistochemical studies have identified evidence of cytokine activation and migration of inflammatory cells into the airways (65). It is likely that these inflammatory responses and mediators are central to the pathogenesis of the inflammation underlying bronchial hyperresponsiveness and asthma.

B. Assessment of Bronchial Responsiveness and Bronchial Inflammation

A wide variety of approaches are available to assess responsiveness to immunological and nonimmunological stimuli (Table 2). As stated previously, the presence and degree of airways hyperresponsiveness is thought to reflect bronchial inflammation in asthma (21,23,25,66–68). The usual methods available to assess bronchial inflammation include the use of investigative bronchoscopy, which provides the ability to examine fluids, cells, and tissue from patients with obstructive airways disease to investigate morphological, biochemical, immunological, and pharmacological function (69,70). Unfortunately, these approaches are far too invasive to use routinely in assessing inflammation in asthma. While this approach may not be feasible, examination of induced sputum may provide a useful noninvasive method to evaluate inflammatory abnormalities in the airways (70). While this method has been described as relatively noninvasive, bronchodilators are usually required prior to sputum induction with hypo- or hypertonic solutions to prevent bronchospasm in asthmatics. In addition, further studies are required to determine whether analysis of induced sputum provides a reliable marker of inflammation that can be used to differentiate the changes found in asthmatic and allergic bronchial inflammation from the sputum of unaffected individuals.

As there are no validated methods to assess bronchial inflammation that can be used on large populations, the use of inhalation challenge testing provides a substitute that may not only indirectly reflect inflammatory changes in the airways but also provides an objective method to assess airways liability in asthma. This is important since bronchodilator reversibility may not be found in asthmatics with normal pulmonary function periods who are not experiencing asthma symptoms. A large number of stimuli can be used to assess bronchial responsiveness (Table 2). In brief, inhalation challenges with methacholine and histamine are the usual techniques in many epidemiological and population-based studies (24,33,40–42). The results of methacholine and histamine bronchial challenges correlate closely (36). However, bronchial challenge with exercise, isocapneic by hyperventilation, or osmotic solutions, may not be positive in all subjects with asthma (71). Recently, challenge with adenosine has been proposed as a sensitive method to assess BHR in asthma that also reflects asthma severity (45,46).

In a specific study, the techniques and methods should be standardized and comparable to accepted protocols for assessing BHR (37,38,40). If a new method is employed, it should be compared to one of the standard protocols. There appears to be little difference in the results of challenges that employ dosimeter or use a tidal breathing method to administer the inhaled agent (36, 38). Short protocols for bronchial challenge may be used since they permit

TABLE 2 Evaluation of Respiratory Function and Bronchial Inflammation in Obstructive Airways Disease

I. Bronchial responsiveness testing
   A. Nonimmunological stimuli
      1. Direct methods
         a. Common inhalation challenge tests
            Methacholine/histamine
         b. Less common inhalation challenge tests
            Prostaglandin D_2, leukotriene D_4
      2. Indirect methods
         a. Common inhalation challenge tests
            Exercise challenge/isocapneic hyperventilation
            Osmotic challenge (hypo- or hypertonic solutions)
            Adenosine
          b. Less common inhalation challenge tests
            Diuretics (furosemide)
            SO_2 exercise challenge
   B. Immunological stimuli
      1. Immediate responses to specific allergen challenge in allergic subjects
      2. Assessment of late-phase responses (1–72 hr) after allergen challenge (airways function and/or bronchial responsiveness to nonimmunological stimuli)
II. Physiological testing
   A. Pulmonary function testing
      1. Spirometry and expiratory flow rates
      2. Bronchodilator response
      3. Airways resistance
   B. Specialized techniques
      Direct measurement of peripheral lung function measurements (bronchoscopy)
III. Investigative bronchoscopy
   A. Bronchial biopsy (morphological and immunohistochemistry studies)
   B. Bronchoalveolar lavage techniques
      1. Cell numbers and differential counts
      2. Inflammatory mediator levels
      3. "In vitro" cell function
      4. Responses to segmental airway challenge (allergen)
IV. Induced sputum studies
   A. Cell differential counts
   B. Inflammatory mediator level

more rapid data acquisition and allow studies to be performed outside the clinical laboratory (72). Some of the short methods may not provide dose-response information but the slope of the stimulus response curve can still be calculated. Usually, the results are expressed as either the PD or PC of the agonist that produces a specific fall in FEV_1 (10%, 15%, or 20%). The slope of the curve can be calculated in subjects who do not achieve a threshold decrease in FEV_1 providing information on bronchial responsiveness in a larger proportion of a study population (14). The major contraindication to inhalation challenge is the degree of airway obstruction. Usually a lower limit of between 60 and 70% predicted FEV_1 is employed by many investigators. However, studies have been performed safely in asthmatic subjects with FEV_1 $\leq 60\%$ predicted (73). If patients with more severe airways obstruction are studied, bronchial reactivity testing may need to be performed in a monitored laboratory setting rather than under nonmedical settings such as at home or at school. Similar methods are available for bronchial reactivity testing in children. A lower age limit of 4–6 years may exist because of inability of younger children to perform spirometry accurately and reproducibly.

C. Relationship of BHR to the Asthma Phenotype

The level of BHR to histamine and cholinergic agonists in asthma correlates with the presence of asthmatic symptoms and the response to treatment (25,26, 35,74,75). High IgE levels are closely correlated with BHR, which may reflect the presence of airway inflammation (76,77). It is well known that corticosteroids, when administered to atopic asthmatics, provide symptomatic relief and reduce the late-phase inflammatory response as well as BHR (78,79). Glucocorticoids have been shown to inhibit the production of IL-1, IL-2, IL-3, TNF, GM-CSF, and other cytokines (80). Also, a significant correlation has been found between numbers of bronchial mucosal cells expressing certain cytokines (GM-CSF) and the level of BHR in asthmatics (60). This suggests that the production of mediators in the bronchial mucosa of symptomatic asthmatic subjects has clinical relevance and may be related to the presence of BHR and asthma.

III. GENETICS OF BHR

There is evidence of heritability of BHR although it has been difficult to develop a specific model of inheritance. Hopp and co-workers have reported an increased incidence of BHR in monozygotic twins when compared to dizygotic twins (81). These same investigators also found that children with BHR, when followed longitudinally (82), have an increased risk of developing asthmatic symptoms, again demonstrating the usefulness of studying BHR in genetic studies. In their segregation analysis of airways responsiveness to methacholine, they were not able to find evidence for a major gene by testing various one-locus models (83). However, such results should not be considered evidence that genetic factors are not important. It is likely that genes at multiple loci are involved and a single-locus model may be a poor approximation to the actual genetic model (84). Also, it is difficult to include the effects of the environment in such models although it is clear that there is a major environmental component that interacts with genetic susceptibility to BHR. Hopefully, further studies will provide insight into the genetic regulation of this response and into the significant epidemiological relationship between total serum IgE levels and BHR (76,77).

IV. GENETICS OF TOTAL SERUM IgE LEVELS

There is strong evidence for an association between total serum IgE levels and BHR (76,77,85,86). Children with elevated IgE levels have an increased risk of developing increased bronchial responsiveness and asthma even when other allergic factors are controlled (87). Approximately 30% of the variance in bronchial responsiveness is explained by an individual's total serum IgE level (76,77). These data suggest that total serum IgE levels and BHR, both important clinical determinants for asthma, may share similar genetic regulatory mechanisms. Thus, investigation of the genetics of asthma must include studies of inheritance of BHR and IgE responses.

The number of genes and modes of inheritances for the regulation of total IgE production are not fully known although there have been significant advances in recent years. Previous segregation analyses of total serum IgE levels provided evidence for a major gene although there were differences in the estimates of the gene frequency and degree of dominance (88–94). In a recent large study of 291 families, Martinez et al. (95) found evidence for codominant inheritance that suggests the presence of three overlapping distributions for total serum IgE levels.

In a recent study of 92 Dutch families ascertained through a parent with clinical asthma who was originally studied approximately 25 years earlier, additional evidence for recessive inheritance of high levels was obtained (96). The estimates of the mean levels for the "low" and "high" phenotypes in this study appear clinically meaningful (38 IU and 437 IU, respectively). Since, in the codominant model, an additional distribution is estimated, similar results to the recessive model were obtained but they were not significantly better. It is important to note that evidence for codominant inheritance in one study and recessive inheritance in another study does not represent conflicting results, but rather reflects the inability to distinguish between two or three underlying distributions that display substantial overlap. As with segregation studies of BHR, there is the problem of trying to approximate multilocus inheritance by a single-locus model. In addition, in the study of the Dutch families, there was a significant residual component, which suggests the presence of additional genes and environmental factors. Further analyses provided evidence for two major loci regulating total serum IgE levels, both inherited in a recessive manner (97).

V. CHROMOSOME 5Q

There are multiple known candidate genes on 5q that regulate IgE production either directly or indirectly and affect the activation and proliferation of cells involved in inflammatory processes associated with BHR, allergy, and asthma. These genes include IL-3, IL-4, IL-5, IL-9, IL-12, IL-13, granulocyte-macrophage colony-stimulating factor (GM-CSF), a receptor for macrophage colony-stimulating factor (CSF-1R), fibroblast growth factor acidic (FGFA), and interferon regulatory factor 1 (IRF1) (98). In addition, there is a β-adrenergic receptor (ADRB2) and a lymphocyte-specific glucocorticoid receptor (GRL1) in this region. The genes for IL-4-related cytokines stimulate B-cell growth and regulate specific immunoglobulin synthesis (99,100). IL-9 and IL-13 enhance IL-4-dependent immunoglobulin synthesis and expression of CD23, an IgE surface binding factor, respectively. GM-CSF, as well as other cellular growth factors such as FGFA, map to chromosome 5q and these factors stimulate proliferation of granulocytes, macrophages, and eosinophils. Thus, this region of 5q contains genes that regulate a large number of factors that are important in the inflammatory processes in asthma as well as in airways hyperresponsiveness and the regulation of serum IgE.

A. Linkage of a Locus Regulating Serum IgE Levels to Chromosome 5q

Linkage studies using DNA markers on 5q have been performed to test for evidence of a major gene for total serum IgE levels or susceptibility to BHR mapping to this region. In the Dutch families ascertained through a parent with asthma 25 years previously, genotyping for highly polymorphic markers on 5q was performed on the first 55 families with DNA available (96). Two methods were used to test for linkage for total serum IgE levels, the sib-pair method and the lod score method using the genetic model obtained from segregation analysis. Genetic analysis showed significant results for marker D5S436 for sib-pair and lod score analysis (Fig. 1). The lod value of 3.56 correlates with greater than 1000:1 odds for linkage of IgE to this chromosomal region. However, from these results, it is not possible to specify one gene candidate within this large region containing multiple candidate genes. In fact, multiple

Chromosome 5q[3']

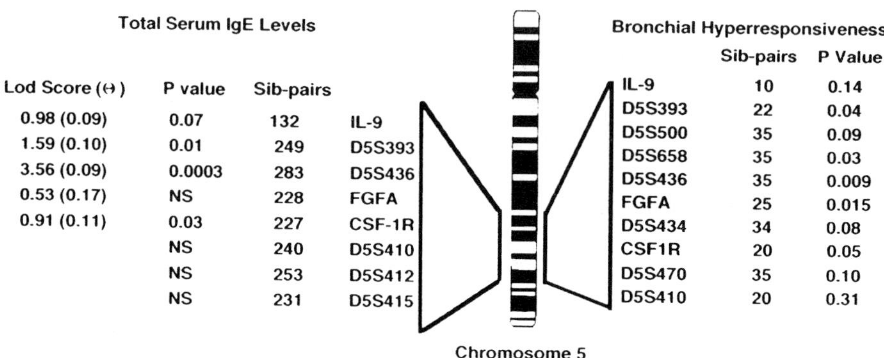

FIGURE 1   Results from linkage analysis for total serum IgE levels and BHR to 5q. For total serum IgE levels, the lod scores and estimated degree of recombination are shown. In addition, the *p* values and number of sib pairs are included for the markers listed on the chromosome. For BHR, the number of sib pairs who are both hyperresponsive and the *p* values are shown.

candidates may well be involved. Marsh and co-workers studied an inbred population and found evidence for a locus regulating total serum IgE production mapping to 5q (101). Doull and co-workers have reported a significant association with the 118 allele at the IL9 locus on chromosome 5q in 131 families selected randomly without regard to allergy and asthma (102).

Xu and co-workers reexamined the IgE linkage in the Dutch cohort using a two-locus segregation and linkage analysis (97). They found that the first locus on chromosome 5q accounted for 50.6% of the variation in the total serum IgE level while a second, unlinked locus explained another 19% of the variation in the Dutch asthma families. Together these two loci accounted for 78.4% of the variation in total serum IgE levels that was observed in these families. These values may overestimate the importance of these loci in the general population since these families were recruited based on a proband with asthma. Further studies are underway to determine the chromosomal location of this second locus.

Since it is reasonable to assume that multiple genes are important in determining susceptibility to asthma or allergy, evidence of linkage may not be seen in all populations. Recently Blumenthal and co-workers (103) studied four large pedigrees originally ascertained for multiple members with atopy. In these families, they were unable to find linkage to 5q. Possibly in these large pedigrees with many atopic members, genes at other loci are more important than those on 5q.

B. Linkage of a Susceptibility Locus for BHR to Chromosome 5q

To further explore the relationship between BHR and IgE levels, the hypothesis that a susceptibility gene for BHR would map to the same chromosomal region as a locus that regulates total serum IgE on chromosome 5q was tested. In the Dutch families previously described, bronchial responsiveness to inhaled histamine was tested in the family members using the method of DeVries et al. (104) that was used for the initial assessment of the probands approximately 25 years ago. The bronchial reactivity testing protocol consists of having each subject inhale increasing concentrations of histamine for 30 sec of tidal breathing starting with a diluent control and continuing until the FEV_1 falls by >20% or the highest concentration of histamine (32 mg/ml) is reached. The raw data were used to calculate the PC of histamine that produced a 20% fall in FEV_1 ($PC_{20}FEV_1$) by extrapolation from the dose-response curve. This value was used for analysis of BHR as a quantitative trait. For analysis of BHR as a qualitative trait, individuals were considered to have BHR if they had a ≥20% decrease in FEV1 at <32 mg/ml histamine.

Serum total IgE levels were strongly correlated ($r = 0.65, p < 0.01$) in pairs of siblings concordant for BHR, suggesting that these traits are coinherited (73). However, there was no significant association ($r = 0.04, p > 0.10$) between PC_{20} values in pairs of siblings concordant for elevated serum total IgE levels. This implies that serum total IgE levels can be influenced by other genetic and environmental factors that may not be common to the development of BHR.

Linkage analyses were performed by estimating the proportion of alleles shared by descent between siblings with BHR, an established approach for the investigation of the genetic basis of complex traits, such as asthma. In contrast to lod score methods, the model of inheritance does not need to be specified. Analysis of affected pairs of siblings demonstrated statistically significant evidence of linkage between BHR and D5S436, D5S658, and several other markers located nearby on chromosome 5q31–q33 (Fig. 1) (73). These data strongly support the hypothesis that one or more genes on chromosome 5q31–q33 determine susceptibility to BHR and regulation of total serum IgE levels.

BHR was also analyzed as a quantitative trait using a regressive approach to identify the relationship between siblings for PC_{20} values and the proportion of marker alleles shared from each parent. For BHR as a quantitative measure and the marker D5S436, the *p* value was highly significant (0.0002). There was still evidence for increased sharing of alleles when total serum IgE levels were included as a covariate ($p < 0.002$). This suggests that evidence for linkage of susceptibility of BHR to 5q is not due to the relationship observed in epidemiological studies between BHR and total serum IgE levels. These results can be interpreted as suggesting that there are multiple genes on 5q important in determining an individual's susceptibility to developing asthma. These data represent an important step toward understanding the interrelationship between allergy (IgE) and BHR.

Specific localization of the postulated genes will be difficult to determine since the allergic and asthmatic phenotypes are closely related and the candidate loci are linked to each other. Future studies will include fine mapping of this region of chromosome 5q31–33 and the examination of known gene candidates on 5q for genetic mutations that determine the biological variability observed in total IgE and bronchial responsiveness. The combination of fine-linkage mapping, physical mapping, and candidate gene analyses should optimize the likelihood for success in identifying the genes important in determining susceptibility to asthma.

Linkages to other chromosomal regions for the BHR have not yet been identified. Clearly, neither BHR nor asthma is inherited in a simple Mendelian fashion and multiple genes are very likely. Currently several groups of investigators are performing genome-wide search to detect additional regions with susceptibility loci.

VI. SUMMARY

The use of associated or subphenotypes is an important strategy for dissecting the complex genetic factors responsible for asthma (84). Thus, studies that explore the genetic basis of susceptibility to BHR and regulation of total serum IgE levels are important in understanding basic physiological processes that lead to the development and progression of asthma. Hopefully, this will eventually lead to more effective therapeutic interventions.

REFERENCES

1. Gergen PJ, Weiss KB. The increasing problem of asthma in the United States. Am Rev Respir Dis 1992; 146:823–824.
2. Meyers DA, Bleecker ER. Approaches to mapping genes for allergy and asthma. Am J Respir Crit Care Med 1995; 152:411–413.
3. Rijcken B, Schouten JHA, Rosner B, Weiss ST. Is it useful to distinguish between asthma and COPD in respiratory epidemiology? Am Rev Respir Dis 1991; 143: 1456–1457.
4. Hughes D. Precise diagnosis of airflow obstruction—does it matter for treatment? SEPCR workshop, Wiesbaden 1989. Eur Respir J 1990; 3:1078–1097.

5. O'Connor GT, Sparrow D, Weiss ST. The role of allergy and nonspecific airway hyperresponsiveness in the pathogenesis of chronic obstructive pulmonary disease. (State of the art). Am Rev Respir Dis 1989; 140:225–252.

6. Braman SS, Kaemerlen JT, Davis SM. Asthma in the elderly: a comparison between patients with recently acquired and long-standing disease. Am Rev Respir Dis 1991; 143:336–340.

7. Orie NGM, Sluiter HJ, de Vries K, Tammeling GJ, Witkop J. The host factor in bronchitis. In: Orie NGM, Sluiter HJ, eds. Bronchitis. Assen, The Netherlands: Roya van Gorcum, 1961:43–59.

8. Sluiter HJ, Koöter GH, de Monchy JGR, Postma DS, de Vries K, Orie NGM. The Dutch hypothesis (chronic non-specific lung disease) revisited. Eur Respir J 1991; 4:479–489.

9. Ciba Guest Symposium: Terminology, definitions, and classification of chronic pulmonary emphysema and related conditions. Thorax 1959; 14:286–299.

10. American Thoracic Society: Definitions and classification of chronic bronchitis, asthma, and pulmonary emphysema. Am Rev Respir Dis 1962; 85:762–768.

11. Medical Research Council: Definition and classification of chronic bronchitis: for clinical and epidemiological purposes. Lancet 1965; 1:775–779.

12. Sheffer AL, Bailey WC, Bleecker ER, Busse WW, Ellis E, Evans D, Fanta CH, Janson-Bjerklie S, Malveaux FJ, Murphy SA, Nelson HS, Shapiro G. Guidelines for the diagnosis and management of asthma. J Allergy Clin Immunol 1991; 88: 425–534.

13. International Consensus Report on Diagnosis and Treatment of Asthma. National Heart, Lung, and Blood Institute, Publication No. 92-3091, 1992.

14. Peat JK, Salome C, Berry G, Woolcock AJ. Relation of dose-response slope to respiratory symptoms in a population of Australian schoolchildren. Am Rev Respir Dis 1991; 144:663–667.

15. Sporik R, Holgate ST, Cogswell JJ. Natural history of asthma in childhood—a birth cohort study. Arch Dis Child 1991; 66:1050–1053.

16. Peat JK, Woolcock AJ, Cullen K. Rate of decline of lung function in subjects with asthma. Eur J Respir Dis 1987; 70:171–179.

17. Sparrow D, O'Connor GT, Rosner B, Segal MR, Weiss ST. The influence of age and level of pulmonary function on nonspecific airway responsiveness: the normative aging study. Am Rev Respir Dis 1991; 143:978–982.

18. Martin AJ, Landau LI, Phelan PD. Lung function in young adults who had asthma in childhood. Am Rev Respir Dis 1980; 122:609–616.

19. Kelly WJW, Hudson I, Phelan PD, Pain MCF, Olinsky A. Childhood asthma in adult life: a further study at 28 years of age. Br Med J 1987; 294:1059–1062.

20. Welty C, Weiss ST, Tager IB, et al. The relationship of airways responsiveness to cold air, cigarette smoking, and atopy to respiratory symptoms and pulmonary function sin adults. Am Rev Respir Dis 1984; 130:198–203.

21. Cartier A, Thomson NC, Frith PA, Roberts RS, Hargreave FE. Allergen-induced increase in bronchial responsiveness to histamine: relationship to the late asthmatic response and change in airway caliber. J Allergy Clin Immunol 1982; 70: 170–177.

22. Hopp RJ, Bewtra A, Nair NM, Townley RG. The effect of age on methacholine response. J Allergy Clin Immunol 1985; 76:609–613.
23. Platts-Mills TAE, Mitchell EB, Nock P, Tovey ER, Moszoro H, Wilkins SR. Reduction of bronchial hyperreactivity during prolonged allergen avoidance. Lancet 1982; 2:675–677.
24. Rijcken B, Schouten JP, Weiss ST, Meinesz AF, de Vries K, van der Lende R. The distribution of bronchial responsiveness to histamine in symptomatic and asymptomatic subjects: a population based analysis of various induces of responsiveness. Am Rev Respir Dis 1989; 140:615–623.
25. Pattemore PK, Asher MI, Harrison A, Mitchell EA, Rea HH, Stewart AW. The interrelationship among bronchial hyperresponsiveness, the diagnosis of asthma, and asthma symptoms. Am Rev Respir Dis 1990; 142:549–554.
26. Clifford RD, Howell JB, Radford M, Holgate ST. Associations between respiratory symptoms, bronchial response to methacholine, and atopy in two age groups of schoolchildren. Arch Dis Child 1989; 64:1133–1139.
27. Tager IB, Weiss ST, Speizer FE. Occurrence of asthma, nonspecific bronchial hyperresponsiveness and atopy: insights from cross-sectional epidemiologic studies. Chest 1987; 91:114S–119S.
28. Boushey HA, Holtzman MJ, Sheller JR, Nadel JA. Bronchial hyperresponsiveness. Am Rev Respir Dis 1980; 121:389–413.
29. Holgate ST, Beasley R, Twentyman OP. The pathogenesis and significance of bronchial hyperresponsiveness in airway disease. Clin Sci 1987; 73:561–572.
30. Tashkin DP, Murray DA, Bleecker ER, van Altena R, Meyers DA, Koeter GM, Postma DS. The lung health study: airway responsiveness to inhaled methacholine in smokers with mild to moderate airflow limitation. Am Rev Respir Dis 1992; 145:301–310.
31. Weiss ST, Tager IB, Weiss JW, Munoz A, Speizer FE, Ingram RH. Airway responsiveness in a population sample of adults and children. Am Rev Respir Dis 1984; 129:898–902.
32. Sears MR, Jones DT, Holdaway MD, et al. Prevalence of bronchial reactivity to inhaled methacholine in New Zealand children. Thorax 1986; 41:283–289.
33. Backer V, Dirksen A, Bach-Mortensen N, Hansen KK, Laursen EM, Wendelboe D. The distribution of bronchial responsiveness to histamine and exercise in 527 children and adolescents. J Allergy Clin Immunol 1991; 88:68–76.
34. Clifford RD, Radford M, Howell JB, Holgate ST. Prevalence of atopy and range of bronchial response to methacholine in 7 and 11 year old schoolchildren. Arch Dis Child 1989; 64:1126–1132.
35. Rijcken B, Schouten JP, Weiss ST, Speizer FE, van der Lende R. The relationship between airway responsiveness to histamine and pulmonary function level in a random population sample. Am Rev Respir Dis 1988; 137:826–832.
36. Chatham M, Bleecker ER, Smith PL, Rosenthal RR, Mason P, Norman PS. A comparison of histamine, methacholine and exercise airways reactivity in normal and asthmatic subjects. Am Rev Respir Dis 1982; 126:235–240.
37. Chai H, Farr RS, Froehlich LA, et al. Standardization of bronchial inhalation challenge procedures. J Allergy Clin Immunol 1975; 56:323–327.

38. Cockcroft DW, Killian DN, Mellon JJA, Hargreave FE. Bronchial reactivity to inhaled histamine: a method and clinical survey. Clin Allergy 1977; 7:235–243.
39. Murray AB, Ferguson AC, Morrison B. Airway responsiveness to histamine as a test for overall severity of asthma in children. J Allergy Clin Immunol 1984; 68: 119–124.
40. Sterk PJ, Fabbri LM, Quanjer Ph, et al. Airway responsiveness: standardized challenge testing with pharmacological, physical and sensitizing stimuli in adults. Report Working Party Standardization of Lung Function Tests. Official Statement European Respiratory Society. Eur Respir J 1993; 6(Suppl 16):53–83.
41. Britton J, Mortagy A, Tattersfield AE. Histamine challenge testing: comparison of three methods. Thorax 1986; 41:128–132.
42. Woolcock AJ, Salome CM, Yan K. The shape of the dose-response curve to histamine in asthmatic and normal subjects. Am Rev Respir Dis 1984; 30:71–75.
43. Peat JK, Salome CM, Bauman A, Toelle BG, Wachinger SL, Woolcock AJ. Repeatability of histamine bronchial challenge and comparability with methacholine bronchial challenge in a population of Australian schoolchildren. Am Rev Respir Dis 1991; 144:338–343.
44. Bascom R, Bleecker ER. Bronchoconstriction induced by distilled water: sensitivity in asthmatics and relationship to exercise-induced bronchospasm. Am Rev Respir Dis 1986; 134:248–253.
45. Cushley MJ, Tattersfield AE, Holgate ST. Inhaled adenosine and guanosine on airway resistance in normal and asthmatic subjects. Br J Clin Pharm 1983; 15: 161–165.
46. Holgate ST, Church MK, Polosa R. Adenosine; a positive modulator of airway inflammation in asthma. Ann NY Acad Sci 1991; 629:227–236.
47. Djakanovic R, Roche WR, Wilson JW. Mucosal inflammation in asthma. Am Rev Respir Dis 1990; 142:434–457.
48. Laitinen LA, Heino M, Laitinen A, Kava T, Haahtela T. Damage of the airway epithelium and bronchial reactivity in patients with asthma. Am Rev Respir Dis 1985; 131:599–606.
49. O'Byrne PM, Hargreave FE, Kirby JG. Airway inflammation and hyperresponsiveness. Am Rev Respir Dis 1987; 136:35–37.
50. Metzger WJ, Zavala D, Richerson HB, Mosely P, Iwamota P, Monick M, Sjoerdsma K, Hunninghake GW. Local allergen challenge and bronchoalveolar lavage of allergic asthmatic lungs. Am Rev Respir Dis 1987; 135:433–440.
51. Kay AB. Mediators and inflammatory cells in allergic disease. Ann Allergy 1987; 59(6):35–42.
52. Cockcroft DW, Ruffin RE, Dolovich J, Hargreave FE. Allergen-induced increase in non-allergic bronchial reactivity. Clin Allergy 1977; 7:503–513.
53. de Monchy JGR, Kauffman HF, Venge P, et al. Bronchoalveolar eosinophilia during allergen-induced late asthmatic reactions. Am Rev Respir Dis 1985; 131:373–376.
54. Metzger WJ, Richerson HB, Worden K, Monick M, Hunninghake GW. Bronchoalveolar lavage of allergic asthmatic patients following bronchoprovocation. Chest 1986; 89:477–483.

55. Liu MC, Bleecker ER, Lichtenstein LM, et al. Evidence for elevated levels of histamine, prostaglandin D2, and other bronchoconstrictor prostaglandins in the airways of subjects with mild asthma. Am Rev Respir Dis 1990; 142:126–132.
56. Bousquet J, Chanez P, Lacoste JY, et al. Eosinophilic inflammation in asthma. N Engl J Med 1990; 323:1033–1039.
57. Broide DH, Lotz M, Cuomo AJ, Coburn DA, Federman EC, Wasserman SI. Cytokines in symptomatic asthma airways. J Allergy Clin Immunol 1992; 89:958–967.
58. Brown PH, Crompton GK, Greening AP. Proinflammatory cytokines in acute asthma. Lancet 1991; 338:590–593.
59. Robinson DS, Ying S, Bentley AM, Meng Q, North J, Durham SR, Kay B, Hamid Q. Relationships among numbers of bronchoalveolar lavage cells expressing messenger ribonucleic acid for cytokines, asthma symptoms, and airway methacholine responsiveness in atopic asthma. J Allergy Clin Immunol 1993; 92:397–403.
60. Ackerman V, Marini M, Vittori E, Bellini A, Vassali G, Mattoli S. Detection of cytokines and their cell sources in bronchial biopsy specimens from asthmatic patients: relationship to atopic status, symptoms, and level of airway hyperresponsiveness. Chest 1994; 105:687–696.
61. Bleecker ER, McCrea KA, Meltzer statistics, Hasday JD. Inflammatory abnormalities in the airways of asthmatics and asymptomatic cigarette smokers. Bronchitis 1994; 5:106–116.
62. Elias JA, Freundlich B, Kern JA, Rosenbloom J. Cytokine networks in the regulation of inflammation fibrosis in the lung. Chest 1990; 97:1429–1445.
63. Djukanovic R, Lai CKW, Wilson JW, et al. Bronchial mucosal manifestations of atopy: a comparison of markers of inflammation between atopic asthmatics, atopic nonasthmatics and healthy controls. Eur Respir J 1992; 5:538–544.
64. Djukanovic R, Roche WR, Wilson JW, et al. State of the art. Mucosal inflammation in asthma. Am Rev Respir Dis 1990; 142:434–457.
65. Djukanovic R, Wilson JW, Britten KM, et al. Quantitation of mast cells and eosinophils in the bronchial mucosa of symptomatic atopic asthmatics and healthy control subjects using immunohistochemistry. Am Rev Respir Dis 1990; 142:863–871.
66. Britton J. Airway hyperresponsiveness and the clinical diagnosis of asthma: histamine or history? J Allergy Clin Immunol 192; 89:19–22.
67. Britton WJ, Woolcock AJ, Peat JK, Sedgwick JT, Lloyd DM, Leeder SR. Prevalence of bronchial hyperresponsiveness in children: the relationship between asthma and skin reactivity to allergens in two communities. Int J Epidemiol 1986; 15:202–209.
68. Josephs LK, Gregg I, Mullee MA, Holgate ST. Nonspecific bronchial reactivity and its relationship to the clinical expression of asthma: a longitudinal study. Am Rev Respir Dis 1989; 140:350–357.
69. Bleecker ER, McFadden ER, co-chairman, National Institute of Health Workshop Summary. Summary and recommendations of a workshop on the investigative use of fiberoptic bronchoscopy and bronchoalveolar lavage in individuals with asthma. J Allergy Clin Immunol 1991; 88:808–814; Eur J Respir Dis 1991; Clin Exp Allergy 1991; Eur Respir J 1992; 5(1):115–121.

70. Fahy JV, Liu J, Wong H, Boushey HA. Cellular and biochemical analysis of induced sputum from asthmatic and from healthy subjects. Am Rev Respir Dis 1993; 147:1126–1131.

71. Chatham M, Bleecker ER, Smith PL, Rosenthal RR, Mason P, Norman PS. A comparison of histamine, methacholine and exercise airways reactivity in normal and asthmatic subjects. Am Rev Respir Dis 1982; 126:235–240.

72. Chatham M, Bleecker ER, Mason P, Smith PL, Norman P. A screening test for airways reactivity—an abbreviated methacholine inhalation challenge. Chest 1982; 82:15–18.

73. Postma DS, Bleecker ER, Amelung PJ, Holroyd KJ, Xu J, Panhuysen CIM, Meyers DA, Levitt RC. Genetic susceptibility to asthma-bronchial hyperresponsiveness coinherited with a major gene for atopy. N Engl J Med 1995; 333:894–900.

74. Kraan J, Koöter GH, van der Mark TW, Sluiter HJ, de Vries K. Changes in bronchial hyperreactivity induced by 4 weeks of treatment with antiasthmatic drugs in patients with allergic asthma: comparison between budesonide and terbutaline. J Allergy Clin Immunol 1985; 76:628–636.

75. Kerrebijn KF, vanEssen-Zandvliet EEM, Neijens HJ. Effect of long-term treatment with inhaled corticosteroids and beta-agonists on the bronchial responsiveness in children with asthma. J Allergy Clin Immunol 1987; 79:653–659.

76. Burrows B, Sears MR, Flannery EM, Herbison GP, Holdaway MD. Relationship of bronchial responsiveness assessed by methacholine to serum IgE, lung function, symptoms, and diagnoses in 11-year-old New Zealand children. J Allergy Clin Immunol 1992; 90:376–385.

77. Sears M, Burrows B, Flannery EM, Herbison GP, Hewitt CJ, Holdaway MD. Relation between airway responsiveness and serum IgE in children with asthma and in apparently normal children. N Engl J Med 1991; 325:1067–1071.

78. Haahtela T, Jarvinen M, Kava T, et al. Comparison of a $beta_2$-agonist, terbutaline, with an inhaled corticosteroid, budesonide, in newly detected asthma. N Engl J Med 1991; 325:388–392.

79. Kerstjens HAM, Brand PLP, Hughes MD, Robinson NJ, Postma DS, Sluiter HI, Bleecker ER, Dekhuijzen R, de Long PM, Menegelers HJI, Overbeek SE, Schoonbrood DSME, and the Dutch CNSLD Group. A comparison of bronchodilator therapy with or without inhaled corticosteroid therapy for obstructive airways disease. N Engl J Med 1992; 327:1413–1419.

80. Schleimer RP. Effects of glucocorticoids on inflammatory cells relevant to their therapeutic applications in asthma. Am Rev Respir Dis 1990; 141(Suppl):S59–69.

81. Hopp RJ, Bewtra AK, Watt GD, Nair NM, Townley RG. Genetic analysis of allergic disease in twins. J Allergy Clin Immunol 1984; 73:265–270.

82. Hopp RJ, Townley RG, Biven RE, Bewtra AK, Nair NM. The presence of airway reactivity before the development of asthma. Am Rev Respir Dis 1990; 141:2–8.

83. Townley RG, Bewtra MD, Wilson AF, Hopp RJ, Elston RC, Nair NM, Watt GD. Segregation analysis of bronchial response to methacholine inhalation in families with and without asthma. J Allergy Clin Immunol 1986; 77:101–107.

84. Lander ES, Schork NJ. Genetic dissection of complex traits. Science 1994; 265: 2037–2048.

85. Burrows B, Martinez FD, Halonen M, Barbee RA, Cline MG. Association of asth-ma with serum IgE levels and skin-test reactivity to allergens. N Engl J Med 1989; 320:271–277.

86. Burrows B, Sears MR, Flannery EM, Herbison GP, Holdaway MD. Relationship of bronchial responsiveness to allergy skintest reactivity, lung function, respiratory symptoms, and diagnosis in 13-year-old New Zealand children. J Allergy Clin Immunol 1995; 95:548–556.

87. Sunyer J, Anto JM, Sabria J, Roca J, Morell F, Rodriguez-Roisin R, Rodrigo MJ. Respiratory pathophysiologic responses: relationship between serum IgE and airway responsiveness in adults with asthma. J Allergy Clin Immunol 1995; 95:699–706.

88. Marsh DG, Bias WB, Ishizaka K. Genetic control of basal serum immunoglobulin E level and its effect on specific reaginic sensitivity. Proc Natl Acad Sci USA 1974; 71:3588–3592.

89. Gerrard JW, Rao DC, Morton NE. A genetic study of immunoglobulin E. Am J Hum Genet 1978; 30:46–58.

90. Blumenthal MN, Manboodiri KK, Mendell N, Gleich G, Elston RC, Yunis E. Genetic transmission of serum IgE levels. Am J Med Genet 1981; 10:219–228.

91. Meyers DA, Bias WB, Marsh DG. A genetic study of total IgE levels in the Amish. Hum Hered 1982; 32:15–23.

92. Meyers DA, Beaty WB, Freidhoff LR, Marsh DG. Inheritance of serum IgE (basal levels) in man. Am J Hum Genet 1987; 41(1):51–62.

93. Meyers DA, Beaty TH, Colyer CR, Marsh DG. Genetics of total serum IgE levels: a regressive model approach to segregation analysis. Genet Epidemiol 1991; 8: 351–359.

94. Hasstedt SJ, Meyers DA, Marsh DG, Skolnick M, King M-C, Bias WB, Amos DB. The inheritance of immunoglobulin E: genetic model fitting. Am J Med Genet 1983; 14:61–66.

95. Martinez FD, Holberg CJ, Halonen M, Morgan WJ, Wright AL, Taussig LM. Evidence for mendelian inheritance of serum IgE levels in Hispanic and non-Hispanic white families. Am J Hum Gen 1994; 55(3):555–565.

96. Meyers DA, Postma DS, Panhuysen CIM, Xu J, Amelung PJ, Levitt RC, Bleecker ER. Evidence for a locus regulating total serum IgE levels mapping to chromosome 5. Genomics 1994; 23:464–470.

97. Xu J, Levitt RC, Panhuysen CIM, Postma DS, Taylor EW, Amelung PJ, Holroyd KJ, Bleecker ER, Meyers DA. Evidence for two unlinked loci regulating total serum IgE levels. Am J Hum Genet 1995; 57:425–430.

98. Chandrasekharappa SC, Rebelsky MS, Firak TA, LeBeau MM, Westbrook CA. A long-range restriction map of the interleukin-4 and interleukin-5 linkage group on chromosome 5. Genomics 1990; 6:94–99.

98a. Marsh DG, Neely JD, Breazeale DR, Ghosh B, Freidhoff LR, Ehrlich-Kautzky E, Shou C, Krishnaswamy G, Beaty TH. Linkage analysis of IL4 and other chromosome 5q31.1 markers and total serum immunoglobulin E concentrations. Science 1994; 264:1152–1156.

99. Kelley J. Cytokines of the lung. Am Rev Respir Dis 1991; 141:765–788.

100. Boulay JL, Paul WE. The interleukin-4-related lymphokines and their binding to hematopoietin receptors. J Biol Chem 1992; 297:20525–20528.
101. Marsh DG, Neely JD, Breazeale DR, Ghosh B, Freidhoff LR, Ehlich-Kautzky E, Schou C, Krishnasawamy G, Beaty TH. Linkage analysis of IL4 and other chromosome 5q31.1 markers and total serum immunoglobulin E concentrations. Science 1994; 264:1162–1166.
102. Doull IJM, Lawrence S, Watson M, Begishvili T, Beasley RW, Lampe F, Holgate ST, Morton NE. Allelic association of gene markers on chromosomes 5q and 11q with atopy and bronchial hyperresponsiveness. Am J Respir Crit Care Med 1996 (in press).
103. Blumenthal MN, Wang Z, Wever JL, Rich SS. Absence of linkage between 5q markers and serum IgE levels in four large atopic families. Clin Exp Allergy 1996; 26 (in press).
104. DeVries K, Goei JT, Booy-Noord H, Orie NGM. Changes during 24 hours in the lung function and histamine hyperreactivity of the bronchial tree in asthmatic and bronchitic patients. Int Arch Allergy 1962; 20:93–101.

14

Genetics of Asthma, Allergy, and Related Conditions

Malcolm N. Blumenthal
University of Minnesota Hospital
Minneapolis, Minnesota

I. INTRODUCTION

Evidence of familial, if not heritable, factors in the causation of asthma and allergies has been noted since ancient times (Chapter 1). Allergies are complex diseases involving multiple steps in which the processes can be either enhanced or attenuated. Many of these steps are under genetic control (Chapters 9–13) while others may involve environmental interactions (Chapters 7 and 8).

Allergies are adverse immune reactions. Immune reactions, either beneficial or adverse, both nonspecific and specific, have been known for many years to be influenced by genetic factors. Species as well as individual differences that appear to be genetic have been reported regarding responses to infections and the development of certain diseases (i.e., allergies, immunodeficiencies, autoimmune diseases, contact sensitization, and transplantations). The first serious modern study of the heredity of asthma and hay fever was undertaken by Cooke and VanderVeer in 1916 (1). On the basis of these earlier studies, it is now generally agreed that genetic factors are involved in the development of asthma and allergy. Our knowledge of the basic biological processes, and of the genetic predisposition that contributes significantly to asthma and allergy, is inadequate. Developing an understanding of asthma and allergies has been difficult in view of the muliple genetic and nongenetic factors that may ultimately determine the clinical picture.

II. BACKGROUND OF EVENTS LEADING TO PRESENT STUDIES OF THE GENETICS OF ASTHMA AND ALLERGIES

Advances in several fields have now made it possible to start understanding the genetics of complex diseases such as asthma and allergies. A better understanding of the pathogenesis of atopic conditions is allowing us to characterize the phenotypes of asthma and allergies. This has consisted of the characterization of IgE, T cells, and cytokines (Chapters 4 and 5). Other advances have been made in molecular genetics (2–6). These include: (1) the discovery of recombinant DNA in the mid-1970s, (2) the cloning of DNA fragments, (3) the discovery that DNA fragments could be separated by electrophoresis, and (4) the development of the polymerase chain reaction, which allows the rapid amplification of short regions of DNA with great ease (4–7; Chapter 2). Statistical methods have improved permitting the analysis of the genetics of complex diseases such as allergies (3,5; Chapter 2). These include methods such as LINKAGE using the lod scores, MASC using nuclear families, regressive model of segregation analysis taking into account environmental factors, transmission/disequilibrium test (TDT), affected-sib-pair analysis, and affected-pedigree-member analysis. All these advances are allowing researchers to define the molecule basis of diseases such as asthma and allergies.

Understanding the molecular basis of inherited diseases ultimately requires researchers to know everything about the gene involved: its chromosomal location, its DNA sequence, how its expression is controlled, and what its product does. For a given disease, there are several routes to this knowledge. The main routes are called forward, reverse or positional genetics, and the candidate gene approach.

The classic human examples of forward genetics are the study of the hemoglobinopathies and inborn errors of metabolism where the defective item is identified and characterized. For asthma, this information is not known. It is possible that studies of the transcriptional control of airway inflammation may provide the necessary information to study its "forward" genetics. The cell adhesion molecules genes, and, in turn, the gene products that control them, are candidates for abnormal expression in inflammation. If the defective factor is known, one can then identify the DNA, the gene sequence, and ultimately its location (2; Chapters 2, 3, and 5).

For many diseases, including asthma and allergies, the underlying defect is not known. Identification of any single gene of unknown function is a complex problem. The human genome comprises 3×10^9 base pairs: thus any specific gene represents only a very small fraction of the total DNA. Here positional (reverse) genetics may be used to characterize the gene. Using this method, the first step is to identify the gene location. We are therefore mapping the chromosomal location of the gene and cloning the gene knowing nothing about it except its location. Once we do this, we can then determine the gene sequence, its DNA structure, and ultimately the gene product that results in production of the disease (2; Chapters 2–6).

The candidate gene approach involves looking at a gene, or genes, already identified that are thought to be involved in the condition you are studying. An example of this would be investigating the gene for IL-4 because we know it is involved in IgE regulation, which appears to be involved in asthma and allergy.

Over the past few years, using these latter methods, the genes for several human diseases have been identified, including cystic fibrosis, Duchenne muscular dystrophy, myotonic dystrophy, and neurofibromatosis. These, however, have all involved diseases caused by a defect in a single major gene. Studies have now been initiated to study the genes for the more complex human diseases such as schizophrenia, bipolar disorder, various autoimmune diseases, cancer, diabetes, and asthma. All these are multifactorial and appear to be genetically heterogeneous. In other words, they involve several genes, along with an array of environmental factors that influence the expression of each of these diseases. Using new methodology and the positional or reverse genetic and candidate gene approaches, we can now identify the genetic components of these more complex conditions.

III. RATIONALE FOR ASTHMA AND ALLERGY GENETIC STUDIES

Asthma and allergic conditions are good models for studying complex diseases resulting from the interaction of genetic with environmental factors. They are common diseases that are increasing in prevalence and there are indications for a cohort effect (Chapters 7 and 8). It is estimated that atopic diseases such as asthma and rhinitis affect approximately 30% of the total population; their clinical picture has been well defined. In addition, the causative allergens can be identified and characterized and the immune response to them (i.e., the specific IgE antibody) can be identified. Finally, a suggested pathogenesis is available to use as a model.

Based on the accumulated data, it is thought that multiple cell types and numerous cellular control mechanisms influence the development of asthma and allergies and their response to treatment. According to current understanding and based on concepts presented in earlier chapters, the following model is being used for investigation of the genetics of asthma and atopic conditions (6–8):

A. Sensitization

Exposure to the allergen (antigen) occurs, following which it is taken up by an antigen-presenting cell (APC) such as a dendritic or B cell. Afterward, through intracellular processing, the allergen (antigen) will be broken down into a specific peptide, which becomes associated with a class II major histocompatibility complex (MHC) molecule selected from an MHC library. The allergen (antigen) peptide-MHC complex then moves to the surface of the APC where it can interact with a subset of T cells, designated CD4$^+$ cells, which have T-cell receptors (TCR) specific for the class II peptide complex chosen from a TCR library. These CD4$^+$ cells may differentiate into either cells called T helper 2 (TH2), which produce largely the cytokine interferon-γ, or to cells called T helper 1 (TH1), which produce mainly IL-4 and a set of associated molecules as the main cytokines. IL-4 appears to be necessary for IgE production. Interferon-γ is a principal regulator of cellular immunity and is associated with a decrease in IgE production. Apparently, in atopic individuals there is preferential development of a disproportionate number of TH2 as opposed to TH1 cells, which interact with the allergen (antigen) binding B-cell clones through the production of cytokines and directly through its action on B cells. This interaction results in signals for the B cells to differentiate and produce antigen-specific antibodies whose Ig has been chosen from a V(h) library for its ability to bind the allergen (antigen). This step may result in two major effects: B cells may mature into plasma cells. In the allergen-specific atopic response, isotope switching occurs followed by the production of allergen-specific IgE. After the specific IgE is formed, it will interact with a cell containing an IgE receptor. Alternatively, this interaction may stimulate new virgin B and T cells to further diversify the immune response.

B. Reexposure

Upon reexposure to the allergen (antigen) it will interact with allergen-specific IgE on the surfaces of cells that will initiate the release of inflammatory mediators. The end-organ response to the released mediators will result in the clinical picture of asthma and atopy.

It is apparent that each of these activities must be coordinated to produce an allergic response. It is equally clear that there are a multitude of steps where the process can be enhanced or attenuated. Many of these steps are under genetic control and many involve environmental interactions. While the specificity of each step may be relatively low, the overall specificity is much greater as a result of sequential gating of independent points of recognition. By studying this proposed mechanism, we should be able to further define the biology of asthma and allergies and develop an understanding of the genetics involved.

IV. APPROACHES TO STUDY GENETICS OF ASTHMA, ALLERGIES, AND RELATED CONDITIONS

Position genetics and the candidate gene approach are being used to study conditions like asthma and other allergies because not enough is known about their biology to do forward genetics. It is therefore important to identify and characterize the phenotype. Position genetics is done by mapping this phenotype by linkage analysis, physical mapping, positional cloning, and ultimately, identification of the gene involved. If an identifiable gene or genes is thought to be involved with the phenotype, the candidate gene approach can be used. The genetic control of these conditions has been studied using asthma- and allergy-related/intermediate phenotypes such as specific immune responses, serum IgE levels, mediator release, bronchial hyperreactivity (Chapters 9–12), as well as the more complex phenotypes such as asthma and atopy.

V. ASTHMA- AND ALLERGY-ASSOCIATED/INTERMEDIATE PHENOTYPES

A. Specific Immune Response

The specific immune response has been studied and its overall mechanism has been defined (Chapter 9). There is growing evidence that the specific immune response is associated with the HLA system, specifically the DR region. As noted in Chapter 9, using atopic populations and purified Amb a V, an association between the IgE and, to a lesser extent IgG, response to Amb a V and HLA DR2*1500 and DW2 has been reported (8–13). No sequence novelty in the polymorphic second exons of the HLA-DRB and DQB genes that play an important role in encoding the antigen-binding portion of MHC class II molecules has been found that is unique to AMb a V responsiveness (12). As reviewed in Chapter 9, it appears that the DRα/β heterodimers are the principal class II molecules involved in Amb a V presentation. Specifically, the presentation was associated with the β_1 sequences at amino acid residues 67, 70, and 71 in HLA-DRB1*1501, *1502. Amb a V responsiveness almost completely predicts HLA-DR2 positivity (14/15, 93%). However, not all HLA DR2-positive individuals are Amb a V reactive. Other allergens' immune responses have been noted to be associated with the HLA-DR system such as Amb t V and Amb a V with DR2, Amb a VI with DR5, Ole e I with DQ2, Para 01 with DRB1*1101, and *Lollium perenne* allergens Lol I, II, and III with DR3 (14).

Another point of restriction involved in the specific immune response is binding of the complex formed by MHC, the critical peptides of the allergen, and the structure of the specific T-cell-receptor complex. A possibly critical relationship exists between the structure determined by the HLA Class II region genes and the availability of selected T-cell-receptor variable region genes that affects the effectiveness of binding of foreign peptides. The arrangement of TCR elements on the α and β chains appears to determine the antigen specificity of the T cell. Renz et al. demonstrated in mice that specific V β-expressing T-cell subpopulations stimulated IgE/IgG1 production and increased airway responsiveness (15). Studies of genomic polymorphisms in humans at the TCR α-β region also suggest that there may be restriction of the IgE responses to particular allergens. Moffatt et al. demonstrated genetic linkage of specific IgE response to the TCR α/δ locus on chromosome 14 (16). Recent communications from Moffatt report that IgE responses to Der p I and Der p II were increased in subjects who had Vα 8.1 allele 2 and were HLA-DDRB1*02-positive (17). At present, evidence suggests that the MHC effect is a necessary, but not sufficient, factor in the development of the specific atoic immune response or the complex phenotype of asthma and allergy. This indicates the need for other factors (genetic or environmental) that completely determine reactivity to specific allergens.

B. IgE Regulation

Our current understanding of the immune system suggests that the up-regulation of IgE synthesis in atopy is due to the induction of IgE isotype utilization at the DNA level in B cells (Chapters 3 and 10). IgE synthesis appears to involve three signals following direct T-B interaction. One is delivered by an IgE isotype-specific signal, provided by the activated CD4 T cell or TH2 cell-derived IL-4. The other two are CD40 ligand (CD4-L) and FcϵRII B-cell activation signals, which require engagement of the TCR with antigenic fragments (peptides) that are recognized on MHC class II molecules on APC. Interferon-γ appears to down-regulate IgE synthesis (7).

Serum IgE level heritability has been demonstrated in twin, family, and population studies (18–24). Family studies reveal a heritability of approximately 50–60%, while in twin studies the concordance in monozygotic twins ranged from 0.36 to 0.88 compared to 0.16 to 0.63 in dyzogotic twins. A major gene appears to be involved. The mode of inheritance and location of the gene have not been well delineated. Dominant, codominant, and recessive modes of inheritances have all been suggested. Studies by Marsh et al. (25) and Meyers et al. (26) present evidence that suggests that one of the genes involved in the synthesis of IgE regulation is located in the 5q31–33 region. This has not been confirmed in another study (27). Rosenwasser et al. reported that analysis of the transcription regulation of IL-4 reveals unique regulatory regions within the IL-4 promotor involved in interaction with standard T-cell-related nuclear transcription factors (28). No direct HLA associations with serum IgE levels have been adequately demonstrated. A study to determine if major structural abnormalities of IGHE, IGHEP1, and IGHEP2 genes might lead to aberrant control and subsequent increase in IgE concentration was performed and no large deletions or duplicatuion could be demonstrated (29).

C. IgE Receptor

The IgE receptors have recently been studied. High-affinity receptors on basophils and mast cells and low-affinity receptors on eosinophils and lymphocytes have been identified and characterized. Using the candidate gene approach, Sandford et al. reported that the gene regulating the β chain of the high-affinity receptor for IgE (FcϵRI-β) is on chromosome 11q13 (30). They described two code variants of FcϵRI-β: l181L and l181L/V183L (originally Leu 181 and Leu 181/183); these variants are rare in the general population. These researchers have recently described a further polymorphism, in the C-terminal cytoplasmic tail of FcϵRI-β (31). Located within exon 7 of FcϵRI-β, the variant results in a change of glutamic acid to glycine at residue 233 (E233G). E233G lies adjacent to the activation motif in FcϵRI-β and introduces a significant hydrophobicity change in this region, which may be of functional importance. The authors suggest that FcϵRI-β belongs to a family of receptors that contain homologous activation motifs that appear capable of autonomously triggering cell activation via protein-tyrosine phosphorylation. This finding has not been confirmed. Other possible candidate genes for study include those for the low-affinity IgE receptor (FcϵRII-β), and its ligand CD40 (Chapters 3 and 10).

D. IgE Receptor/IgE/Allergen Interactions

The mechanisms of the IgE receptor-IgE and allergen-IgE interactions and the regulation of the release of mediators and cytokines are just being characterized. The genetics of the regulation of the release of mediators or cytokines involving the interaction of IgE with cells and their ability to release mediating substances have not been extensively investigated. The phenotype of histamine release following the anti-IgE challenge of peripheral blood basophils has been reported in a twin study by Marone et al. (32), and a nuclear family study by Roitman-Johnson and Blumenthal (33), to be influenced by genetic factors.

E. End-Organ Response

The pathogenesis of the end-organ responses to mediators also has not been well characterized. Bronchial hyperreactivity, one of the main end-organ responses studied, is poorly defined genetically. It should be realized that the bronchial reactivity may be a result of a variety of different steps ranging from the stimulus; receptors; state of the smooth muscle; and airway characteristics, including its circumference, external diameters, wall thickness, and secretion. Familial factors have been reported to be involved in the development of bronchial hyperresponsiveness (BHR), defined principally as the bronchial response to methacholine and histamine inhalation challenge. Many studies provided evidence of heritability of bronchial hyperreactivity, but there was distinct heterogeneity (34; Chapter 12). Recently evidence has been presented suggesting that regions of 5q31–33 that may be important in the regulation of total serum IgE may also be involved in the development of BHR in allergy and asthma (35). Genetic polymorphism of the β_2-adrenergic receptors in asthma has been studied and shown conflicting results. Evidence has been presented that certain cases of human asthma may have mutations of G-protein-coupled β_2 receptors (36,37). It was reported that four polymorphic loci have been found within the open reading frame of the β_2-adrenergic receptor (β2AR) gene in asthmatic and nonasthmatic populations.

Inflammation, a major component of asthma, is just being characterized in asthma (Chapter 11). Chemical mediators (i.e., cytokines), cell adhesion molecules, as well as other mediators of the inflammatory response (i.e., heat shock proteins) have been identified and are now being characterized and localized to specific chromosomal regions. The activation of transcription factors as well as the role of the TGF-β, EGF, ICAM, CD-23, HLA-DR, TNF, IL-10, IL-4, UK6, and IL-5 are a few of the many areas probably involved in the pathogenesis of asthma which are being investigated.

F. Summary

Many steps are hypothesized for the development of asthma and allergies. It is evident that the specific immune response to certain aeroallergens is genetically influenced by a gene(s) located on *chromosome 6* at the DR loci. The T-cell receptors may play a role in the specific IgE response. One report relates it to be on *chromosome 14* (16,17). Regulation of IgE is heritable and due to a major gene. Its mode of inheritance and the characterization of the gene(s) involved are under intense study, especially on *chromosome 5q*. The IgERI has been suggested in one study to be under genetic control due to a gene on *chromosome 11q* and related to the development of atopy (30,31). Histamine release and bronchial hyperreactivity appear to have heritability, but their mode of inheritance and whether there is a major gene involved and the location of the gene is not well established at present (32,33). One study has noted the gene for bronchial hyperreactivity may be on *chromosome 5q* near the gene suggested to be responsible for IgE levels (35). Phenotypes of the inflammatory processes in asthma are just now being studied. It is clear that both genetic and environmental factors are important in the phenotype seen.

VI. COMPLEX PHENOTYPES

The general expression of allergic disease has been noted to be familial and have heritability for many years. Early investigators emphasized the familial nature of asthma, allergy, and atopic diseases and provided evidence of a genetic predisposition (Chapter 1; 8,38). Depending on the study, as many as 40–80% of patients with allergic rhinitis or bronchial asthma have been noted to have a positive family history of allergy as opposed to 20% or less of nonallergic subjects. It is well established that there is heritability of asthma. The relative risk of allergic conditions has been difficult to estimate in view of problems of definition and the fact that it is influenced by the population prevalence of the disease under study, which, in the case of allergy, is high. For hay fever and asthma the heritability has been in the range of 0.36–0.79. It appears that the incidence of allergic disease in children roughly doubles with each parent who is allergic or has asthma. The problems of definition of phenotypes in these early studies are apparent. Recently, investigators have been attempting to study the phenotypes of complex diseases such as atopy and asthma using updated parameters to define the phenotypes and more sophisticated molecular genetic and statistical approaches to their analysis.

A. Atopy

Atopy may be defined using a variety of different parameters including IgE responses. It has been estimated that between 10 and 30% of the general poulation has some form of atopic disease. Cookson et al. investigated families looking at not only total serum IgE levels, but also the specific IgE response to allergens as determined by skin testing and the radio allergosorbent test (RAST) (39). They defined atopy as an elevated serum IgE level and/or an elevated specific IgE as measured by RAST or skin test. They suggested that atopy, as defined by the ability to produce IgE response using these parameters, is inherited as an autosomal dominant trait and is linked to chromosome 11q. Similar linkage was noted by Collee et al. (40), Shirakawa et al. (41), and Hizawa et al. (42). Rich et al. investigated the same complex phenotypes of atopy with respect to their genetics and environmental determinants (43). Using the definition of Cookson et al., as well as several other different phenotypes, no evidence for linkage was found in three large pedigrees using the dominant mode of inheritance. Lympany et al. (44,45). Hizawa et al. (46), Brereton et al. (47), and Amelung et al. (48), in separate studies, also could not confirm Hopkin and Cookson's observations. Recently, Cookson et al.

suggested that the 11q13-linked atopy gene is inherited preferentially from the maternal side, possibly due to either paternal genetic imprinting or maternal modification of the infants' IgE responses through the placenta or breast milk (49). Investigation by Walter et al. of the IGHE gene of the immunoglobulin heavy-chain constant region on chromosome 14 identified a deletion of approximately 120 kb of the IGH constant region in one of five atopic patients (50). These studies have not been confirmed by other groups.

B. Asthma

It has been estimated that between 3 and 15% of the general population has asthma. The incidence varies with definition and geographical location. Although most individuals feel they can easily recognize asthma, the exact definition or phenotype used for studies has been difficult to determine (8,38; Chapter 6). Most of the studies have been based on questionnaire data stressing symptoms and physician's diagnosis. The majority do not have the advantage of definitions using pulmonary function or other more objective data. In recent studies the phenotypes of asthma have consisted of symptoms such as coughing, wheezing, and shortness of breath as well as evidence of bronchial hyperreactivity as demonstrated by reversibility and/or a bronchial challenge with an agent such as histamine or methacholine. Others have suggested using IgE responsiveness as a parameter. Morton (in Chapter 6) defines asthma as a disorder characterized by wheezing and BHR, for which atopy is the major cause. Atopy is defined as a condition characterized by a persistent and heritable immunoglobulin E response to protein allergens. Using these definitions, Morton found the two traits are correlated and multivariate, including total and specific IgE titer, skin prick tests, medical history, and tests of bronchial reactivity. Studies by Burrow et al. (51) and Sears et al. (52) have stressed the relationship between IgE levels and asthma whether the latter is defined as atopic or idiopathic (intrinsic). Recent investigations suggest that BHR is accompanied by bronchial inflammation and an atopic diathesis in patients with asthma (Chapter 11).

The complex as well as the less complex phenotypes of asthma have been investigated with regard to their genetics and relationship to known genetic markers. Early studies, including those of Sennertus and Floyer in the late 17th century and the more systematic studies of Cooke and VanderVeer, presented evidence of a hereditary factor (Chapter 1). Asthma tends to cluster in families. The relative risk for asthma has been estimated to be between 3 and 6. Twin studies reveal a concordance rate for asthma in monozygotic twins between 12 and 89% and in dizygotic twins between 4.8 and 33%. Family and twin studies suggest the heritability of asthma to be in the range of 36–72%. Evidence appears to indicate that the major gene(s) for asthma and bronchial hyperreactivity is different than the gene for IgE. The accumulated data suggest that significant genetic components are involved in the pathogenesis of asthma. Characterizations of the gene(s) is being performed using both the candidate and positional approaches. The main areas studied using the candidate gene approach have been C6, C5, C7, and C14.

1. Chromosome 6

This chromosome has been studied because of its relationship to the HLA system and its role in the activation of T cells and the specific immune response. In addition, there is now data suggesting that tumor necrosis factor (TNF) plays a significant role in the pathogenesis of asthma (53). The gene for TNF-α is located within the class III region of the MHC. Studies suggest that linkage disequilibrium may exist within the TNF locus and the MHC and several extended haplotypes. Markers on the C6 chromosome have yielded conflicting results regarding the location of the gene regulating asthma. In early studies of the MHC class I and II regions, Thorsby and Lie (54), Morris et al. (55), and Turner et al. (56) all noted an increase in HLA-B8. On the other hand, Rachelefsky et al. (57) found an increase in HLA-A2, but a decrease in HLA-B8, in patients with bronchial asthma. Geerts et al. could find no changes in the B8 frequencies in asthma (58). Preliminary studies by Morrison suggested that polymorphisms within the class III MHC, possibly with the TNF gene cluster, may be associated with asthma (59). All these studies stress the importance of having a well-defined phenotype. In view of the problems of defining asthma, investigators directed their attention to phenotypes involving known triggers of asthma.

 a. Mite-Sensitive Asthma.   The phenotype of mite-sensitive allergic asthma has been investigated in relationship with HLA antigens. Caraballo and Hernandez studied HLA haplotype segregation in families with mite-sensitive allergic asthma (60). They studied 20 families with allergic asthma and *D. fariniae* sensitivity and eight families with intrinsic or no allergic asthma. Genetic analysis was performed using the affected sib pair method. Their results suggest the existence of an HLA-linked recessive gene controlling the IgE immune responsiveness to mite alleregens and conferring susceptibility to allergic asthma. Hsieh et al. also found an association of house dust mite reactivity to the HLA-DQw2 in Chinese children with asthma (61).

 b. ASA-Sensitive Asthma.   Associations of aspirin-sensitive asthma were reported by Mullarkey et al. (62) with HLA-DQw2 but not confirmed in a study by Lympany et al. (63). Perichon and Krishnamoorthy found no association between ASA and DQ antigens but did show an increased occurrence of the DPB1*0101 allele (64).

c. TDI-Sensitive Asthma. Isothiocyanates have been noted to be associated with antigens of the HLA system (65). Allele DQB1*0503 and allelic combination DQB1*0201/0301 have been reported to be associated with susceptibility to the isothiocyanate sensitivity. Conversely, allele DQB1*0501 and the DQA1*0101-DQB1*0501-DR1 haplotype conferred significant protection to exposed healthy control subjects. These results are consistent with the hypothesis that immune mechanisms are involved in isothiocyanate-induced asthma and that specific genetic factors may increase or decrease the risk of developing it in exposed workers. These investigators suggested that an amino acid substitution in the DQB1 antigen may be directly involved in the pathogenesis of isothiocyanate sensitivity.

d. Ragweed-Sensitive Asthma. The general expression of certain diseases has been noted to be associated with the presence of the extended HLA haplotypes. It is suggested that different extended haplotypes contain a different pattern of chromosomal deletions and insertions, some of which may influence the level of gene expression. As a result, certain combinations of alleles, especially of the D/DR and complement loci, are seen to be highly associated with a disease. Blumenthal et al. have studied the association of ragweed allergic rhinitis and bronchial asthma with the extended HLA haplotype (10). Total serum IgE concentrations and titers of IgE-specific anti-Amb a V were measured in 144 patients with ragweed pollen allergy. MHC haplotypes were determined for 50 of these patients and 28 nonatopic controls.

Total IgE levels were unimodally distributed in all study groups and were higher in the atopic patients in general compared with nonatopics. Although anti-Amb a V IgE levels were all low in the nonatopic patient population, a group in the atopic group had high levels of IgE Amb a V. It was noted that those with asthma had distinctly higher levels than those with rhinitis only and the nonatopic population. The frequencies of HLA-DR2 and the extended MHC haplotype B7, SC31, DR2 were significantly increased among the patients with asthma and high titers of IgE anti-Amb a V. Conversely, this group had decreased frequencies of HLA-DR3 and the extended haplotype HLA-B8, SC01, DR3 compared with patients with only rhinitis, who had an increased number with the extended haplotype HLA-B8, SC01, DR3 and low levels of IgE Amb a V. These findings are consistent with a dominant MHC-linked gene of genes on HLA-B7, SC31, DR2 controlling the IgE immune response to Amb a V and predisposing to asthma.

2. Chromosome 5q

This chromosome contains many genes that are implicated in bronchial inflammation associated with asthma, including (1) granulocyte-macrophage colony-stimulating factor, fibroblast growth factor acidic, other colony-stimulating factors and receptors; (2) the lymphocyte-specific glucocorticoid receptor 1, and the β₂-adrenergic receptors; (3) a cluster of cytokines, IL-3, IL-4, IL-9, and IL-13; and (4) the genes possibly related to IgE regulation (Chapter 11).

Four polymorphic loci within the open reading frame of the β₂-adrenergic receptor (β2AR) gene in asthmatic and nonasthmatic populations have been reported. These occurred at amino acid positions 16, 27, 34, and 164 corresponding to Arg/Gly, Gln/Glu, Met/Val, and Thr/Ile, respectively (66). This genetic polymorphism of the β₂-adrenergic receptors showed no evidence for differences in the frequency of polymorphisms in asthmatics versus normals. However, severe, oral-corticosteroid-dependent asthmatics and those requiring immunotherapy were more likely to have the Gly 16 polymorphism. The Arg 16→IL-3 results in a receptor with decreased affinity for β-agonists and depressed functional coupling to Bs. The Arg 16→Gly receptor displays enhanced agonist-promoted down-regulation. Gln 27→Blu displays resistance to down-regulation. The Gly 16 variant is associated with nocturnal asthma and the Glu 27 variant is associated with decreased BHR (35,36,63). Ohe et al. (67) have reported a two-allele polymorphism in the Japanese population, which can be detected by the presence or absence of a BanI restriction enzyme site within the β₂-adrenergic receptor gene. One allele was associated with an increased prevalence of asthma and decreased airway and peripheral blood leukocyte responsiveness to β-agonists in their asthmatic families. Therefore, mutations of the β-adrenergic receptor may modulate the severity of symptoms in asthmatic patients.

As discussed previously, Postma et al. have presented information suggesting that regions of 5q31–33 are important in the regulation of total serum IgE and BHR in allergy and asthma (35), and Rosenwasser et al. suggest that a polymorphism within the IL-4 promoter may be associated with biological functions seen in asthma (28).

3. Chromosome 7

Associations of asthma and BHR have been reported with heterozygosity for cystic fibrosis (73,74), while others suggest that heterozygosity for the CF allele ΔF508 may give protection (75).

4. Chromosome 14

Associations of allotypes with asthma have been investigated. The gene for the Ig heavy chain is on chromosome 14. An investigation of Gm allotypes revealed nonatopic bronchial asthma showed a significantly increased frequency of the phenotypes containing the Gm(a,″,g) haplotype, named the Gm(a,″,g/a,″,g) and Gm(a,″,g/f,″,b), and an increased number of individuals were homozygous G2m(″,″) on the IgG2 locus. Individuals with atopic asthma showed a preponderance of the haplotype with the alternative allotypes on all IgG subclass loci, namely Gm(f,n,b) (76). These results emphasize the presence of qualitatively and quantitatively different IgG molecules in nonatopic and atopic bronchial asthma patients and suggest that the investigation of IgG genes and IgG molecules is important. G2m(",") homozygosity may be a marker of nonatopic bronchial asthma (76).

α_1-**Antitrypsin** The association between α_1-antitrypsin deficiency and asthma has been suggested since 1969. Several studies have suggested that the gene variants for α_1-antitrypsin, which plays an important role in the pathogenesis of chronic obstructive lung disease, may be associated with asthma (68). As many as 75 molecular variants have been distinguished by isoelectric focusing. The variants are named according to their mobility, with those moving toward the anode ahead of normal M type being given letters below M and those moving slower being given letters above M. Reports from several groups have indicated an increased prevalence of the slow variants S and/or Z in asthmatic patients. Children with more severe and steroid-dependent asthma had more Z hetero-zygotes than non-steroid-dependent and less severe asthmatics. The frequency of the presence of various phenotypes of α_1-antitrypsin was studied in patients with intrinsic asthma and with ASA-sensitive asthma and compared to people representative of the general population. The MZ and SZ phenotype is more frequent in intrinsic asthmatics ($p < 0.00001$) and MZ in ASA-sensitive asthma ($p < 0.0005$) than in the control group. No differences were found between the intrinsic asthmatics and ASA-sensitive asthma (69). This study suggests that α_1-antitrypsin deficiency may be important in the pathogenesis of inflammatory processes and in the clinical manifestations characteristic of patients with intrinsic asthma and ASA-sensitive asthma. A recent study found evidence that the occurrence of the M1(ala213) allele of α_1-antitrypsin in white individuals living in Africa was higher in asthmatics (70). There also have been reports that suggest an association between low levels of α-antichymotrypsin and asthma (71,72). These and other associations have been observed but there has been a lack of adequate confirmation of them.

5. Chromosome 16

Several investigations suggest a decreased asthma prevalence in familial Mediterranean fever (FMF) heterozygote patients. These results have not been consistent or significant. It has been suggested that identification of the FMF gene on 16p may provide an insight into asthma (77).

Position genetics studies are now in progress to identify genes associated with bronchial asthma. To date no published or replicated sites or genes have been identified.

C. Allergic Rhinitis/Hay Fever

It is estimated that 10–41% of the general population has allergic rhinitis. Allergic rhinitis has been reported to be associated with asthma and atopic dermatitis. Many early investigators, including Bostock, Elliotson, Wyman, and Mackenzie, as well as Cooke and VanderVeer (1,18,78), have demonstrated in population, twin, and family studies a hereditary diathesis. It appears that there is a genetic predisposition to develop hay fever or allergic rhinitis, which is independent of the general susceptibility to allergy. Few studies of the genetics of allergic rhinitis have been performed using newer methodology. The HLA system has been studied without any definite findings. Kitano et al. noted that subjects with *D. fariniae* and allergic rhinitis showed a positive association with HLA-DQ3 and a negative association with HLA-A2. HLA-DQB1*0303 was increased in patients with mite allergy (79).

D. Urticaria and Angioedema

Urticaria and angioedema are thought to involve a variety of complex cellular and humoral factors. Many etiological factors have been suggested, and the majority are without a definite known etiology. Several familial, if not hereditary, syndromes of urticaria and angioedema have been reported. Hereditary angioedema (HAE), probably the best defined of the genetic syndromes of this type (80–85; Chapter 1), was described in the last part of the 19th century by Quincke, Dinkelacher, Valentin, Strubing, and Osler. It is associated with an autosomal dominant deficiency of C1 esterase inhibitor activity. The C1 INH gene is located on human chromosome 11 region q11–q13. It is comprised of seven exons and at least seven introns. The C1 INH gene also contains several copies of Alu sequences that are highly repetitive DNA sequences dispersed throughout the human genome. Expression of C1 INH is enhanced by androgens, IFN-γ, and, to a lesser extent, IFN-α, TNF-α, IL-6, and M-CSF. Two subtypes of HAE have been defined on the basis of apparent protein abnormalities. HAE type I, comprising about 85% of patients with HAE, is characterized by decreased level of functionally normal C1 INH in plasma. The underlying molecular event is suggested to be the apparent lack of function of one C1 INH allele in the genome. It is suggested by genomic sequence analysis that there are partial deletions or insertions within the C1 INH gene and that repetitive Alu sequences in the C1 INH gene play a primary role in this process. In 80–85% of type I HAE patients, however, a polymorphism is not seen. In these cases, it is suggested that small mutations are present in regions of the C1 INH gene that are required for either proper transcription or translation. Type II HAE accounts for 15% of the cases of HAE and is characterized by normal or increased levels of C1 INH, but the protein has reduced functional activity. The underlying molecular changes responsible for the functional defects may be of two types: mutation in the reactive 100 p of the C1 INH molecules and mutation outside the reactive 100 p. C1 INH cleavage by C1s or C1r takes place between C1 INH residues Arg and Thr. Thus binding and cleavage of C1 INH by the target proteases requires an intact Arg-Thr peptide bond and proper folding of the C1 INH reactive loop. Point mutations affecting the nucleotides that code for Arg in one study were responsible for about 70% of all cases of type II HAE analyzed. Mutations are reported more often for type II than for type I HAE. Less well defined syndromes (all of which appear to be autosomal dominant conditions) are familial cold urticaria, a syndrome of cold intolerance; hereditary vibratory angioedema; and Muckle-Wells syndrome, which is characterized by recurrent urticaria, periodic arthritis, sensorineural deafness, general signs of inflammation, and secondary amyloidosis (Chapter 1; 85,86). A C3b inactivator deficiency has been described which appear to be autosomal recessive (87).

E. Eczema/Atopic Dermatitis

The word "eczema" has never been satisfactorily defined (Chapter 1). It has different interpretations in different areas and has gradually lost its medical significance as it may be a general term used to refer to a variety of types of chronic as well as acute dermatitis. Atopic dermatitis is a chronic dermatitis that possesses distinctive features in respect to localization of the lesion, personal and family history of allergy, and a characteristic, though often erratic, course. It has been estimated that between 1 and 3% of the general population has atopic dermatitis. It appears to be a multifactorial disease brought about by various familial and environmental influences, and it seems to be increasing in frequency. The magnitude of the concordance rates indicates that genetic factors are important in the development of atopic dermatitis. It has been suggested that the inheritance of atopic dermatitis is autosomal dominant (88). Despite these relationships with a family history of atopy, 10% of family members of patients with atopic dermatitis do not have such a history (38,88). Associations between atopic dermatitis and the HLA system have been reported (89,90). In 19 families studied (91) Scholz et al. observed that there is evidence of an increased association of HLA-A and HLA-A9 with atopic dermatitis. Ozawa et al. (92) noted that patients with atopic dermatitis and bronchial asthma and allergic rhinitis had an increase in HLA-B12 and -B40 but noted no difference in the HLA antigen frequencies in patients with atopic dermatitis alone. Svejgaard et al. noted that the frequency of HLA-DR7 was decreased in patients with atopic dermatitis when uncorrected, but when corrected for multiple variables no negative association was observed (93). Goudemand et al. showed an increased BW35 among 27 patients (94). Recently Saeki et al. also found associations with HLA antigens but none remained significant after *p* values were corrected (95). Others have found no associations with the HLA system (96). Kuwata et al. studied the polymorphism of transporter associated with antigen-processing genes in atopic dermatitis (97). They reported that the gene frequency of TAP1 637Asp exhibited a tendency to increase in patients with atopic dermatitis. They suggested that this may contribute to the pathogenesis of atopic dermatitis in combination with HLA-DRB1*1302DQ B1*0604.

In view of the suggestion that atopy was associated with chromosome site 11q13, this region was studied in 95 multiplex families through probands with active atopic eczema. Linkage analyses between atopy and markers on 11q13 excluded a major susceptibility locus for atopy in this region. There was no significant deviation from the expected proportions of alleles shared by affected sib pairs. The families were then analyzed according to parental atopic phenotype. A positive lod score (0.8) in 19 families with unaffected fathers, in contrast to markedly negative scores for other combinations of affected parental phenotype, was observed. The possibility of a maternal influence on the inheritance of atopy was not excluded (98).

F. Allergic Contact Dermatitis

Allergic contact dermatitis is a result of sensitization to a wide variety of contactant material usually thought to be mediated by a cellular nonatopic mechanism. The antigens or contactants are simple substances (haptens), which include poison ivy, metals such as nickel, and cosmetics as well as medications (99). They form covalent derivatives with skin proteins. The antigen involved with contact dermatitis is taken in by the antigen-presenting cells where they combine with MHC molecule. These in turn interact with the T cells, which sets in motion the release of mediators ultimately resulting in the contact dermatitis. There does not appear to be more allergic contact dermatitis in atopic compared to nonatopic populations. Human family and twin studies as well as animal studies have suggested that genetic factors play a role in the development of contact sensitization (100). There is an increased concordance rate of nickel sensitivity in monozygotic compared to dizygotic twins. Heritability with nickel sensitization has been noted to be about 60% (101).

Human studies carried out investigating the HLA system and contact dermatitis have yielded conflicting results. Emtestam et al. (102) described an association in nickel-sensitive subjects with an HLA-DQA restriction fragment length polymorphism (RFLP) (4.5-kb TaqI band, DQA1*0501). They could not confirm this association in another population of subjects. Liden et al. have suggested HLA factors such as B7 may be involved (103). Janonovic et al. (104) reported a statistically significant increase of A1 antigen frequency and decrease of A28 antigen frequency, as well as the absence of B13 and

BW41 antigens, in a group of subjects with contact dermatitis. No significant correlation between HLA class III polymorphisms (BF, C4A, C4B) and atopic contact dermatitis was found by Orecchia et al. (105).

Experimental studies in animals have shown that there is a genetic predisposition for responses to specific haptens involved in contact dermatitis. It has been demonstrated in animals that the MHC class II molecules play an important role during the sensitization phase of allergic contact dermatitis (100,106,107). Several studies using an animal model present evidence that there is an augmented participation of MHC class II molecules in the endocytotic processes, which is mediated by reactive substances like contact allergens and might contribute to the processing and presentation of these compounds (108).

VII. ENVIRONMENTAL INFLUENCES ON THE ASTHMA AND ALLERGY PHENOTYPES

Although the genetic composition of the subject is an important factor determining the development of asthma and allergy, interactions with environmental factors, almost by definition, are needed. As summarized in Chapters 7 and 8, environmental factors play a major role in the development of asthma and allergies; however, the mechanisms involved are still largely unknown. Sensitization to allergens is essential for the development of an allergy. It appears that the age of exposure (i.e., allergen exposure in early life), the type of allergen (i.e., mites, cockroach, dogs, and cats being associated with asthma), and the allergen load (i.e., low levels are more likely to induce specific IgE production than high levels) are a few of the environmental factors that influence expression of the allergy. Infections will also influence the various clinical phenotypes of allergies. Parasitic infections, for example, will increase the IgE levels. Others have reported an inverse relationship between parasitic disease and high IgE levels with asthma and allergies in non-Westernized countries. IgE levels are influenced by viral infections, especially infectious mononucleosis and cytomegalovirus infections. The relationship between rhinovirus and asthma is not clear. Other factors, such as age, sex, air pollution including tobacco smoke, and psychological factors, all appear to influence the various phenotypes of allergies and asthma. It is possible that environmental factors may modulate the genetic factors as well as the resulting clinical picture.

VIII. PAST AND FUTURE DIRECTIONS OF THE GENETICS OF ASTHMA AND ALLERGY RESEARCH

Asthma and allergies have been noted since ancient times to have a familial, if not a genetic, component (Chapter 1). It has been only in the last part of the

20th century that technology has developed enough in a variety of areas to enable us to define the biology and genetic components of such complex diseases. Examples include the characterization of IgE, cytokines, TH1, and TH2 cells (Chapters 3, 10, and 11), and the development of DNA technology and a sophisticated statistical methodologies (Chapters 2, 4, and 6). With these advances we are characterizing the genetics of asthma and allergies, especially with regard to its DNA basis (Chapters 9–12). As a result, we are starting to see the "blueprints" of the development of these immunologically related adverse conditions.

The allergic reaction appears to require the interaction of environmental factors with a series of steps that are genetically regulated (Chapters 9–11). For example, to develop atopic asthma after an environmental allergen exposure, the interaction of the peptide of the allergen with the HLA system is regulated by a gene(s) on chromosome 6 (HLA-DR). Another gene, possibly on chromosome 14, controls the antigen peptide HLA class II interaction with the T cell. In addition, there is a genetic control reported in some studies on chromosomes 5q and 14q, which determines and regulates the IgE produced from the interaction of the T cells with the B cells. One study suggested that the β-chain of the high-affinity receptor for IgE is on chromosome 11q. The release of mediating substances and the end-organ response to the mediators also appear to be under genetic control. BHR as well as the inflammatory reactions in asthma appear to have heritability. Recently investigations suggested that this may be related to a gene(s) on chromosome 5. Certain types of asthma have been reported to be related to markers on chromosome 6. Other genetic controls, such as variants of genes for β-adrenergic receptor, TNF, α-antitrypsin, and cystic fibrosis, may influence the development of asthma. The condition of atopy has been reported by one group, but not confirmed by others, to be regulated by a gene on 11q.

It is now apparent that an allergic reaction such as an atopic condition involves a variety of steps with both genetic and nongenetic controls. We suggest a gating hypothesis in which the multigene system, controlling these various restriction points, can remain very flexible and accommodating at each point but may lead to an overall restricted response. Therefore, the specificity at each step may be low but the overall specificity will be much greater as a result of sequential gating by the independent control points. In atopic asthma the genetic controls at each different step may appear to be normal. It is only the sequential nature of these independent points of restriction that will ultimately select a subpopulation from an apparently normal population that will exhibit an allergic response such as atopic asthma.

Identification of the errant DNA will provide us with the reason asthma and allergies develop as well as a drug (the corrected DNA) to correct the error. Even if we obtain the genetic DNA blueprint of asthma and allergies, it should be realized that nongenetic factors in the environment may play a major role in their development (Chapters 7 and 8). A critical question is the importance of the genetic versus the other factors in determining the presence of asthma and allergies. It may be that different populations have different blueprints and, as a result, different responses to their environment. If this is so, it may be difficult to predict what is going to happen in which individual. Although at present it appears we might be able to predict who will develop asthma and allergies, we still do not know enough to be sure. It may be that developoment of truth, as Aristotle suggested, is a result of the method of probable reasoning, as opposed to the demonstrative methods of science (109). Therefore, caution should be used in interpretation of the results emerging from genetic studies.

What influence do nongenetic factors have on the blueprints of asthma and allergies? It may be that only a small portion of asthma may be inherited within families in patterns that can be predicted according to present-day genetic rules. It should be stressed that progress is uneven and unexpected findings will be seen. Mendel's early findings were thought to apply to most human disease. Present-day studies regarding genetics, however, indicate that major-change single Mendelian traits are rarely seen in human DNA.

Many ethical problems are developing as the results of the performance of genetic studies. These include potential economic problems resulting from the possibility of loss of insurfance once a person is identified as having asthma or allergies as well as the psychological effects of knowing you may develop a disease. Genetic research and therapy is also seen by some as "interfering with the will of God," and therefore to be avoided.

The rapid explosion of information permitting the understanding of complex diseases such as asthma and allergies has generated much interest by the scientific community and the general population (110–113). Against the background explored in this volume, the following three questions formulated by the British biostatistician Bradford Hill should be addressed. What is wrong? Who is going to develop it? What can be done about it?

IX. WHAT IS WRONG?

Human beings are the results of genetic information expressed within a specific environment. It is apparent it is the interaction between these which determines the ultimate clinical picture. The first step in finding out what is wrong includes defining the biology of asthma and allergies in terms of the DNA and the role of nongenetic factors. Looking for a gene from scratch is overwhelming but is possible through methods such as forward and positional genetics as well as the candidate gene approach. As reviewed in this book, much information has been defined. Information of this type will provide a better understanding of these conditions and what went wrong.

X. WHO IS GOING TO GET IT?

If we know the mechanism and how the genes interact with environmental factors, it should be possible to identify who is predisposed to develop asthma and allergies. The most immediate effects of information regarding the genetic basis of asthma will be screening of subjects to determine who is susceptible. At our present state of knowledge it may be difficult to decide whether an individual should be tested to see if he/she has a tendency to develop asthma and allergies if very little can be done about preventing it. We will probably be able to detect the flaws in DNA before they can be fixed. Furthermore, a person may have the DNA for asthma but have minimal disability from it. Therefore information will be needed to predict not only who will develop asthma or allergies, but also the severity or extent of the disability. Although without question this information will ultimately be extremely helpful, there may be problems with the use of this knowledge. These include issues such as insurance companies refusing to cover these individuals, whether individuals will change their life-styles based on incomplete information, and the psychological ramification of knowing that one is going to develop a disease. Many ethical problems may develop if we can identify who is going to be affected. This information will affect such decisions as whether to have children, occupational choices, and following unproven methods to prevent asthma.

XI. HOW CAN WE FIX IT?

The ideal treatment of asthma and allergies will be to identify the errant DNA and then replace it with the proper molecular thread. There are, however, many known and yet-to-be-identified problems with gene therapy. In addition, some individuals will object to this type of therapy on an ethical basis. Other management procedures will include avoidance of offending environmental factors or interfering with the pathways activated as a result of the interaction of the genetic and environmental factors.

XII. SUMMARY

The search for the genes involved in the control of asthma and allergy is just beginning. We are starting to sort out the genetic control of these conditions. To date, much of the information has been fragmentary and not confirmed. It should be stressed that findings need to be replicated. At the present time it appears that alleles at multiple single loci are involved in the complex etiology of asthma or allergies, either directly in which asthma or allergies are defined as a complex phenotype, or by their action on simple or intermediate phenotypes that are associated with the clinical syndrome. The identification of these genetic controls has many implications for the management of asthma and allergic diseases. This includes a better understanding of their pathogenesis; redefinition of asthma and allergic conditions; improved diagnostic measures; and more specific modes of management of these conditions ranging from genetic manipulation, to avoidance of environmental risk factors, to manipulation of pathways involved in their production. In addition, studies with regard to the genetics of asthma and allergic diseases will give us basic knowledge regarding the factors that determine the type of health we all enjoy during our lifetime.

ACKNOWLEDGMENT

This work was supported in part by NIH Grant HL49609.

REFERENCES

1. Cooke RA, VanderVeer A. Human sensitization. J Immunol 1916; 1:201–305.
2. Davies KE, Read AP, eds. Molecular Badsis of Inherited Diseases, 2nd ed. Oxford: IRL Press, 1988.
3. Connor JM, Ferguson-Smith MA. Essential Medical Genetics, 3rd ed. Oxford: Blackwell Scientific Publications, 1991.
4. Weber JL, May PM. Abundant class of human DNA polymorphisms which can be typed using the polymerase chain reaction. Am J Hum Genet 1989; 44:388–396.
5. Cooper ND, Schmidtke J. Molecular genetic approaches to the analysis and diagnosis of human inherited disease: an overview. Ann Med 1992; 24:29–42.
6. Abbas, Lichtman AH, Pober JS. Cellular and Molecular Immunology. Philadelphia: WB Saunders, 1991:186–203.
7. Sutton BJ, Gould HJ. The human IgE network. Nature 1993; 366:421–428.
8. Blumenthal MN. Family, twin and population studies of allergic responsiveness. In: Marsh DG, Lockhart A, Holgate ST, eds. The Genetics of Asthma. Oxford: Blackwell Scientific Publications, 1993:133–141.
9. Marsh DG, Meyers DA, Freidhoff LR, et al. HLA-Dw2: a genetic marker for human immune response to short ragweed pollen allergen Ra5. II. Response after ragweed immunotherapy. J Exp Med 1982; 155:1452–1463.
10. Blumenthal MN, Marcus-Bagley D, Adweh Z, et al. Extended major: HLA-DR2, [HLA-B7, SC31, DR2] and [HLA-B8, SC01, DR3] haplotypes distinguish subjects with asthma from those with only rhinitis in ragweed pollen allergy. J Immunol 1992; 148:411–416.
11. Coulter KM, Dorval G, Goodfriend L. Genetic control of IgE antibody responses in humans: the Amb V (Ra 5) model. In: Marsh DG, Blumenthal MN, eds. Genetic and Environmental Factors in Clinical Allergy. Minneapolis: University of Minnesota Press, 1990:124–131.

12. Zwollo P, Ehrlich-Kautzky E, Scharf S, et al. Sequencing of HLAD in responders and nonresponders to short ragweed allergen Amb A V. Immunogenetics 1991; 33:141–151.

13. Marsh DG. Immunogenetic and immunochemical factors determining immune responsiveness to allergens: studies in unrelated subjects. In: Marsh DG, Blumenthal MN, eds. Genetic and Environmental Factors in Clinical Allergy. Minneapolis: University of Minnesota Press, 1990:97–123.

14. Marsh DG, Blumenthal MN, Ishikawa T, et al. HLA and specific immune responsiveness to allergens. In: Tsuji K, Aizawa M, Sasazuki T, eds. HLA 1991: Proceedings of the 11th International Histocompatibility Workshop. New York: Oxford University Press, 1992:765–771.

15. Renz H, Saloga J, Bradley KL, Loader JE, Greenstein JL, Larsen G, Gelfand EW. Specific V β T cell subsets mediate the immediate hypersensitivity response to ragweed allergy. J Immunol 1993; 151:1907–1917.

16. Moffatt MF, Hill MR, Cornelis F, Schou C, Faux JA, Young RP, James AL, Ryan G. le Souef P, Musk AW, et al. Genetic linkage of T-cell receptors and α/δ complex to specific IgE response. Lancet 1994; 343:1597–1600.

17. Moffatt MF. HLA and TCR related genes and atopy and asthma. Presented at Genetics of Asthma, Oxford, 1995.

18. Blumenthal MN, Bonini S. Immunogenetics of specific immune responses to allergens in twins and families. In: Marsh DG, Blumenthal MN, eds. Genetics and Environmental Factors in Clinical Allergy. Minneapolis: University of Minnesota Press, 1990:132–142.

19. Hanson B, McGue M, Roitman-Johnson B, Segal NL, Bouchard TC, Blumenthal MN. Atopic disease and immunoglobulin E in twins reared apart and together. Am J Hum Genet 1991; 48:873–879.

20. Blumenthal MN, Namboodiri M, Gleich G, et al. Genetic transmission of serum IgE levels. Am J Genet 1981; 10:219–228.

21. Marsh DG, Chase GA, Freidhoff LR, Meyers DA, Bias WB. Association of HLA antigens and total serum immunoglobulin E level with allergic response and failure to respond to ragweed allergen Ra3. Proc Natl Acad Sci USA 1979; 76:2903–2907.

22. Gerrard JW, Rao DC, Morton NE. A genetic study of immunoglobulin E. Am J Hum Genet 1978; 30:46–58.

23. Rao DC, Lalonel JM, Morton NE, Gerrard JW. Immunoglobulin E revisited. Am J Hum Genet 1980; 32:620–625.

24. Blumenthal MN, Yunis E, Mendell N, Elston RC. Preventative allergy: genetics of IgE-mediated diseases. J Allergy Clin Immunol 1986; 78:962–968 (review).

25. Marsh DG, Neely JD, Breazeale DR, Ghosh B, Freidhoff LR, Ehrlich-Kautzky E, Schou C, Krishnaswamy G, Beaty TH. Linkage analysis of IL-4 and other chromosome 5q31.1 markers and total serum immunoglobulin E concentrations. Science 1994; 264:1152–1156.

26. Meyers DA, Postma DS, Panhuysen CIM, Xu J, Amelung PF, Levitt RC, Bleecker ER. Evidence for a locus regulating total serum IgE levels mapping to chromosome 5. Genomics 1994; 23:464–470.

27. Blumenthal MN, Wang Z, Weber J, Rich SS. Absence of linkage between 5q markers and serum IgE levels in four large atopic families. Clin Exp Allergy 1996 (in press).

28. Rosenwasser L, Klemm DJ, Dresback JK, Inamura H, Mascali J, Klinnert M, Borish L. Promoter polymorphisms in the chromosome 5 gene cluster in asthma and atopy. Clin Exp Allergy 1995; 25:74–78.

29. Fujii H, Kondo N, Agata H, et al. Genetic analysis of IgE and the IgHE, IgHEP1, and IGHEP2 in atopic families. Int Arch Allergy Immunol 1995; 106:62–68.

30. Sandford AO, Shirakawa TS, Moffatt MF, Daniels SE, Ra C, Faux JA, Young RP, Nakamura Y, Lathrop GM, Cookson, et al. Localization of atopy and the β sub unit of the high-affinity Immunoglobulin E receptor (FcεR1) on chromosome 11q. Lancet 1993; 341:332–334.

31. Shirakawa T, Airong L, Dubowitz M, et al. Association between atopy and variants of the β sub unit of the high-affinity immunoglobulin E receptor. Nature Genet (to be published).

32. Marone G, Poto S, Celestino D, Bonini S. Human basophil releasability. III. Genetic controls of the human basophil releasability. J Immunol 1986; 137:3588–3592.

33. Roitman-Johnson B, Blumenthal MN. Family analysis of histamine release. J Allergy Clin Immunol 1988; 81:232.

34. Hopp RJ, Nair NM, Bewtra AK, Townley RG. Genetic aspects of bronchial hyperreactivity. In: Marsh DG, Blumenthal MN, eds. Genetics and Environmental Factors in Clinical Allergy. Minneapolis: University of Minnesota Press, 1990: 143–152.

35. Postma DS, Bleecker ER, Amelung PJ, Holroyd KJ, Jianfeng X, Panhuysen CIM, Meyers DA, Levitt RC. Genetic susceptibility to asthma—bronchial hyperresponsiveness coinherited with a major gene for atopy. N Engl J Med 1995; 333:894–900.

36. Bai TR, Zhou D, Aubent J, et al. Expression of β2 adrenergic receptor mRNA in peripheral lung in asthma and chronic obstructive pulmonary disease. Am J Respir Cell Mol Biol 1993; 8:325.

37. Reihsaus E, Innis M, MacIntyre N, Ligget S. Mutation in the gene encoding for the β2 adrenergic receptor in normal and asthma subjects. Am J Respir Cell Mol Biol 1993; 8:334.

38. Freidhoff L. Epidemiology of atopic allergy. In: Marsh DG, Blumenthal MN, eds. Genetics and Environmental Factors in Clinical Allergy. Minneapolis: University of Minnesota Press, 1990:53–72.

39. Cookson WO, Sharp PA, Faux JA, Hopkin JM. Linkage between immunoglobulin E responses underlying asthma and rhinitis and chromosome 11q. Lancet 1989; 1: 1292–1295.

40. Collee JM, ten Kate LP, de Vries, et al. Allele sharing on chromosome 11q in sibs with asthma and atopy. Lancet 1993; 342:936.

41. Shirakawa T, Hashimoto T, Furuyama J, Morimoto K. Linkage between severe atopy and chromosome 11q13 in Japanese families. Clin Genet 1994; 46:228–232.

42. Hizawa N, Yamaguchi E, Furuya K, et al. Association between high serum total IgE level and D11595 of chromosome 11q13 in Japanese subjects. J Med Genet 1995; 32:363–369.

43. Rich SS, Roitman-Johnson B, Greenberg B, et al. Genetic analysis of atopy in three large kindreds: no evidence of linkage to D11S97. Clin Exp Allergy 1992; 22:1070–1076.

44. Lympany P, Welsh K, MacCochrane G, et al. Genetic analysis using DNA polymorphism of the linkage between chromosome 11q13 and atopy and bronchial hyperresponsiveness to methacholine. J Allergy Clin Immunol 1992; 89:619–628.

45. Lympany P, Welsh KI, Cochrane GM, et al. Genetic analysis of the linkage between chromosome 11q and atopy. Clin Exp Allergy 1992; 1085–1092.

46. Hizawa N, Yamaguchi E, Ohe M, et al. Lack of linkage between atopy and locus 11q13. Clin Exp Allergy 1992; 22:1065–1069.

47. Brereton HM, Ruffin RW, Thompson PJ, Turner DR. Familial atopy in Australian pedigrees: adventitious linkage to chromosome 8 is not confirmed nor is there evidence of linkage to high-affinity IgE receptor. Clin Exp Allergy 1994; 24:868–877.

48. Amelung PJ, Panhuysen CIM, Postma DS, Levitt RC, Koeter GH, Francomano CA, Bleecker ER, Meyers DA. Atopy and bronchial hyperresponsiveness: exclusion of linkage to markers on chromosomes 11q and 6q. Clin Exp Allergy 1992; 22:1077–1084.

49. Cookson WOCM, Young RP, Sandford AJ, Moffatt MF, Shirakawa T, Sharp PA, Faux JA, et al. Maternal inheritance of atopic responsiveness on chromosome 11q. Lancet 1992; 340:381–384.

50. Walter MA, Chambers C, Zimmerman B, Cox D. A multigene deletion in the immunoglobulin heavy chain region in a highly atopic individual. Hum Genet 1990; 85:643–647.

51. Burrows B, Martinez F, Halonen, et al. Association of asthma with serum IgE level and skin test reactivity to allergens. N Engl J Med 1989; 320:271.

52. Sears M, Burrows B, Flannery G, et al. Relationship between airway responsiveness and serum IgE in children with asthma and in apparently normal children. N Engl J Med 1991; 325:1067.

53. Virchow JC, Walker C, Hafner D, Kortsik C, Werner P, Matthys H, Kroegel C. T cells and cytokines in bronchoalveolar lavage fluid after segmented allergen provocation in atopic asthma. Am J Respir Crit Care Med 1995; 151:960–968.

54. Thorsby E, Lie SO. Relationship between the HLA system and susceptibility to disease. Transplant Proc 1971; 1303.

55. Morris MJ, Vaughan H, Lane DJ, Morrs PJ. HLA in asthma. In: de Weck AL, Blumenthal MN, eds. HLA and Allergy: Monographs in Allergy 11. Basel: S Karger, 1977:30.

56. Turner MN, Brostoff J, Wells SR, Soothill JF. Histocompatibility antigens in atopy with special reference to eczema and hayfever. In: de Weck AL, Blumenthal MN, eds. HLA and Allergy: Monographs in Allergy 11. Basel: S Karger, 1977:19.

57. Rachelefsky GS, Terasaki PI, Katz RM, Siegel SC. B lymphocyte and histocompatibility antigens in extrinsic asthma. In: de Weck AL, Blumenthal MN, eds. HLA and Allergy: Monographs in Allergy 11. Basel: S Karger, 1977:35.

58. Geerts SJ, Pöttgens H, Limburg M, van Rood JJ. Predisposition for atopy or allergy linked to HLA. Lancet 1975; 1:461.

59. Morrison J. Class III MHC polymorphisms and asthma. In: Genetics of Asthma. Broadway, Worcestershire: Wellcome Trust, 1995:47.

60. Caraballo LR, Hernandez M. HLA haplotype segregation in families with allergic asthma. Tissue Antigens 1990; 35:182–186.

61. Hsieh KH, Shien CC, Hsieh RP, Liu WJ. Association of HLA-DQW2 with Chinese childhood asthma. Tissue Antigens 1991; 38:181–182.

62. Mullarkey M, Thomas P, Hansen J, et al. Association of aspirin-sensitive asthma with HLA-DQW2. Am Rev Respir Dis 1986; 133:261–263.

63. Lympany P, Welsh KI, Christie PE, Schmitz-Schumann M, Kemeny DM, Lee TH. An analysis with sequence-specific oligonucleotide probes of the association between aspirin-induced asthma and antigens of the HLA system. J Allergy Clin Immunol 1993; 92:114–123.

64. Perichon B, Krishnamoorthy R. Asthma and HLA system. Allergie Immunol 1991; 23:301–307.

65. Bignon J, Aron Y, Jo L, et al. HLA class II alleles in isocyanate-induced asthma. Am J Respir Crit Care Med 1994; 149:7–15.

66. Liggett S. Adrenergic receptor polymorphism. In: Genetics of Asthma. Broadway, Worcestershire: Wellcome Trust, 1995:45.

67. Ohe M, Munakata M, Hizawa N, et al. Beta$_2$ adrenergic receptor genetic restriction fragment length polymorphism and bronchial asthma. Thorax 1995; 50:353–359.

68. Colp C, Lieberman J. Asthma and α-1 antitrypsin. In: Weiss E, Stein M, eds. Bronchial Asthma, 3rd ed. 1993:1185–1187.

69. Prados M, Monteseirin F, Carranco M, Aragon R, Conde A, Conde J. Phenotype of α-1-antitrypsin in intrinsic asthma and ASA-triad patients. Allergol Immunol Pathol 1995; 23(1):24–28.

70. Gaillard M, Zwi S, Noguiera C, Ludewick H, et al. Ethnic differences in the occurrence of the M1 (ala 213) haplotype of α 1-antitrypsin in asthmatic and non-asthmatic black and white South Africans. Clin Genet 1994; 45(3):122–127.

71. Lindmark S, Svenonius E, Eriksson S. Heterozygous α 1-antichymotrypsin and PiZ α 1-antitrypsin deficiency: prevalence and clinical spectrum in asthmatic children. Allergy 1990; 45:197–203.

72. Lindmark B. Asthma and heterozygous α 1-antichymotrypsin deficiency: a possible association. J Intern Med 1990; 227:115–118.

73. Warner JO, Norman A, Soothill J. Cystic fibrosis heterozygosity in the pathogenesis of allergy. Lancet 1976; 1:990–991.

74. Gyukovits K, Markus V, Mittera I. Cystic fibrosis heterozygosity in childhood bronchial asthma. Lancet 1977; 1:203.

75. Schroeder SA, Gaughan DM, Swift M. Protection against bronchial asthma by CFTR-δ 508 mutation: a heterozygote advantage in cystic fibrosis. Nature Med 1995; 1:703–705.

76. Oxelus VA, Hultquist C, Husby S. GM allotype as indicators of non-atopic bronchial asthma. Int Arch Allergy Immunol 1993; 101:66–71.

77. Brenner-Ullman A, Melzer-Ofin H, Daniels M, Shohat M. Possible protection against asthma in heterozygotes for familial Mediterranean fever. Am J Med Genet 1994; 53:172–175.

78. Vaughan WT. Practice of Allergy. Revised by Black JH, 3rd ed. St. Louis: CV Mosby, 1957.

79. Kitano V, Sadanaga Y, Ishikawa T. Genetic regulation of allergic rhinitis. Acta Pediatr Jpn 1985; 29:654–657.

80. Oltvai ZN, Wong E, Atkinson J, Tung K. C-1 inhibitor deficiency: molecular and immunologic basis of hereditary and acquired angioedema. Lab Invest 1991; 65: 381–388.
81. Quincke H. Über akutes umschriebenes H-autoderm. Monatsschr Prakt Dermatol 1892; 1:129.
82. Wolffler W. Hereditary angioedema. Am J Med Sci 1888; 95:362.
83. Siddique Z, McPhaden AR, Whaley K. Characterisation of nucleotide sequence variants and disease-specific mutations involving the 3´ end of the C1-inhibitor gene in hereditary angio-oedema. Hum Hered 1995; 45:98–102.
84. Verpy E, Couture-Tosi E, Eldering E, et al. Crucial residues in the carboxy-terminal end of C1 inhibitor revealed by pathogenic mutants impaired in secretion or function. J Clin Invest 1995; 95:350–359.
85. Kaplan AP. Urticaria and angioedema. In: Middleton E, Reed CE, Ellis F, eds. Allergy Principles and Practices, 4th ed. St. Louis: CV Mosby, 1993:1553–1580.
86. Black JT. Amyloidosis, deafness, urticaria, and limb pain: a hereditary syndrome. Ann Intern Med 1969; 70:989–994.
87. Alpers C, Abramson N, Johnston R, Jandel J, Rosen F. Increased susceptibility to infection associated with abnormality of complement-mediated function and of the third component of complement (C3). N Engl J Med 1970; 282:349–353.
88. Evans R. Epidemiology and natural history of asthma, allergic rhinitis and atopic dermatitis (eczema). In: Middleton E, Reed CE, Ellis EF, Adkinson NF, Yunginger JW, eds. Allergy Principles and Practices, 4th ed. St. Louis: CV Mosby, 1993: 1109–1136.
89. de Weck A, Blumenthal MN, Yunis E, Jeannet M. HLA in allergy. In: Dausset J, Svejgaard A, eds. HLA and Disease. Baltimore: Williams & Wilkins, 1977:196–211
90. de Weck AL, Blumenthal MN, eds. HLA and Allergy. Basel: S Karger, 1977.
91. Scholz S, Ziegler E, Wüstner H, et al. HLA family studies in patients with atopic dermatitis. In: de Weck AL, Blumenthal MN, eds. HLA and Allergy. Monographs in Allergy 11. Basel: S Karger, 1977:44.
92. Ozawa A, Ohkido M, Tsuji S. Some recent advances in HLA and skin disease. J Am Acad Dermatol 1981; 4:205–230.
93. Svejgaard E, Jakobsen B, Svejgaard A. Studies of HLA-ABC and DR antigens in pure atopic dermatitis and atopic dermatitis combined with allergic respiratory disease. Acta Dermatol Venereol 1985; 114(Suppl):72–76.
94. Goundemand J, Defrenne C, Desmons F. HLA antigens and atopic dermatitis. In: de Weck AL, Blumenthal MN, eds. HLA and Allergy. Monographs in Allergy 11. Basel: S Karger, 1977:24–29.
95. Saeki H, Kuwata S, Nakagawa H, et al. HLA and atopic dermatitis with high serum IgE levels. J Allergy Clin Immunol 1994; 94:575–583.
96. Larson F, Grunnet N. Investigations in atopic dermatitis. Tissue Antigens 1987; 29:1–6.
97. Kuwata S, Yanagisawa M, Saeki H, et al. Polymorphisms of transporter associated with antigen processing genes in atopic dermatitis. J Allergy Clin Immunol 1994; 94:565–574.

98. Coleman R, Trembath RC, Harper JI. Chromosome 11q13 and atopy underlying atopic eczema. Lancet 1993; 341:1121–1122.

99. Maibach MI, Epstein E, Lahti A. Contact skin allergy. In: Middleton E, Reed CE, Ellis EF, Adkinson NF, Yunginger JW, eds. Allergy Principles and Practice, Vol II, 3rd ed. St Louis: CV Mosby, 1988:1429–1468.

100. Chase MW. Inheritance in guinea pigs of the susceptibility to skin sensitization with simple chemical compounds. J Exp Med 1941; 73:711–726.

101. Menne T, Holm NY. Nickel allergy in a female twin population. Int J Dermatol 1992; 22:22–28.

102. Emtestam L, Zetterquist H, Olerup O. HLA-DR, -DQ and -DP alleles in nickel, chromium, and/or cobalt-sensitive individuals: genomic analysis based on restriction fragment length polymorphisms. J Invest Dermatol 1993; 100:271–274.

103. Liden S, Beckman L, Cedergren B, Goransson K, Nyquist H. HLA antigens in allergic contact dermatitis. Acta Dermatol Venereol 1978; 58(Suppl):53–56.

104. Jovanovic M, Poljacki M, Milakov J, et al. Phenotyping: personal contribution to research on increased susceptibility of individual HLA phenotype combinations in predisposition to contact allergies. Med Pregl 1993; 46:221–224.

105. Orecchia G, Perfetti L, Finco O, et al. Polymorphisms of HLA class III genes in alleregic contact dermatitis. Dermatology 1992; 184:254–259.

106. Geczy A, de Weck AL. Genetic control of sensitization to chemically defined antigens and its relationship to histocompatibility antigens in guinea pigs. In: Contact Hypersensitivity in Experimental Animals. Basel: S Karger, 1974:83–88.

107. Kohler J, Martin S, Pflugfelder U, et al. Cross-reactive trinitrophenylated peptides as antigens for class II major histocompatibility complex-restricted T cells and inducers of contact sensitivity in mice: limited T cell receptor repertoire. Eur J Immunol 1995; 25:92–101.

108. Becker D, Neiss U, Neiss S, et al. Contact allergens modulate the expression of MHC class II molecules on murine epidermal Langerhans cells by endocytotic mechanisms. J Invest Dermatol 1992; 98:700–705.

109. Farrington B. Aristotle: Founder of Scientific Philosphy. London: Weidenfeld & Nicolson (Educational), 1965.

110. McKusick VA, Claiborne R, eds. Medical Genetics. New York: HP Publishing Co., 1973.

111. Weiss K. Genetic variation and human disease. Cambridge: Cambridge University Press, 1993.

112. The genetic revolution. Time 1994; 143:46–57.

113. Biotechnology and genetics. Economist 1995; 334:3–18.

Index

Adhesion molecules, 268-270
Alleles, 20
    associations, 56-57, 123-124, 127
Allergens:
    as diagnostic tools, 96
Allergic response:
    cellular components, 66-72
    modification of, 78-80
Allergic rhinitis:
    definition and history, 11
    genetics, 341
    HLA, 341
Allergy (*see also* Analysis, Epidemiology):
    definition, 10
    environmental influences, 180-181, 183-
        184, 344-345
    evaluation, 91-107
    genetics, 14, 38-42, 327-348
    geographical variations, 181-183
    history, 1-2, 10-15
        anaphylaxis, 11-12
        asthma, 11
        atopic dermatitis, 12-13
        atopy, 10-11
        eczema, 12
        rhinitis, 11

[Allergy]
    urticaria, 12
    model, 329-331
    phenotypes, 309
    psychological factors, 179-180
    socio-economic factors, 179-
        180
Allergy associated phenotype (*see* Pheno-
        type)
Analysis (*see also* Family studies; Genetics,
        studies), 21-38, 47-62, 111-135
    ascertainment, 127-129
    association/disequilibrium, 56-77, 111-
        135
    extended pedigrees, 51-52
    heredity and risks, 57
    isolated populations, sample designs, 52
    linkage analysis and mapping, 58-60 (*see
        also* Linkage)
    mixed models, 118-119
    molecular genetics, 54-56
    monocytes, 253-256
    multifactorial inheritance, 26-27
    multiple pairwise tests, 120-121
    multipoint tests, 121
    multivariate traits, 112-114

[Analysis]
　　nuclear families, sample designs 50-51
　　qualitative traits, 124-127
　　quantitative traits, 114-124
　　risk factors, 57, 141-147, 153-157, 171-
　　　　195
　　sample designs, 49-52
　　segregation analysis, 57-58
　　sib pair analysis, 121-122, 127
　　single locus models, 117-118
　　statistical methods, 111-132
　　twins, 50 (*see also* Twin studies)
　　unrelated individuals, 50
Anaphylaxis (*see* Allergy)
Angioedema:
　　genetics, 341-342 (*see also* Genetics)
Antibodies:
　　history, 6-7
Antigen Presenting Cell (APC), 202-205
Arachidonic acid:
　　metabolism, 265-268
Arthus reaction, 9
ASA (aspirin):
　　asthma, 338, 340
Ascertainment (*see* Analysis)
Asthma, 1,11, 41-42, 112, 141-168, 241, 331
　　　　(*see also* Analysis; Epidemiology;
　　　　Inflammation; Risk factors; Pheno-
　　　　types)
　　analysis, 112, 331
　　atopy, 142-143
　　climatic factors, 147
　　definition, 1
　　epidemiological trends, 147-156
　　evaluation, 91-107
　　genetics, 38-42, 141-142, 307-318, 327-
　　　　348
　　geographical variations, 145
　　incidence, 139
　　infections, 147
　　inflammation, 244-247, 308
　　model, 329-331
　　mortality, 150-153
　　natural history, 139-141
　　phenotype, 309, 313, 336-341
　　physiology, 281-305
　　pollution, 145-146
　　prevalence, 139
　　risk factors, 141-147, 308
　　seasonal variations, 147

[Asthma]
　　socio-economic factors, 146-147, 151-
　　　　156
Asthma- and allergy-associated phenotypes
　　　　(*see* Phenotype)
Atopic dermatitis, 72-74
　　chromosome 11, 343
　　definition, history, 12
　　genetics, 342-43
　　HLA (*see also* Chromosome 6), 342-343
Atopy, 10, 241-243
　　analysis, 112-114
　　genetics, 335-336
　　model, 329-331

B-cells, 71-72
　　epitope, 205-207
Basophils:
　　degranulation, 101
　　diagnostic methods, 102
Bronchial hyperreactivity (BHR), 308-318
　　　　(*see also* Phenotype; Asthma;
　　　　Provocation tests)
　　chromosome 5q, 317-318, 333-334
　　genetics, 40, 313-314, 317-318, 333-
　　　　334
　　mechanism, 75-78, 310
　　phenotype, 313
Blood gas analysis, 288-289
Bronchial-associated lymphoid tissue
　　　　(BALT), 75-78
BHR (*see* Bronchial hyperreactivity)
Bronchial provocation tests (*see* Provocation
　　　　tests)

Candidate gene (*see also* Analysis; Chromo-
　　　　some), 53-54, 131
CD4
　　age, 176-178
　　in IgE production, 217-218
　　infections, 178-179
　　variations in susceptibility, 175-
　　　　180
CD23, 66, 218-219
CD40:
　　biology, 67-68
　　function, 218
Cell interaction, 254-256
Cellular composition of allergic response,
　　　　66-72

Cellular immunity:
  history, 8-9
Chemical mediators, 256-268
Chromosome, 20
  abnormalities, 22-23
  chromosome 5:
    α_1-antitrypsin, 339-340
    asthma, 339-340 (*see also* Asthma,
      genetics)
    bronchial hyperreactivity, 317-318,
      333-334, 339 (*see also* Bronchial
      hyperreactivity)
    immunoglobulin E, 315-318, 332-333,
      339 (*see also* Immunoglobulin)
    genes, 315-318
  chromosome 6:
    asthma, 337-338
    immune response specific (*see also*
      Immune response)
  chromosome 7:
    asthma, 340 (*see also* Asthma,
      Genetics)
    bronchial hyperreactivity, 340 (*see
      also* Bronchial hyperreactivity)
    cystic fibrosis, 340
  chromosome 11:
    atopy, 335-336 (*see also* Atopy)
    hereditary angioedema, 341-342 (*see
      also* Hereditary
      angioedema)
    immunoglobulin E receptor (*see also*
      Immunoglobulin, regulation)
  chromosome 14:
    asthma, 340 (*see also* Asthma;
      Genetics)
    atopy, 336 (*see also* Atopy)
    Gm allotype, 340
    Ig heavy chain, 340
    immunoglobulin heavy chain constant
      region, 336, 340
  chromosome 16:
    familial Mediterranean gene, 340-341
      (*see also* Asthma)
Clinical evaluation, 91-107
  allergens, 96
  allergy, 91-107
  asthma, 91-107
  basophil, 101
  clinical history, 95, 139-141
  cytokines, 103

[Clinical evaluation]
  eosinophil, 102
  IgE tests, 98-100, 174-175
  immune complex, 104
  immune system, 91-107
  inflammation, mediators of, 102-103
  interleukins, 103
  lung function, 205-206
  lymphocyte, 101-102
  mast cells/basophil, 102
  non-IgE immunoglobulin, 104
  provocation tests, (*see* provocation tests)
  skin test, 96-98
  specific IgE, 98-100
  questionnaires, 95
Commingling, 115 (*see also* Analysis)
Complement, 7-8
  system, 271 (*see also* Inflammation)
Conjunctival provocation tests (CPT) (*see*
      Provocation tests)
Contact dermatitis:
  chromosome 6, 343-344 (*see also*
      Chromosome 6)
  genetic, 343-344 (*see also* Genetics)
  HLA, 343-344 (*see also* HLA)
Corticosteroid, 80
Cyclosporin, 80
Cycloxygenose, 265-268
Cystic fibrosis (*see* Chromosome 7)
Cytokines, 68-70, 257-265 (*see also* Asthma;
      Genetics; Inflammation; Mediator)
  anticytokines/anticytokine receptor,
      79
  diagnostic methods, 103
  genetic control, 258-259, 264-265
  IgE inhibiting, 215-217
  IgE promoting, 213-215
  IgE synthesis, 68-70, 212-217
  inflammation, 244, 257-265
  inhibitory, 78-79, 215-217
  junction, 257-265
  stimulatory, 213-215

Diagnosis (*see* Clinical evaluation)
Disequilibrium studies, 30, 56-57
DNA, 19-20, 54-56

Eczema (*see also* Atopic dermatitis):
  definition and history, 12
  genetics, 342-343

Environment:
   asthma and allergy, 153-156, 171-195,
      344-345
   tobacco smoking, 144-145, 184-185
Eosinophil, 250-252, 254-256 (*see also*
      Asthma; Clinical evaluation)
Eosinophil cationic protein (ECP), 94
Epidemiology, 137-169, 171-195 (*see also*
      Allergy; Asthma)
Evolution, 3

Familial aggregate, 29-30
Family studies, 31-38
Food allergy, 74-75

Gastrointestinal tract, 74-75, 221-223
Gene, 19-20
Gene mapping, 33-38, 58-60 (*see* Analysis)
Genetics, 2-4 (*see also* Allergy; Asthma)
   allergy, 14, 327-348
      approaches, directions, 329, 331, 345-
         348
      history, 14, 327-329
   analysis, 111-132
   asthma, 14, 327-348
      approaches, directions, 329, 331, 345-
         348
      history, 14, 327-329
   history, 1-4
   human, 19-42
   human diseases, (*see* Single gene dis-
         orders; Chromosome, abnormalities)
   interaction, 129-130 (*see also* Analysis)
   markers, 54
   multi-discipline approach, 15
   polygenetic traits, multi-factoral inheri-
         tance, analysis, 20-27
   research, 345-346
      future of, 345-346
   studies (*see also* Analysis):
      allergy, 38-39 (*see also* Allergy)
      asthma, 38-39, 41-42 (*see also*
         Asthma)
      bronchial hyperreactivity (BHR), 40
         (*see also* Bronchial hyperreactivity)
      immunoglobulin E level, 40-41 (*see
         also* Immunoglobulin)
      mediator release, 39-40 (*see also*
         Mediator)
      specific IgE, 39

[Genetics]
   tools, 47-60
   twins, 27-29
Gut-associated lymphoid tissue (GALT), 74-
      75

Hay fever (*see* Allergic rhinitis, Atopy)
Heat shock protein, 271-272 (*see also* In-
      flammation)
Hereditary angioedema (HAE) (*see* Angio-
      edema)
Heredity, 1-4
Histamine, 256-257
Histamine challenges (*see* Provocation tests)
Histamine release (*see also* Genetics,
      studies, mediator release)
HLA (*see* Major histocompatibility complex
      [MHC])

IgA, 74-75
Immune response (specific):
   animal, 221-222
   HLA, 39, 198-204, 207-208, 331-332 (*see
      also* Genetics)
   T cell, 204-208, 332 (*see also* T cell)
Immune sensitization, 330
Immune system:
   allergy, 13
   atopy, 13
   evaluation, 91-107
   non-infectious factors, 9
Immunity:
   mechanism, 6
Immunogenetics:
   history, 9-10
Immunoglobulin (IgE), 7, 220-221
   animal model, 76-78
   biology, 64-68
   CD40, 67-68 (*see also* CD40)
   chromosome 5, 339, 332-333, 315-318
   chromosome 5q, 315-318
   environment, 344-345 (*see also*
      Environment)
   genetics, 40-41, 314-315
   genetics, specific immune response,
      39
   immune recognition, 198-200
   interaction with receptors, 65-66
   mechanisms, 63-64
   methods, 98-100

[Immunoglobulin]
    mode of inheritance, 332-333 (*see also* Genetics)
    modulation by cytokines, 68
    production, cognate signals, 217-219
    receptors, 268-270
        chromosome 11, 333
        FCeRI, 65-66, 73
        FceRII, 66-67, 218
    regulation, 63-80, 307-318, 332-333 (*see also* Immunoglobulin, synthesis; Genetics)
    structure, 64-65
    synthesis, 63-64, 66-67, 211-239 (*see also* Cytokines)
    T-cell independent synthesis, 71
Immunology:
    history, 4-10
Immunosuppression, 80
    corticosteroids, 80
    cyclosporin, 80
Indoor climate, 185-186
Infection:
    allergy, 178-179, 229-230
    asthma, 178-179, 229-230
Inflammation, 241-272 (*see also* Cytokines)
    asthma, 244-247
    cells, 247-256
    cytokines, 244, 257-265
    diagnostic methods, 102-103
    genetic control, 243-244
    genetics in mice, 243-244
    regulation, 219-220, 229-230
Inheritance patterns, 21
Integins, 268-270
Intermediate phenotypes (*see* Asthma- and allergy-associated phenotypes)

Leukotriens, 265-268
Linkage, 33-38, 58-60, 120-123, 126-127, 129 (*see also* Analysis)
Lipoxygenase, 265-268
Logarithm of the odds (LODS), 34-35, 120-122 (*see also* Analysis)
Lung, 75-78
Lung function, 105-107, 281-300
    airway closure, 286-288
    airway resistance, 282-284
    breathing, 284
    genetic influence, 298-299

[Lung function]
    lung perfusion, 288-291
    mechanics, 282-294
    spirometry, 285-286
    ventilation distribution, 286-288
Lymphocyte function tests, 105-106
Lymphocytes, 101-102

Macrophages, 253-254 (*see also* Asthma)
Major histocompatibility complex (MHC), 30-31
    asthma, genetics (*see* Asthma, genetics)
    extended haplotype, 338
    HLA, 198-200, 201-208
    IgE response, 198-200, 201-208, 217-218
    immune response specific, 197-208, 331-332 (*see also* Immune response)
Mast cells, 249-250 (*see also* Asthma)
    diagnostic methods, 102
Mediator (*see also* Heat shock protein; Complement, system):
    cytokines, 257-265
    genetics, 39-40, 333
    histamine, 256-257
    leukotriens, 265-268
Mendelian inheritance, 21-22
Meta-analysis, 130-131 (*see also* Analysis)
Methacholine challenges, 311-313 (*see also* Provocation tests, bronchial)
Mite sensitivity (*see* Asthma; chromosome 6; HLA)

Nasal provocation test (NPT) (*see* Provocation tests)
Neutrophil, 252-253, 254-256 (*see also* Asthma)

Oligogenic models, 119-120 (*see also* Analysis)

Path analysis, 116 (*see also* Analysis)
Phenotype, 48-49
    asthma and allergy associated, (intermediate), 331-335
    atopy, 335-336 (*see also* Genetics)
    BHR, 48-49
    Immunoglobulin E, 49 (*see also* Immunoglobulin E)
    qualitative measures, 48-49
    quantitative measures, 49

[Phenotype]
  complex:
    allergy, 335-344
    asthma, 309, 319
Pollution, 180-181
Polygene traits, 24-26
Positional cloning, 54-56
Prevention, 186-188
Provocation tests:
  bronchial, 105-106
    histamine, 311-313
    methacholine challenge, 311-313
  conjunctival, 105
  food challenge, 106-107
  nasal provocation, 105
Purified allergens, 331-332 (*see also*
    Immune response)
  immune response, 197-208, 331-332

Qualitative traits, 124-127 (*see also*
    Analysis)
Quantitative traits, 114-124 (*see also*
    Analysis)

Ragweed, 197-198, 201-208
  asthma genetics, 338
  HLA, genetics, 338 (*see also* HLA)
Receptors:
  anticytokine, 79
  FCeRI, 65-66, 73
  FCeRII, 66, 218
Regression models (*see* Analysis)
Rhinitis (*see* Allergic rhinitis)
Risk factors: (*see also* Analysis)
  prenatal, 186

Sensitivity, 92-94
Sensitization, 221-230, 329-331
  gastrointestinal tract, 74-75, 221-223
  identification of susceptible individuals,
    173-175

[Sensitization]
  local, 72-74, 92
  lung, 75-78
  skin, 72-74
Serum sickness, 9
Single-gene disorders, 23-24
Single-locus models (*see* Analysis)
Skin-associated lymphoid tissues (SALT),
    72-74
Skin tests, 96-98
Specificity, 92-94
Statistical methods (*see* Analysis)

T cell, 247-249 (*see also* asthma):
  epitope:
    purified allergens, 204-205 (*see also*
      Immune response; Purified
      allergens)
  independent IgE synthesis, 71-72
  IgE biology, 66-79
  receptor (TCR):
    immune response specific, 332 (*see
      also* chromosome 14)
T-helper cells:
  compartmentalization, 69-70
  cytokine profiles, 69-70
  in disease, 70-71
  heterogenesity, 212

Target organ:
  sensitization/immune system, 72-78
TDI:
  asthma, 338
  HLA, 338
Tolerance:
  environmental influence, 225
  inhalent allergens, 223-225
  oral, 222-223

Urticaria, 12
  genetics, 341-342

About the Editors

MALCOLM BLUMENTHAL is Professor and Director of the Asthma and Allergy Program, Department of Medicine, University of Minnesota Hospital, Minneapolis. The author, coauthor, or editor of nearly 150 books, book chapters, articles, and abstracts, he is a Fellow of the American Academy of Allergy and Immunology, the American College of Allergy and Immunology, the American College of Physicians, and the American College of Chest Physicians. A member of the American Thoracic Society and the American Association of Immunology, among others, Dr. Blumenthal received the B.A. degree (1954) in sociology and zoology, and the M.D. degree (1958) from the University of Minnesota, Minneapolis.

BENGT BJÖRKSTÉN is Professor and Chairman of the Department of Pediatrics at University Hospital, Linköping, Sweden, as well as adjunct Professor of Pediatrics at Tartu University, Estonia. The author of over 400 original papers, congress abstracts, and book chapters and reviews, he is editor-in-chief of *Pediatric Allergy and Immunology*, the President of the Scandinavian Pediatric Federation, and Corresponding Fellow of the American Academy of Allergy and Immunology. Dr. Björkstén received the M.D. degree (1967) from the University of Lund, Sweden.